Molecular Pathology Library

Series Editor:

Philip T. Cagle
Houston, TX
USA

More information about this series at http://www.springer.com/series/7723

Chen Liu
Editor

Precision Molecular Pathology of Liver Cancer

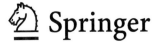 Springer

Editor
Chen Liu
Department of Pathology and Laboratory Medicine
Rutgers Robert Wood Johnson Medical School
and New Jersey Medical School
Newark, New Jersey
USA

ISSN 1935-987X   ISSN 1935-9888   (electronic)
Molecular Pathology Library
ISBN 978-3-319-88543-8   ISBN 978-3-319-68082-8   (eBook)
https://doi.org/10.1007/978-3-319-68082-8

Printed on acid-free paper

This Springer imprint is published by Springer Nature
The registered company is Springer International Publishing AG
The registered company address is: Gewerbestrasse 11, 6330 Cham, Switzerland

Preface

Hepatocellular carcinoma (HCC) is the predominant primary malignant cancer in the liver. It is one of the most common and malignant cancers in the world. There are 700,000 deaths due to HCC every year. The cancer incidence is increasing in many countries, including the United States. Unfortunately, the treatment options are very limited compared to other human cancers. Many clinical trials have been conducted over the years, but the results are generally disappointing. The high failure rate for clinical trials is partially attributed to lack of adequate biomarkers for patient selection. Developing molecular markers is paramount for early diagnosis and optimal treatment of HCC. This book provides the most updated knowledge on the advancement of molecular pathogenesis, molecular diagnosis, and therapy development. The authors are experts in the topics they have contributed. Besides reviewing the current available knowledge, the authors also discuss their prospective for future developments in precision/personalized medicine approach for HCC.

Newark, New Jersey, USA   Chen Liu

Contents

Contributors

Naziheh Assarzadegan, M.D. Department of Pathology, Immunology, and Laboratory Medicine, University of Florida, Gainesville, FL, USA

Cuong Bach, Ph.D. Department of Biological Sciences, Hunter College of The City University of New York, New York, NY, USA

Tony S. Brar, M.D. Gastroenterology, Hepatology and Nutrition, University of Florida, Gainesville, FL, USA

Roniel Cabrera, M.D. Division of Gastroenterology, Hepatology, and Nutrition, University of Florida, Gainesville, FL, USA

Darren R. Carpizo, M.D. Rutgers Cancer Institute of New Jersey, New Brunswick, NJ, USA

Joydeep Chakraborty, M.D. Division of Gastroenterology, Hepatology, and Nutrition, University of Florida, Gainesville, FL, USA

Amy Leigh Collinsworth, M.D. Department of Pathology, Immunology and Laboratory Medicine, University of Florida, Gainesville, FL, USA

Dan Delitto, M.D. Department of Pathology and Laboratory Medicine, Rutgers New Jersey Medical School and Robert Wood Johnson Medical School, Newark, NJ, USA

Michael Feely, M.D. Department of Pathology, Immunology, and Laboratory Medicine, College of Medicine, University of Florida, Gainesville, FL, USA

Joseph R. Grajo, M.D. Department of Radiology, University of Florida, Gainesville, FL, USA

Stephanie H. Greco, M.D. Rutgers Cancer Institute of New Jersey, New Brunswick, NJ, USA

Eric Hilgenfeldt, M.D. Gastroenterology, Hepatology and Nutrition, University of Florida, Gainesville, FL, USA

Division of Gastroenterology, Department of Internal Medicine, Carolinas Medical Center, Charlotte, NC, USA

Jeannette Huaman, Ph.D. Department of Biological Sciences, Hunter College of The City University of New York, New York, NY, USA

Department of Biology, The Graduate Center of The City University of New York, New York, NY, USA

Adeodat Ilboudo, Ph.D. Department of Biological Sciences, Hunter College of The City University of New York, New York, NY, USA

Junfang Ji, Ph.D. Life Sciences Institute, Zhejiang University, Hangzhou, China

Jesse Kresak, M.D. Department of Pathology, Immunology, and Laboratory Medicine, University of Florida, Gainesville, FL, USA

Niya Liu, Ph.D. Life Sciences Institute, Zhejiang University, Hangzhou, China

Chen Liu, M.D., Ph.D. Department of Pathology and Laboratory Medicine, New Jersey Medical School, Rutgers, The State University of New Jersey, Newark, NJ, USA

Department of Pathology and Laboratory Medicine, Rutgers New Jersey Medical School and Robert Wood Johnson Medical School, Newark, NJ, USA

Olorunseun O. Ogunwobi, M.D., Ph.D. Department of Biological Sciences, Hunter College of The City University of New York, New York, NY, USA

Department of Biology, The Graduate Center of The City University of New York, New York, NY, USA

Joan and Sanford I. Weill Department of Medicine, Weill Cornell Medicine, Cornell University, New York, NY, USA

Kien Pham, Ph.D. Department of Pathology and Laboratory Medicine, Rutgers New Jersey Medical School and Robert Wood Johnson Medical School, Newark, NJ, USA

Williams Puszyk, Ph.D. Department of Pathology, Immunology, and Laboratory Medicine, University of Florida, Gainesville, FL, USA

Keith Robertson, Ph.D. Department of Molecular Pharmacology and Experimental Therapeutics, Mayo Clinic Comprehensive Cancer Center, Mayo Clinic, Rochester, MN, USA

Naziya Samreen, M.D. Department of Radiology, University of Florida, Gainesville, FL, USA

Consuelo Soldevila-Pico, M.D. Gastroenterology, Hepatology and Nutrition, University of Florida, Gainesville, FL, USA

Kristen Spencer, M.D. Rutgers Cancer Institute of New Jersey, New Brunswick, NJ, USA

Beau Toskich, M.D. Department of Radiology, University of Florida College of Medicine, Gainesville, FL, USA

Xin Wei Wang, M.D., Ph.D. Liver Carcinogenesis Section, Laboratory of Human Carcinogenesis, Center for Cancer Research, National Cancer Institute, Bethesda, MD, USA

Xiyang Wei, Ph.D. Life Sciences Institute, Zhejiang University, Hangzhou, China

Lanjing Zhang, M.D., M.S., F.C.A.P., F.A.C.G. Department of Pathology, University Medical Center of Princeton, Plainsboro, NJ, USA

Rutgers Cancer Institute of New Jersey, New Brunswick, NJ, USA

Department of Chemical Biology, Ernest Mario School of Pharmacy, Rutgers University, Piscataway, NJ, USA

Faculty of Arts and Sciences, Department of Biological Sciences, Rutgers University, Newark, NJ, USA

Etiology and Pathogenesis of Hepatocellular Carcinoma

Tony S. Brar, Eric Hilgenfeldt, and Consuelo Soldevila-Pico

1.1 Introduction

Worldwide, hepatocellular carcinoma (HCC) ranks as the third leading cause of cancer-related deaths [1, 2]. Historically, HCC has been more prevalent in the developing world; however, in the last two decades the incidence has nearly doubled in developed countries; this has been largely due to liver cirrhosis [2, 3]. The 5-year survival rate of HCC in the United States is only 8.9% [4]. Even with aggressive conventional therapy, this malignancy is the second most lethal cancer after pancreatic adenocarcinoma [4]. This review summarizes the etiology and pathogenesis of HCC.

1.2 Etiology

HCC has been associated with various risk factors including viral hepatitis, cirrhosis (with any underlying etiology including nonalcoholic fatty liver disease (NAFLD)), and toxin-mediated disease (Fig. 1.1). There are two main hepatitis viruses associated with the development of HCC: hepatitis B virus (HBV) and hepatitis C virus (HCV) [5]. The major toxins that predispose to HCC include alcohol and aflatoxin-B1 [6]. During the last 10 years, there has been a clear delineation of the nature of the genetic alterations in HCC, including homozygous deletions in chromosome 9 (CDKN2A) and high-level DNA amplifications in chromosome 11q13 (FGF19/CNND1) and 6p21 (VEGFA) [7]. Associated with an increased telomerase expression, the most frequent mutations affect TERT promoter [7]. CTNNB1 and TP53 are the next most prevalent mutations [7]. Other etiological factors have been proposed to develop into HCC but at a much lower frequency.

T.S. Brar, M.D. • E. Hilgenfeldt, M.D. • C. Soldevila-Pico, M.D. (✉)
Gastroenterology, Hepatology and Nutrition, University of Florida, Gainesville, FL, USA
e-mail: Tony.Brar@medicine.ufl.edu; Consuelo.SoldevilaPico@medicine.ufl.edu

© Springer International Publishing AG 2018
C. Liu (ed.), *Precision Molecular Pathology of Liver Cancer*,
Molecular Pathology Library, https://doi.org/10.1007/978-3-319-68082-8_1

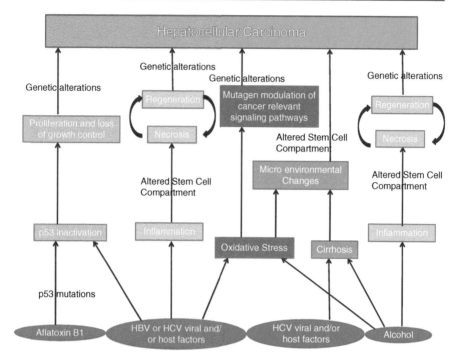

Fig. 1.1 Hepatocarcinogenesis mechanisms. The various risk factors are shown. Hepatitis B virus (HBV) and hepatitis C virus (HCV)

1.3   Virus-Induced Hepatocarcinogenesis

As mentioned previously, the two major viral contributors to HCC are HBV and HCV. Worldwide, HBV infects over two billion individuals and accounts for more than 300,000 deaths annually [8], and close to half of all HBV-related deaths are attributable to HCC [8]. A strong correlation between elevated serum HBV DNA levels and incidence of HCC has been described [9]. The prevalence of HCV is much lower than that of HBV [10]. There are over 170 million individuals worldwide infected with HCV [11], but only 2.5% develop HCC. However, over 20% of chronic cases result in liver cirrhosis [12]. Both viral and host factors are involved in driving hepatocarcinogenesis.

1.3.1   HBV

Classified as a member of the *Hepadnaviridae* family, HBV is a partially double-stranded hepatotropic DNA virus [13]. During the transformation process, there is direct involvement of HBV. To illustrate, HBV genomic integration has been linked to host DNA microdeletions, which target cancer-related genes such as mitogen-activated protein kinase 1 (MAPK1), platelet-derived growth factor receptor-beta (PDGFR-β), and telomerase reverse transcriptase (TERT) [14]. There are several other mechanisms that have demonstrated the direct involvement of HBV in the development of HCC [15]. The expression of growth control genes (JNK, ERK, Raf, Ras, MAPK, and SRC tyrosine kinases) can be altered by protein x (HBx) transcriptional activation [16]. Lastly, tumor-suppressor p53 can be bound and inactivated in vitro by HBx; this compromises DNA damage checkpoints and increases cellular survival and proliferation [17].

There are several ways in which host-viral interactions play a role. HBV mutations may result in retention of the virus within the hepatocyte, allowing the virus to escape the host's system, leading to liver disease [18]. An alternative mechanism involves the generation of free radicals which activate stellate cells through the induction of oxidative stress, thus stimulating survival-signaling pathways [19] creating a pro-carcinogenic state in the liver. Most HBV infections are acute; however, 10% of adults have reduced clearance leading to chronic active infection [20]. This creates sustained cycles of necrosis-inflammation-regeneration [4]. This process can lead to genomic instability through the propagation of oncogenic lesions and telomere erosion [21].

1.3.2 HCV

As a member of the *Flaviviridae* family, HCV is a non-cytopathic positive-stranded RNA genome [22]. There are several important distinctions between HCV and HBV that are relevant to hepatocarcinogenesis. First, HCV is a RNA virus so it cannot integrate into host genomes as it has no DNA intermediate [23]. Second, HCV is much more likely to yield chronic infection: 80% of HCV vs. 10% of HBV [24]. This can be attributed to high rates of replication errors, which result in immune avoidance by HCV [25]. Lastly, after 10 years of infection, about 10% of HCV-infected patients develop liver cirrhosis, a percentage that is almost 20 times larger than that of HBV-infected patients [24].

Core proteins and HCV RNA impair important steps involved with T-cell activation and dendritic cell functions [26]. NS5A nonstructural protein and HCV core protein are involved with evasion from immune-mediated cell killing [27]. This process involves interactions with various factors that include but are not limited to tumor necrosis factor-alpha (TNF-α) receptor and interferon-alpha (IFNα) [28]. Furthermore, NS3 and NS4A HCV proteins cleave and activate components through their protease function that is vital in signaling an immune response [29, 30]. HCV core proteins have been shown to modulate cell proliferation by interacting with components of the MAPK signaling pathway which includes Raf, MEK, and ERK [31]. The p53-regulated pathways that control tumor angiogenesis, cell-cycle progression, response to hypoxic and genotypic stresses, and cellular survival are inactivated by NS5A through sequestration of the perinuclear membrane [32, 33]. An oxidative stress-mediated mechanism is likely involved with HCV-induced HCC due to the carcinogenic potential of the HCV core proteins that lead to hepatic steatosis [34].

1.4   NAFLD Cirrhosis-Induced Hepatocarcinogenesis

The rise in NAFLD can be associated with the increase in the prevalence of diabetes mellitus and obesity [6]. It has been estimated that close to two thirds of the diabetic and obese population ultimately develop NAFLD [35]. Globally, the most common etiology for chronic liver disease is NAFLD [35]. NAFLD can be viewed as a spectrum of disease ranging from an accumulation of fat greater than 5% of liver weight known as simple steatosis to an aggressive form with fibrosis and necroinflammation nonalcoholic steatohepatitis (NASH) [36]. Up to 20% of the patients who develop NASH are likely to advance to cirrhosis and are at risk for complications of end-stage liver disease [37]. One of these complications is HCC.

There are numerous mechanisms underlying the pathogenesis of NASH-related HCC (Fig. 1.2). Pro-inflammatory cytokines including IL-6 and TNF-α and free fatty acids are produced with insulin resistance which is associated with NAFLD [38]. Pro-oncogenic pathways are promoted by TNF-α that specifically involve mammalian target of rapamycin complex (mTOR), c-Jun amino acid-terminal kinase (JNK), and nuclear factor κB [39, 40]. A decreased carcinogenic response occurs with weight loss through reduced levels of IL-6 and TNF-α [41]. Continued malignant transformation is likely with prolonged upregulation of the IL-6/STAT3 axis [42].

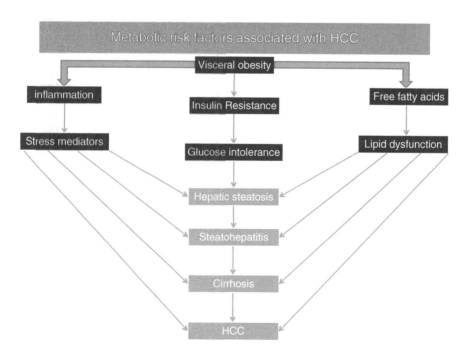

Fig. 1.2 Metabolic pathogenetic pathways to hepatocellular carcinoma (HCC)

Insulin-like growth factor-1 (IGF-1) is produced through the upregulation by insulin resistance [43]. HCC development is linked to IGF-1-promoted processes such as activating mitogen-activated protein kinases (MAPK) and the expression of proto-oncogenes c-jun and c-fos in vitro [43]. A MAPK, JNK, is downregulated by weight loss [44]. The role of phosphorylated JNK in the development of HCC is demonstrated by histopathological analysis revealing that over 70% of HCC tissue specimens stain positive for the protein kinase [44]. The frequency of TERT promoter mutations rapidly increased during the different steps of the transformation of premalignant lesions into HCC on cirrhosis [45]. Consequently, somatic TERT promoter mutation is a new biomarker predictive of transformation of premalignant lesions into HCC [45].

1.5 Toxin-Mediated Hepatocarcinogenesis

1.5.1 Alcohol Induced

Chronic alcohol use is an important risk factor for the development of HCC [46]. Chronic alcohol use causes activation of monocytes through the production of inflammatory cytokines [47]. Circulating endotoxin concentrations are increased, activating Kupffer cells and resulting in the release of many cytokines and chemokines (including prostaglandin E2, IL6, TNF-α, interleukin-1β); these factors have an adverse effect on the survival of hepatocytes [48]. An increased sensitivity to TNF-α in the setting of chronic alcohol exposure leads to stellate cell activation, chronic hepatocyte destruction-regeneration, cirrhosis, and eventually HCC [49].

Other alcohol-induced oxidative stress mechanisms include changes in hepatocarcinogenesis signaling pathways with the loss of protective effects of IFNγ, reduced STAT1 (signal transducer and activator of transcription 1) tyrosine phosphorylation, and diminished STAT1-directed activation of IFNγ signaling, which result in subsequent hepatocyte damage [50]. Fibrosis and/or cirrhosis can be the result of oxidative stress [51] creating a permissive HCC microenvironment that has a pro-carcinogenic effect which has been shown in PDGF transgenic mice [52]. The fibrotic response involves elevated collagen synthesis and cell proliferation that occurs with oxidative stress induction of cultured stellate cells with isoprostane treatment [53]. In the injured liver, the main source of collagen deposition are the stellate cells [54].

1.5.2 Aflatoxin-B1 Induced

An increased risk for the development of HCC also occurs with ingestion of the fungal toxin aflatoxin-B1 [55]. Cooperating mutational activation of oncogenes such as HRAS and associated with a particular p53 mutation, aflatoxin-B1 functions as a specific mutagen [56]. The major difference between this etiology and alcohol-induced and HCV-induced hepatocarcinogenesis is that there is no clear connection between the development of cirrhosis and aflatoxin-B1 exposure [57]. The primary drivers of HCC development are the mutational activities of the toxin itself. It is important to note that HBV infection coexists with aflatoxin-B1 exposure and there is a tenfold increased risk of developing HCC compared with exposure to just one of these factors [58].

1.6   Common Themes

After review of the major etiologies present in the development of HCC, it is evident there are common pathogenetic processes and pathways. To illustrate, p53 mutation or inactivation is consistent with aflatoxin-B1, HBV, and HCV-induced HCC [59]. Furthermore, characteristics inherent to alcohol-, HBV-, and HCV-induced hepatocarcinogenesis such as oxidative stress, inflammation, and continuous cycles of necrosis and regeneration suggest the importance of these fundamental mechanisms in the development of HCC [60]. HBV and HCV activate the MAPK pathway, indicating its pathogenetic relevance. Epidermal growth factor (EGF), hepatocyte growth factor (HGF), platelet-derived growth factor (PDGF), and vascular endothelial growth factor (VEGF) participate in the activation of RAS/MAPK signaling pathway playing a key role in cell proliferation [61]. The abnormal activation of RAS/MAPK pathway results from an aberrant upstream signals from EGFR and IGF [62]. VEGF, PDGF, and FGF are important proangiogenic factors that play a role in neovascularization, invasiveness, and metastatic potential of HCC [63]. VEGFR-1 and VEGFR-2 are expressed on the endothelial cells and initiate the cascade. PDGF is helpful for angiogenesis by recruiting pericytes and smooth muscle cells around nascent vessel sprouts [64]. As VEGF, FGF, and PDGF expression correlates with metastatic potential of tumor cells, inhibitors of VEGF, FGF, and PDGF signaling pathways are useful as therapeutic agents [65].

The drug discovery industry will find the common molecular changes among the different etiologies to be very important [4]. This will hold the largest plausibility for investment and increase the probability of deploying and developing the agents necessary that would benefit particularly the underserved populations [66] (Table 1.1).

Table 1.1 Hepatocarcinogenesis mechanisms with respect to etiology

Etiologies	Mechanism
HBV, HCV, aflatoxin-B1	p53 inactivation or mutation
HBV, HCV, alcohol	Inflammation, necrosis/regeneration
HBV, HCV, alcohol	Oxidative stress
HCV, alcohol	Liver cirrhosis

1.7 Molecular Mechanisms

The neoplastic evolution of HCC follows through a several staged histologic mechanism that is not as properly defined as that of other cancer types. First step toward HCC involves regenerating hepatocytes that have hyperplastic nodules with normal cytological features [67]. Abnormal liver architecture is noted when there is increased thickening of the trabeculae, nuclear crowding, and clear cell changes [68]. This occurs when the hyperplastic nodules progress to premalignant dysplastic nodules [69]. Metastatic potential is achieved, and these dysplastic nodules gain the capacity to invade the vessels and surrounding fibrous stroma [70]. Several key tumor-suppressor genes and oncogenes are deregulated through many epigenetic and genetic alterations that occur during the pathway to HCC, and they include cyclooxygenase 2 (COX2), E-cadherin, p16(INK4α), MET and its ligand hepatocyte growth factor (HGF), ErbB receptor family members, B-catenin, and TP53 [71].

1.7.1 Methylation

Deviant DNA methylation forms have been documented in the development of human HCC [72]. In the earliest stages of hepatocarcinogenesis, methylation has played a vital role in the tumor progression [73]. There are specific hypermethylation events that targeted apoptosis-associated speck-like protein (ASC), COX2, E-cadherin, p16(INK4α), and deleted in liver cancer 1 (DLC1) [74–77]. Abnormal apoptotic activity has been shown to play a role in the pathogenesis of HCC, and agents have been in developmental phases targeting pro-apoptotic receptors. Apoptosis can occur intrinsically or extrinsically. In HCC some pro-apoptotic molecules like p53, PTEN, and Bax are downregulated, and anti-apoptotic signals like Snail, B-catenin, NF-Kb, and Ras/ERK are overexpressed, leading to imbalance and evasion of apoptosis [61, 78]. The significance of hypermethylation of some of these genes has shown relevance in silencing these key genes, which would provide an alternate route for the development of anti-oncological medications [79, 80].

1.7.2 MET and HGF

In advanced HCC, there have been reports of overexpression of the MET receptor [81]. This role has actually been confirmed in mouse models. One of the most lethal hepatocyte mitogens, MET ligand HGF, in developed HCCs by one and a half years of age [82]. Tumor regression by impaired cell proliferation and apoptosis resulted from the termination of transgene expression and hepatic-driven expression of the inducible activated MET transgene leading to HCC [83]. IGF-I and IGF-II have a limited role in the pathogenesis of HCC, but downregulation of tumor-suppressor IGFBP-1, IGFBP-2, IGFBP-3, and IGFBP-4 was found to be associated with HCC

[84]. Overexpression of IGF-1 and IGF-2 receptors and downregulation of IGF binding proteins contribute to proliferation of cancer cells, anti-apoptosis, and invasive behavior [65, 78]. Some agents are in developmental stages targeting IGF-1 receptors.

1.7.3 ErbB Receptor Family

There are four members of the ErbB family of receptor tyrosine kinases (ERBB1–ERBB4) that have been involved in the process of several different types of human cancers [85]. There is in fact overexpression of ERBB3 about 85% of HCC cases, ERBB1 (epidermal growth factor receptor (EGFR)) in about 70%, ERBB4 in 60%, and ERBB2 (also known as HER2) in 20% [86]. Dedifferentiation and tumor size, intrahepatic metastasis, and high proliferation index were some of the more aggressive presentations that were correlated with ERBB3 and ERBB1 expression [86, 87]. Gefitinib inhibits ERBB1, and this shows further support of its involvement in hepatocarcinogenesis [88]. This results in apoptosis, cell-cycle arrest, and growth inhibition [88]. Erlotinib, another ERBB1 inhibitor, also showed clinical efficacy with evidence by disease control with about 60% of participating patients and about 35% remained progression-free after 6 months of treatment [89]. Further evidence of ErbB family of receptor involvement comes from studies in mice. Mice transgenic for transforming growth factor-alpha (TGFα) (a ligand for ErbB receptors and a member of the EGF family) have been shown to develop HCC [90, 91]. In TGFα-deficient mice, there are smaller hepatic neoplasms, whereas hepatocarcinogen treatment increases HCC development in the TGFα transgenic strain [92, 93]. HBV transgenic strains can also cooperate with TGFα to effectively increase the incidence of HCC [94].

1.7.4 B-Catenin

A crucial downstream component of the Wnt signaling pathway is B-catenin. Aberrant Wnt/B-catenin signaling activity has been demonstrated in up to one third of cases of HCC secondary to HCV. The pathway is dysregulated primarily as a result of mutations in CTNNB1 or AXIN1 or altered expression of Wnt receptors inducing changes in oncogenes like CCDN1, Cmyc, or BIRC [95, 96]. The pathway can be exploited as a target for treatment of HCC. Increased nuclear expression and B-catenin mutations have been detected in human HCC [97].

There are some reports that indicate that B-catenin mutations and overexpression have related to HCC progression and others that showed early-stage HCC [98–100]. More frequently mutations and overexpression of B-catenin occur in HCV-related HCC compared with HBV-related HCC [98, 101]. However, in hepatoma cells, the HBx protein stabilizes B-catenin and as a result is implicated in HBV-related HCC [102]. There has been an association of increased nuclear p53 expression and loss of E-cadherin with the accumulation of nuclear B-catenin [103].

In HCCs that are not characterized by genomic instability, there have been suggestions that B-catenin mutations are in fact typical. Detected by their elevated loss of heterozygosity (LOH), human HCCs with increased rates of genomic instability demonstrate decreased mutations of B-catenin [104]. While studies in the mouse show that there is a high genomic instability or high rate of B-catenin mutations in HCCs [105]. This indicated that the Wnt signaling pathway might represent another route to hepatocarcinogenesis [104, 105].

1.7.5 p53 Tumor Suppression

It is widely accepted that deficiency of p53 participates in the pathogenesis of HCC, but there still remains some issue as to whether a p53 mutation contributes to cancer progression, initiation, or both, and this remains an active area of investigation [106]. In an HBx transgenic mouse model, p53 was involved with constraining progression to HCC by the functional inactivation of p53 by HBx (through sequestration in the cytoplasm) but not in altered foci (initiation foci) [15, 107]. Full genetic inactivation of p53 is associated with progression to late-stage disease as is evidenced by mutations in p53 being detected only in larger HCCs [108]. There has been an increased association with advanced malignances (greater than 40%) with p53 mutations in HBV- and HCV-related HCCs as compared to regenerative nodules (less than 7%) [109]. Even though this pattern might indicate some role of progression, it does not exclude the chance that the p53 mutant generative nodules initiated the productive carcinogenic process [109]. Also, conventional sequencing approaches may not detect rare p53 mutant cells that are more common in regenerative nodules [110]. Furthermore, in regions of low aflatoxin-B1 exposure, there are p53 mutations in very late stages of HCC, but in regions of high aflatoxin-B1 exposure, the p53 mutations are in very early-stage HCC lesions [111].

Depending on the sequence of events, it is likely that a p53 mutation can either operate in HCC initiation or progression. In the presence of aflatoxin-B1, initiation of tumor can be driven by the mutation with other cooperating events with other etiologies, specifically those that provoke telomere erosion, oxidative stress, and regeneration; the loss of p53 has a more prominent role in HCC progression [112]. This can contribute to HCC genomic instability which is facilitated by the continued proliferative potential occurring by activated DNA damage signaling [113]. This is evident in liver tumor progression with telomere-induced chromosomal instability. The p53 heterozygosity through germline mutation allows progression of HCC in mice with short telomeres in chronic liver disease [114].

Conclusion

It is evident that HCC is an enigmatic and aggressive disease that is driven by various etiologies ranging from viruses to metabolic disorders. There are many opportunities to study further in the areas relating to the environment, genetic, and cell biology mechanisms of hepatocarcinogenesis that are applicable to the differing etiologies. It is clear that early diagnosis and treatment are essential due to the high levels of genomic instability in chronic disease and the lethality of HCC. As we continue to further our understanding of human HCC and the mechanisms involved, the field will gain a solid foundation that can help to refine animal models and truly comprehend the entire range of human disease.

References

1. Singal AG, El-Serag HB. Hepatocellular carcinoma from epidemiology to prevention: translating knowledge into practice. Clin Gastroenterol Hepatol. 2015;13(12):2140–51.
2. Njei B, Rotman Y, Ditah I, Lim JK. Emerging trends in hepatocellular carcinoma incidence and mortality. Hepatology. 2015;61(1):191–9.
3. El-Serag HB, Kanwal F. Epidemiology of hepatocellular carcinoma in the United States: where are we? Where do we go? Hepatology. 2014;60(5):1767–75.
4. Farazi PA, DePinho RA. Hepatocellular carcinoma pathogenesis: from genes to environment. Nat Rev Cancer. 2006;6(9):674–87.
5. Nault J-C. Pathogenesis of hepatocellular carcinoma according to aetiology. Best Pract Res Clin Gastroenterol. 2014;28(5):937–47.
6. Khan FZ, Perumpail RB, Wong RJ, Ahmed A. Advances in hepatocellular carcinoma: nonalcoholic steatohepatitis-related hepatocellular carcinoma. World J Hepatol. 2015;7(18):2155–61.
7. Zucman-Rossi J, Villanueva A, Nault JC, Llovet JM. Genetic landscape and biomarkers of hepatocellular carcinoma. Gastroenterology. 2015;149(5):1226–39.e4.
8. Lavanchy D. Hepatitis B virus epidemiology, disease burden, treatment, and current and emerging prevention and control measures. J Viral Hepat. 2004;11(2):97–107.
9. Wong GL. Optimal surveillance program for hepatocellular carcinoma—getting ready, but not yet. World J Hepatol. 2015;7(18):2133–5.
10. Chen CJ, Yang HI, Su J, Jen CL, You SL, Lu SN, et al. Risk of hepatocellular carcinoma across a biological gradient of serum hepatitis B virus DNA level. JAMA. 2006;295(1):65–73.
11. Chisari FV. Unscrambling hepatitis C virus-host interactions. Nature. 2005;436(7053):930–2.
12. Bowen DG, Walker CM. Adaptive immune responses in acute and chronic hepatitis C virus infection. Nature. 2005;436(7053):946–52.
13. Onofrey S, Aneja J, Haney GA, Nagami EH, DeMaria A, Lauer GM, et al. Underascertainment of acute hepatitis C virus infections in the U.S. surveillance system: a case series and chart review. Ann Intern Med. 2015;163(4):254–61.
14. Murakami Y, Saigo K, Takashima H, Minami M, Okanoue T, Bréchot C, et al. Large scaled analysis of hepatitis B virus (HBV) DNA integration in HBV related hepatocellular carcinomas. Gut. 2005;54(8):1162–8.
15. Feitelson MA, Sun B, Satiroglu Tufan NL, Liu J, Pan J, Lian Z. Genetic mechanisms of hepatocarcinogenesis. Oncogene. 2002;21(16):2593–604.
16. Tarn C, Lee S, Hu Y, Ashendel C, Andrisani OM. Hepatitis B virus X protein differentially activates RAS-RAF-MAPK and JNK pathways in X-transforming versus non-transforming AML12 hepatocytes. J Biol Chem. 2001;276(37):34671–80.
17. Park YM. Clinical utility of complex mutations in the core promoter and proximal precore regions of the hepatitis B virus genome. World J Hepatol. 2015;7(1):113–20.
18. Baran B. Nucleos(t)ide analogs in the prevention of hepatitis B virus related hepatocellular carcinoma. World J Hepatol. 2015;7(13):1742–54.
19. Galli A, Svegliati-Baroni G, Ceni E, Milani S, Ridolfi F, Salzano R, et al. Oxidative stress stimulates proliferation and invasiveness of hepatic stellate cells via a MMP2-mediated mechanism. Hepatology. 2005;41(5):1074–84.

20. Lok AS, Heathcote EJ, Hoofnagle JH. Management of hepatitis B: 2000—summary of a workshop. Gastroenterology. 2001;120(7):1828–53.
21. Lee JE, Oh BK, Choi J, Park YN. Telomeric 3′ overhangs in chronic HBV-related hepatitis and hepatocellular carcinoma. Int J Cancer. 2008;123(2):264–72.
22. Tada T, Kumada T, Toyoda H, Kiriyama S, Tanikawa M, Hisanaga Y, et al. Long-term prognosis of patients with chronic hepatitis C who did not receive interferon-based therapy: causes of death and analysis based on the FIB-4 index. J Gastroenterol. 2016;51(4):380–9.
23. Rehermann B, Bertoletti A. Immunological aspects of antiviral therapy of chronic hepatitis B virus and hepatitis C virus infections. Hepatology. 2015;61(2):712–21.
24. Rehermann B, Nascimbeni M. Immunology of hepatitis B virus and hepatitis C virus infection. Nat Rev Immunol. 2005;5(3):215–29.
25. Kogiso T, Hashimoto E, Ikarashi Y, Kodama K, Taniai M, Torii N, et al. Spontaneous clearance of HCV accompanying hepatitis after liver transplantation. Clin J Gastroenterol. 2015.
26. Pachiadakis I, Pollara G, Chain BM, Naoumov NV. Is hepatitis C virus infection of dendritic cells a mechanism facilitating viral persistence? Lancet Infect Dis. 2005;5(5):296–304.
27. Melén K, Fagerlund R, Nyqvist M, Keskinen P, Julkunen I. Expression of hepatitis C virus core protein inhibits interferon-induced nuclear import of STATs. J Med Virol. 2004;73(4): 536–47.
28. Park KJ, Choi SH, Choi DH, Park JM, Yie SW, Lee SY, et al. 1Hepatitis C virus NS5A protein modulates c-Jun N-terminal kinase through interaction with tumor necrosis factor receptor-associated factor 2. J Biol Chem. 2003;278(33):30711–8.
29. Foy E, Li K, Sumpter R, Loo YM, Johnson CL, Wang C, et al. Control of antiviral defenses through hepatitis C virus disruption of retinoic acid-inducible gene-I signaling. Proc Natl Acad Sci U S A. 2005;102(8):2986–91.
30. Li K, Foy E, Ferreon JC, Nakamura M, Ferreon AC, Ikeda M, et al. Immune evasion by hepatitis C virus NS3/4A protease-mediated cleavage of the Toll-like receptor 3 adaptor protein TRIF. Proc Natl Acad Sci U S A. 2005;102(8):2992–7.
31. Chen WC, Tseng CK, Chen YH, Lin CK, Hsu SH, Wang SN, et al. HCV NS5A up-regulates COX-2 expression via IL-8-mediated activation of the ERK/JNK MAPK pathway. PLoS One. 2015;10(7):e0133264.
32. Dixit U, Pandey AK, Liu Z, Kumar S, Neiditch MB, Klein KM, et al. FUSE binding protein 1 facilitates persistent hepatitis C virus replication in hepatoma cells by regulating tumor suppressor p53. J Virol. 2015;89(15):7905–21.
33. EI-Emshaty HM, Gadelhak SA, Abdelaziz MM, Abbas AT, Gadelhak NA. Serum P53 Abs in HCC patients with viral hepatitis—type C. Hepatogastroenterology. 2014;61(134):1688–95.
34. Moriya K, Nakagawa K, Santa T, Shintani Y, Fujie H, Miyoshi H, et al. Oxidative stress in the absence of inflammation in a mouse model for hepatitis C virus-associated hepatocarcinogenesis. Cancer Res. 2001;61(11):4365–70.
35. Raff EJ, Kakati D, Bloomer JR, Shoreibah M, Rasheed K, Singal AK. Diabetes mellitus predicts occurrence of cirrhosis and hepatocellular cancer in alcoholic liver and non-alcoholic fatty liver diseases. J Clin Transl Hepatol. 2015;3(1):9–16.
36. Berzigotti A, Saran U, Dufour JF. Physical activity and liver diseases. Hepatology. 2016;63(3):1026–40.
37. Perumpail RB, Wong RJ, Ahmed A, Harrison SA. Hepatocellular carcinoma in the setting of non-cirrhotic nonalcoholic fatty liver disease and the metabolic syndrome: US experience. Dig Dis Sci. 2015;60(10):3142–8.
38. Dongiovanni P, Romeo S, Valenti L. Genetic factors in the pathogenesis of nonalcoholic fatty liver and steatohepatitis. Biomed Res Int. 2015;2015:460190.
39. Stickel F, Hellerbrand C. Non-alcoholic fatty liver disease as a risk factor for hepatocellular carcinoma: mechanisms and implications. Gut. 2010;59(10):1303–7.
40. Marra F, Gastaldelli A, Svegliati Baroni G, Tell G, Tiribelli C. Molecular basis and mechanisms of progression of non-alcoholic steatohepatitis. Trends Mol Med. 2008; 14(2):72–81.

41. Bougoulia M, Triantos A, Koliakos G. Effect of weight loss with or without orlistat treatment on adipocytokines, inflammation, and oxidative markers in obese women. Hormones (Athens). 2006;5(4):259–69.

42. Zhao H, Guo Y, Li S, Han R, Ying J, Zhu H, et al. A novel anti-cancer agent Icaritin suppresses hepatocellular carcinoma initiation and malignant growth through the IL-6/Jak2/Stat3 pathway. Oncotarget. 2015;6(31):31927–43.

43. Sasaki Y. Insulin resistance and hepatocarcinogenesis. Clin J Gastroenterol. 2010;3(6):271–8.

44. Chang Q, Zhang Y, Beezhold KJ, Bhatia D, Zhao H, Chen J, et al. Sustained JNK1 activation is associated with altered histone H3 methylations in human liver cancer. J Hepatol. 2009;50(2):323–33.

45. Nault JC, Calderaro J, Di Tommaso L, Balabaud C, Zafrani ES, Bioulac-Sage P, et al. Telomerase reverse transcriptase promoter mutation is an early somatic genetic alteration in the transformation of premalignant nodules in hepatocellular carcinoma on cirrhosis. Hepatology. 2014;60(6):1983–92.

46. Raffetti E, Portolani N, Molfino S, Baiocchi GL, Limina RM, Caccamo G, et al. Role of aetiology, diabetes, tobacco smoking and hypertension in hepatocellular carcinoma survival. Dig Liver Dis. 2015;47(11):950–6.

47. McClain CJ, Hill DB, Song Z, Deaciuc I, Barve S. Monocyte activation in alcoholic liver disease. Alcohol. 2002;27(1):53–61.

48. Wang F, Yang JL, Yu KK, Xu M, Xu YZ, Chen L, et al. Activation of the NF-κB pathway as a mechanism of alcohol enhanced progression and metastasis of human hepatocellular carcinoma. Mol Cancer. 2015;14:10.

49. Kawaguchi Y, Mizuta T. Interaction between hepatitis C virus and metabolic factors. World J Gastroenterol. 2014;20(11):2888–901.

50. Osna NA, Clemens DL, Donohue TM. Ethanol metabolism alters interferon gamma signaling in recombinant HepG2 cells. Hepatology. 2005;42(5):1109–17.

51. Takaki A, Yamamoto K. Control of oxidative stress in hepatocellular carcinoma: helpful or harmful? World J Hepatol. 2015;7(7):968–79.

52. Campbell JS, Hughes SD, Gilbertson DG, Palmer TE, Holdren MS, Haran AC, et al. Platelet-derived growth factor C induces liver fibrosis, steatosis, and hepatocellular carcinoma. Proc Natl Acad Sci U S A. 2005;102(9):3389–94.

53. Comporti M, Arezzini B, Signorini C, Sgherri C, Monaco B, Gardi C. F2-isoprostanes stimulate collagen synthesis in activated hepatic stellate cells: a link with liver fibrosis? Lab Invest. 2005;85(11):1381–91.

54. Thompson AI, Conroy KP, Henderson NC. Hepatic stellate cells: central modulators of hepatic carcinogenesis. BMC Gastroenterol. 2015;15:63.

55. Kew MC. Aflatoxins as a cause of hepatocellular carcinoma. J Gastrointestin Liver Dis. 2013;22(3):305–10.

56. Riley J, Mandel HG, Sinha S, Judah DJ, Neal GE. In vitro activation of the human Harvey-ras proto-oncogene by aflatoxin B1. Carcinogenesis. 1997;18(5):905–10.

57. De Minicis S, Marzioni M, Benedetti A, Svegliati-Baroni G. New insights in hepatocellular carcinoma: from bench to bedside. Ann Transl Med. 2013;1(2):15.

58. Kew MC. Synergistic interaction between aflatoxin B1 and hepatitis B virus in hepatocarcinogenesis. Liver Int. 2003;23(6):405–9.

59. Hao PP, Li H, Lee MJ, Wang YP, Kim JH, Yu GR, et al. Disruption of a regulatory loop between DUSP1 and p53 contributes to hepatocellular carcinoma development and progression. J Hepatol. 2015;62(6):1278–86.

60. Sakurai T, He G, Matsuzawa A, Yu GY, Maeda S, Hardiman G, et al. Hepatocyte necrosis induced by oxidative stress and IL-1 alpha release mediate carcinogen-induced compensatory proliferation and liver tumorigenesis. Cancer Cell. 2008;14(2):156–65.

61. Lachenmayer A, Alsinet C, Chang CY, Llovet JM. Molecular approaches to treatment of hepatocellular carcinoma. Dig Liver Dis. 2010;42(Suppl 3):S264–72.

62. Calvisi DF, Ladu S, Gorden A, Farina M, Conner EA, Lee JS, et al. Ubiquitous activation of Ras and Jak/Stat pathways in human HCC. Gastroenterology. 2006;130(4):1117–28.
63. Torimura T, Sata M, Ueno T, Kin M, Tsuji R, Suzaku K, et al. Increased expression of vascular endothelial growth factor is associated with tumor progression in hepatocellular carcinoma. Hum Pathol. 1998;29(9):986–91.
64. Conway EM, Collen D, Carmeliet P. Molecular mechanisms of blood vessel growth. Cardiovasc Res. 2001;49(3):507–21.
65. Huynh H. Molecularly targeted therapy in hepatocellular carcinoma. Biochem Pharmacol. 2010;80(5):550–60.
66. Hlady RA, Tiedemann RL, Puszyk W, Zendejas I, Roberts LR, Choi JH, et al. Epigenetic signatures of alcohol abuse and hepatitis infection during human hepatocarcinogenesis. Oncotarget. 2014;5(19):9425–43.
67. Sakamoto M. Pathology of early hepatocellular carcinoma. Hepatol Res. 2007;37(Suppl 2):S135–8.
68. Sciarra A, Di Tommaso L, Nakano M, Destro A, Torzilli G, Donadon M, et al. Morphophenotypic changes in human multistep hepatocarcinogenesis with translational implications. J Hepatol. 2016;64(1):87–93.
69. Lu XF, Zhou YJ, Zhang L, Ji HJ, Li L, Shi YJ, et al. Loss of Dicer1 impairs hepatocyte survival and leads to chronic inflammation and progenitor cell activation. World J Gastroenterol. 2015;21(21):6591–603.
70. Hsieh YH, Chang YY, Su IJ, Yen CJ, Liu YR, Liu RJ, et al. Hepatitis B virus pre-S2 mutant large surface protein inhibits DNA double-strand break repair and leads to genome instability in hepatocarcinogenesis. J Pathol. 2015;236(3):337–47.
71. Nishida N, Kudo M. Alteration of epigenetic profile in human hepatocellular carcinoma and its clinical implications. Liver Cancer. 2014;3(3–4):417–27.
72. Fan H, Zhao Z, Cheng Y, Cui H, Qiao F, Wang L, et al. Genome-wide profiling of DNA methylation reveals preferred sequences of DNMTs in hepatocellular carcinoma cells. Tumour Biol. 2016;37(1):877–85.
73. Lee S, Lee HJ, Kim JH, Lee HS, Jang JJ, Kang GH. Aberrant CpG island hypermethylation along multistep hepatocarcinogenesis. Am J Pathol. 2003;163(4):1371–8.
74. Murata H, Tsuji S, Tsujii M, Sakaguchi Y, Fu HY, Kawano S, et al. Promoter hypermethylation silences cyclooxygenase-2 (Cox-2) and regulates growth of human hepatocellular carcinoma cells. Lab Invest. 2004;84(8):1050–9.
75. Kubo T, Yamamoto J, Shikauchi Y, Niwa Y, Matsubara K, Yoshikawa H. Apoptotic speck protein-like, a highly homologous protein to apoptotic speck protein in the pyrin domain, is silenced by DNA methylation and induces apoptosis in human hepatocellular carcinoma. Cancer Res. 2004;64(15):5172–7.
76. Wong CM, Lee JM, Ching YP, Jin DY, Ng IO. Genetic and epigenetic alterations of DLC-1 gene in hepatocellular carcinoma. Cancer Res. 2003;63(22):7646–51.
77. Maeta Y, Shiota G, Okano J, Murawaki Y. Effect of promoter methylation of the p16 gene on phosphorylation of retinoblastoma gene product and growth of hepatocellular carcinoma cells. Tumour Biol. 2005;26(6):300–5.
78. Villanueva A, Newell P, Chiang DY, Friedman SL, Llovet JM. Genomics and signaling pathways in hepatocellular carcinoma. Semin Liver Dis. 2007;27(1):55–76.
79. Vacchelli E, Pol J, Bloy N, Eggermont A, Cremer I, Fridman WH, et al. Trial watch: tumor-targeting monoclonal antibodies for oncological indications. Oncoimmunology. 2015;4(1):e985940.
80. Perini MV, Starkey G, Fink MA, Bhandari R, Muralidharan V, Jones R, et al. From minimal to maximal surgery in the treatment of hepatocarcinoma: a review. World J Hepatol. 2015;7(1):93–100.
81. Daveau M, Scotte M, François A, Coulouarn C, Ros G, Tallet Y, et al. Hepatocyte growth factor, transforming growth factor alpha, and their receptors as combined markers of prognosis in hepatocellular carcinoma. Mol Carcinog. 2003;36(3):130–41.

82. Sakata H, Rubin JS, Taylor WG, Miki T. A Rho-specific exchange factor Ect2 is induced from S to M phases in regenerating mouse liver. Hepatology. 2000;32(2):193–9.
83. Horiguchi N, Takayama H, Toyoda M, Otsuka T, Fukusato T, Merlino G, et al. Hepatocyte growth factor promotes hepatocarcinogenesis through c-Met autocrine activation and enhanced angiogenesis in transgenic mice treated with diethylnitrosamine. Oncogene. 2002;21(12):1791–9.
84. Breuhahn K, Longerich T, Schirmacher P. Dysregulation of growth factor signaling in human hepatocellular carcinoma. Oncogene. 2006;25(27):3787–800.
85. Bekaii-Saab T, Williams N, Plass C, Calero MV, Eng C. A novel mutation in the tyrosine kinase domain of ERBB2 in hepatocellular carcinoma. BMC Cancer. 2006;6:278.
86. Ito Y, Takeda T, Sakon M, Tsujimoto M, Higashiyama S, Noda K, et al. Expression and clinical significance of erb-B receptor family in hepatocellular carcinoma. Br J Cancer. 2001;84(10):1377–83.
87. Berasain C, Avila MA. The EGFR signalling system in the liver: from hepatoprotection to hepatocarcinogenesis. J Gastroenterol. 2014;49(1):9–23.
88. Höpfner M, Sutter AP, Huether A, Schuppan D, Zeitz M, Scherübl H. Targeting the epidermal growth factor receptor by gefitinib for treatment of hepatocellular carcinoma. J Hepatol. 2004;41(6):1008–16.
89. Philip PA, Mahoney MR, Allmer C, Thomas J, Pitot HC, Kim G, et al. Phase II study of Erlotinib (OSI-774) in patients with advanced hepatocellular cancer. J Clin Oncol. 2005;23(27):6657–63.
90. Jhappan C, Stahle C, Harkins RN, Fausto N, Smith GH, Merlino GT. TGF alpha overexpression in transgenic mice induces liver neoplasia and abnormal development of the mammary gland and pancreas. Cell. 1990;61(6):1137–46.
91. Sandgren EP, Luetteke NC, Palmiter RD, Brinster RL, Lee DC. Overexpression of TGF alpha in transgenic mice: induction of epithelial hyperplasia, pancreatic metaplasia, and carcinoma of the breast. Cell. 1990;61(6):1121–35.
92. Webber EM, Wu JC, Wang L, Merlino G, Fausto N. Overexpression of transforming growth factor-alpha causes liver enlargement and increased hepatocyte proliferation in transgenic mice. Am J Pathol. 1994;145(2):398–408.
93. Russell WE, Kaufmann WK, Sitaric S, Luetteke NC, Lee DC. Liver regeneration and hepatocarcinogenesis in transforming growth factor-alpha-targeted mice. Mol Carcinog. 1996;15(3):183–9.
94. Lee SY, Song KH, Koo I, Lee KH, Suh KS, Kim BY. Comparison of pathways associated with hepatitis B- and C-infected hepatocellular carcinoma using pathway-based class discrimination method. Genomics. 2012;99(6):347–54.
95. Mínguez B, Tovar V, Chiang D, Villanueva A, Llovet JM. Pathogenesis of hepatocellular carcinoma and molecular therapies. Curr Opin Gastroenterol. 2009;25(3):186–94.
96. Taniguchi K, Roberts LR, Aderca IN, Dong X, Qian C, Murphy LM, et al. Mutational spectrum of beta-catenin, AXIN1, and AXIN2 in hepatocellular carcinomas and hepatoblastomas. Oncogene. 2002;21(31):4863–71.
97. Sempoux C, Paradis V, Komuta M, Wee A, Calderaro J, Balabaud C, et al. Hepatocellular nodules expressing markers of hepatocellular adenomas in Budd-Chiari syndrome and other rare hepatic vascular disorders. J Hepatol. 2015;63(5):1173–80.
98. Thorgeirsson SS, Grisham JW. Molecular pathogenesis of human hepatocellular carcinoma. Nat Genet. 2002;31(4):339–46.
99. Peng SY, Chen WJ, Lai PL, Jeng YM, Sheu JC, Hsu HC. High alpha-fetoprotein level correlates with high stage, early recurrence and poor prognosis of hepatocellular carcinoma: significance of hepatitis virus infection, age, p53 and beta-catenin mutations. Int J Cancer. 2004;112(1):44–50.
100. Wang XH, Meng XW, Sun X, DU YJ, Zhao J, Fan YJ. Wnt/b-catenin signaling pathway affects the protein expressions of caspase-3, XIAP and Grp-78 in hepatocellular carcinoma. Zhonghua Gan Zang Bing Za Zhi. 2011;19(8):599–602.

101. Yam JW, Wong CM, Ng IO. Molecular and functional genetics of hepatocellular carcinoma. Front Biosci (Schol Ed). 2010;2:117–34.
102. Cha MY, Kim CM, Park YM, Ryu WS. Hepatitis B virus X protein is essential for the activation of Wnt/beta-catenin signaling in hepatoma cells. Hepatology. 2004;39(6):1683–93.
103. Prange W, Breuhahn K, Fischer F, Zilkens C, Pietsch T, Petmecky K, et al. Beta-catenin accumulation in the progression of human hepatocarcinogenesis correlates with loss of E-cadherin and accumulation of p53, but not with expression of conventional WNT-1 target genes. J Pathol. 2003;201(2):250–9.
104. Gross-Goupil M, Riou P, Emile JF, Saffroy R, Azoulay D, Lacherade I, et al. Analysis of chromosomal instability in pulmonary or liver metastases and matched primary hepatocellular carcinoma after orthotopic liver transplantation. Int J Cancer. 2003;104(6):745–51.
105. Calvisi DF, Factor VM, Ladu S, Conner EA, Thorgeirsson SS. Disruption of beta-catenin pathway or genomic instability define two distinct categories of liver cancer in transgenic mice. Gastroenterology. 2004;126(5):1374–86.
106. You J, Yang H, Lai Y, Simon L, Au J, Burkart AL. ARID2, p110α, p53, and β-catenin protein expression in hepatocellular carcinoma and clinicopathologic implications. Hum Pathol. 2015;46(7):1068–77.
107. Kim CM, Koike K, Saito I, Miyamura T, Jay G. HBx gene of hepatitis B virus induces liver cancer in transgenic mice. Nature. 1991;351(6324):317–20.
108. Wu H, Ng R, Chen X, Steer CJ, Song G. MicroRNA-21 is a potential link between nonalcoholic fatty liver disease and hepatocellular carcinoma via modulation of the HBP1-p53-Srebp1c pathway. Gut. 2016;65(11):1850–60.
109. Minouchi K, Kaneko S, Kobayashi K. Mutation of p53 gene in regenerative nodules in cirrhotic liver. J Hepatol. 2002;37(2):231–9.
110. Honda M, Takehana K, Sakai A, Tagata Y, Shirasaki T, Nishitani S, et al. Malnutrition impairs interferon signaling through mTOR and FoxO pathways in patients with chronic hepatitis C. Gastroenterology. 2011;141(1):128–40, 40.e1–2.
111. Aguilar F, Harris CC, Sun T, Hollstein M, Cerutti P. Geographic variation of p53 mutational profile in nonmalignant human liver. Science. 1994;264(5163):1317–9.
112. Gori M, Barbaro B, Arciello M, Maggio R, Viscomi C, Longo A, et al. Protective effect of the Y220C mutant p53 against steatosis: good news? J Cell Physiol. 2014;229(9):1182–92.
113. Kew MC. The role of cirrhosis in the etiology of hepatocellular carcinoma. J Gastrointest Cancer. 2014;45(1):12–21.
114. Farazi PA, Glickman J, Horner J, Depinho RA. Cooperative interactions of p53 mutation, telomere dysfunction, and chronic liver damage in hepatocellular carcinoma progression. Cancer Res. 2006;66(9):4766–73.

Histologic Classification of Hepatocellular Carcinoma and Its Clinical Implications

2

Amy Leigh Collinsworth

Hepatocellular carcinoma (HCC) is the most common type of primary hepatic malignancy. The focus of this chapter is to review the histologic classification of HCC and the clinical implications of the various subtypes. Conventional HCC is the most common subtype, and the assigned nuclear grade is considered to have impact on prognosis. Many of the subtypes are so rare, including lymphoepithelioma-like and diffuse cirrhosis-like, that we have not yet accumulated enough data to assign prognostic significance. For the scirrhous variant, reports are conflicting as to whether they behave differently than conventional HCC [1]. While it may seem that assigning a histologic subtype may be an exercise in futility, we are making advances in the molecular classification that may potentially bring together histologic patterns with the molecular profile and ultimately result in a targeted treatment strategy.

2.1 Conventional Hepatocellular Carcinoma (HCC)

Some tumors form an expansile mass well demarcated from the surrounding background liver with or without a capsule (Fig. 2.1). Other tumors show an infiltrating edge at the tumor margin [2]. Vascular invasion is frequent in HCC with involvement of the portal vein, hepatic veins, or vena cava. Bile duct invasion is infrequent. Grossly HCC displays a variety of colors: cream-colored, yellow, green, brown, or mixed.

Histologically, the tumor cells of HCC resemble normal liver cells to a variable extent depending on the degree of differentiation. Nuclei are prominent with

A.L. Collinsworth, M.D.
Department of Pathology, Immunology and Laboratory Medicine,
University of Florida, Gainesville, FL, USA
e-mail: acolli@ufl.edu

© Springer International Publishing AG 2018
C. Liu (ed.), *Precision Molecular Pathology of Liver Cancer*,
Molecular Pathology Library, https://doi.org/10.1007/978-3-319-68082-8_2

Fig. 2.1 HCC arising in the background of cirrhosis

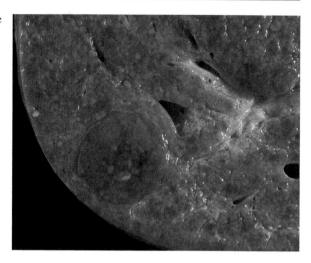

prominent nucleoli and cells have a high nuclear-cytoplasmic (N:C) ratio. There is typically some degree of nuclear pleomorphism and hyperchromasia, but this is highly variable. Cell membranes are usually distinct, and the cytoplasm is eosinophilic and finely granular (Fig. 2.2a, b) [2].

The cells of HCC can contain cellular products that mimic normal liver cell function. Bile canaliculi are almost always present and can be highlighted by an immunohistochemical (IHC) stain for polyclonal CEA (Fig. 2.2c). Bile pigment is seen in approximately 50% of tumors. Cytoplasmic fat and/or glycogen can be abundant and produce a clear cell appearance. Approximately 20% of tumors contain Mallory-Denk bodies and/or hyaline globules of alpha-1-antitrypsin.

Tumor cells grow in a pattern that mimics the cell plates of normal liver resulting in a classic trabecular growth pattern with thickened cell plates separated by capillarized sinusoids. The cells lining the thickened trabeculae phenotypically resemble capillary endothelial cells and can be highlighted with an immunohistochemical (IHC) stain for CD34 which would not stain normal hepatic sinusoidal endothelium (Fig. 2.2d). Both polyclonal CEA and CD10 show a canalicular staining pattern in HCC (Fig. 2.2c). Often the center of the trabeculae contains a dilated canaliculus producing a "pseudoglandular" appearance (Fig. 2.2b) [2]. Other than the scirrhous and fibrolamellar variants, fibrous stroma is not usually observed.

Stains can be a useful adjunct in both confirming hepatocellular differentiation and in distinguishing malignant from benign hepatocellular neoplasms. Multiple IHC stains are currently available to confirm hepatocellular differentiation including HepPar-1, arginase, and glypican-3. Glypican-3 is also useful to differentiate benign versus malignant hepatocellular tumors as it is found in 70–90% of HCCs and has not been reported in adenomas or normal hepatocytes [3].

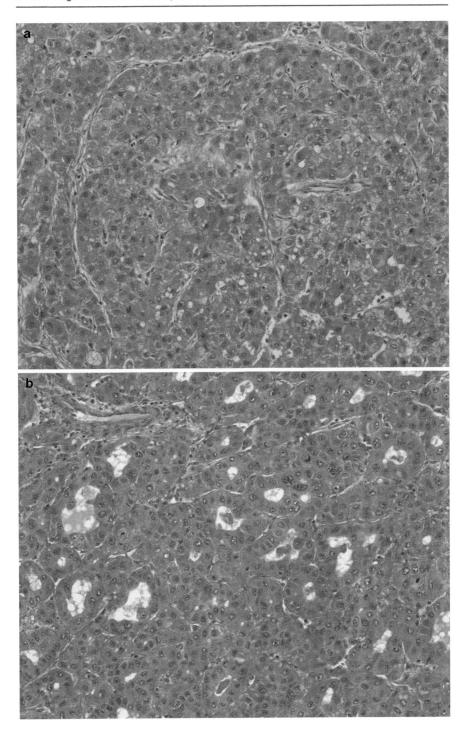

Fig. 2.2 Histological features of HCC. Immunohistochemical stain for polyclonal CEA (**c**) and CD34 (**d**)

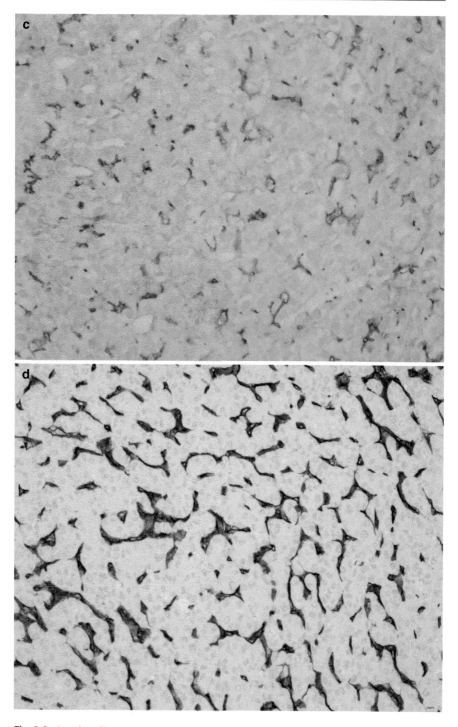

Fig. 2.2 (continued)

2.2   Small HCC

Small HCCs, less than 2 cm, are divided into two groups. The first group is termed early HCC which are grossly nodular, very well-differentiated, and difficult to discern from a high-grade dysplastic nodule. The second group, called progressed HCC, shows a distinctly nodular pattern and is easily recognized as HCC, typically moderately differentiated, and often with evidence of vascular invasion. Making this distinction has clinical implications because compared to progressed HCC, early HCC has a better 5-year survival rate [3, 4].

In an effort to increase reproducibility of applying diagnostic criteria to these small lesions, the International Consensus Group for Hepatocellular Neoplasia (ICGHN) published a summary of their recommendations in a 2009 consensus paper. They found the greatest degree of interobserver variability in differentiating high-grade dysplastic nodules from early HCC. Increased diagnostic agreement was achieved by recognizing stromal invasion as a criterion for diagnosis of HCC. Diagnosing stromal invasion is subjective and may require ancillary stains including reticulin and Victoria blue stains as well as immunohistochemical stains for CK7 or CK19 which aids in differentiating from pseudoinvasion [4].

2.3   Special Histologic Subtypes

2.3.1   Fibrolamellar HCC

Fibrolamellar HCC (FHCC) is a variant with clinicopathologic features that are distinct from classic HCC. This variant has no gender predilection and typically occurs in children and young adults in a non-cirrhotic liver. Two-thirds of cases involve in the left lobe [5]. FHCC is associated with fewer chromosomal alterations and genomic heterogeneity compared to HCC. Serologic markers that are typically elevated in HCC such as alpha-fetoprotein (AFP) are normal or mildly elevated in FHCC [6].

Grossly, FHCC are yellow to pale tan and firm and many have a central scar (Fig. 2.3). Histologically, the tumor cells are large and polygonal with hyperchromatic eosinophilic macronucleoli and abundant mitochondria-rich cytoplasm. Lamellar, collagenous stroma is typical but can be scant on a biopsy (Fig. 2.4a, b). Cytoplasmic "pale bodies" are frequent and represent hyaline bodies containing fibrinogen (Fig. 2.4c). Characteristically, PAS-positive globular hyaline cytoplasmic inclusions can be found and typically contain α1-antitrypsin (Fig. 2.4d). FHCC is more frequently positive for cytokeratin 7 (CK7) than classic HCC [2].

The prognosis of FHCC is similar to classic HCC that arises in a non-cirrhotic liver but better than HCC arising in a cirrhotic liver [5]. The prognosis may be due in part to the younger age at presentation, non-cirrhotic background, and lack of other comorbidities. Surgical resection remains the mainstay of treatment due to a lack of alternative therapy [6].

Fig. 2.3 Fibrolamellar HCC. Gross photo showing a mass in the background of normal liver

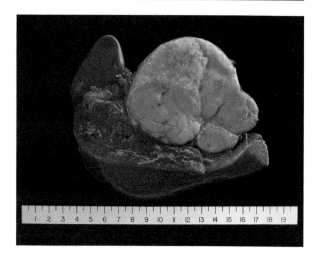

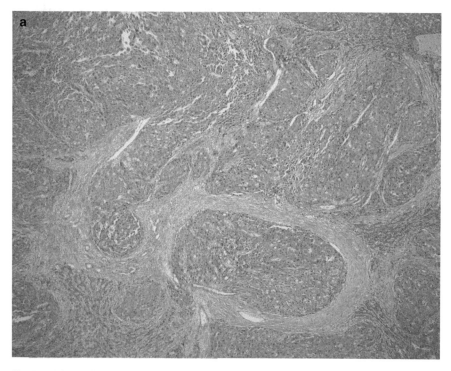

Fig. 2.4 Histologic features of Fibrolamellar HCC

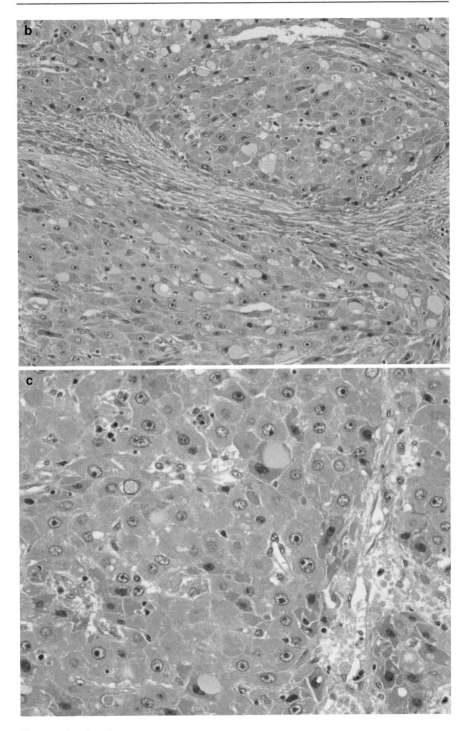

Fig. 2.4 (continued)

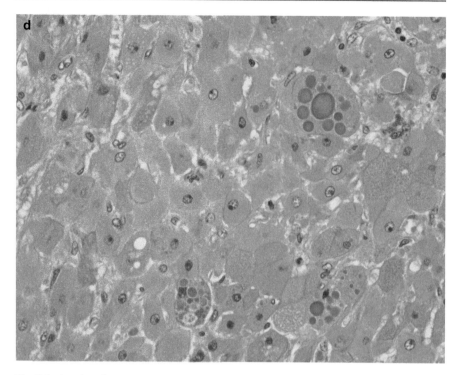

Fig. 2.4 (continued)

2.3.2 Scirrhous HCC

The scirrhous variant of HCC (ScHCC) is rare, comprising less than 5% of all HCCs. Radiologic findings are atypical and often show peripheral enhancement in the arterial phase and persistent enhancement in the venous phase [1]. Most cases arise in a subcapsular location. Histologically, ScHCC shows marked sinusoidal fibrosis with atrophy of the tumor trabeculae [5].

ScHCC needs to be differentiated from FHCC, cholangiocarcinoma, and metastatic adenocarcinoma due to the widely different therapeutic and prognostic implications [1]. ScHCC is frequently negative for HepPar-1 (Fig. 2.5d), may lack canalicular pCEA staining, and frequently expresses adenocarcinoma markers including CK7, CK19, and EPCAM. Two newer immunohistochemical markers, glypican-3 (Fig. 2.5b) and arginase-1 (Fig. 2.5c), can aid in the differentiation of ScHCC from intrahepatic cholangiocarcinoma [1]. Arginase-1 has higher sensitivity for hepatocellular differentiation than HepPar-1. Glypican-3 is expressed in greater than 80% of HCC, but it is not a specific marker of hepatocellular differentiation (Fig. 2.5) [1].

Studies are conflicting regarding the prognostic significance of this subtype with data showing a mixture of better, similar, and worse prognoses than classic HCC [1].

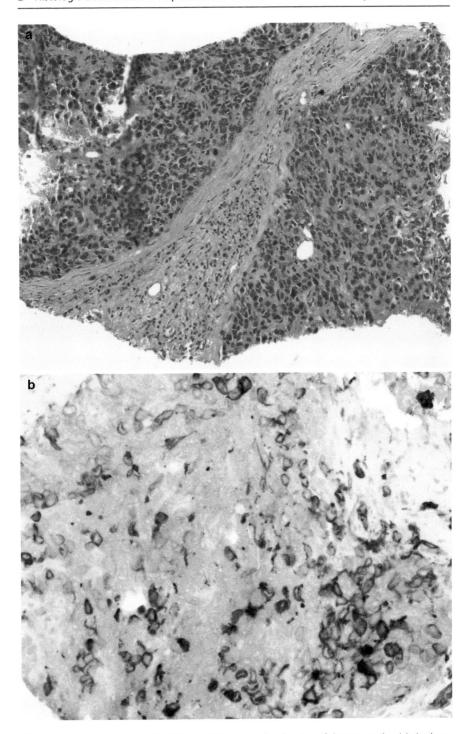

Fig. 2.5 Scirrhous variant of HCC. (**a**) H&E stain; (**b**) Glypican 3 immunostain; (**c**) Arginase immunostain; (**d**) Hepar 1 immunostain

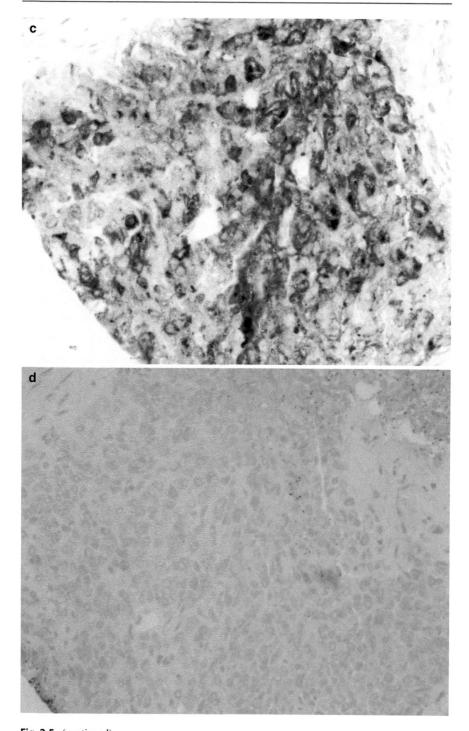

Fig. 2.5 (continued)

2.3.3   Steatohepatitic HCC

The influence of nonalcoholic fatty liver disease (NAFLD) on the development of HCC is an active area of research. NAFLD is considered the chief hepatic manifestation of obesity, diabetes mellitus, and syndromes related to insulin resistance [7]. While multiple studies support the role of NAFLD in hepatocarcinogenesis, there is a subset of SH-HCC that arise in the absence of background steatosis and/ or steatohepatitis that may be caused by tumor-specific pathways and genetic alterations [8].

Steatohepatitic HCC (SHCC) has histologic features similar to nonneoplastic steatohepatitis, including steatosis, hepatocyte ballooning, Mallory-Denk bodies, inflammation, and pericellular fibrosis [7]. One study showed two distinct patterns of fibrosis on the trichrome stain, a pericellular fibrosis similar to the pattern seen in steatohepatitis and a trabecular pattern consisting of thicker fibrous bundles with a haphazard arrangement [7]. Typically SHCC has an infiltrative growth pattern with some areas of conventional HCC but more distinctive areas of SHCC.

2.3.4   Lymphoepithelioma-Like HCC (LEL-HCC)

Lymphoepithelioma-like carcinomas (LELC) have been reported in many organs including nasopharynx, salivary glands, lungs, stomach, trachea, lacrimal glands, ureters, urinary bladder, uterus, vagina, ovaries, breast soft tissues, and skin. The WHO has recognized lymphoepithelioma-like HCC (LEL-HCC) as a variant of HCC. LEL-HCC is extremely rare with less than 20 cases reported showing features of HCC rather than cholangiocarcinoma [9, 10]. LEL-HCC is characterized by areas of poorly differentiated or undifferentiated HCC associated with a marked lymphoplasmacytic infiltrate that may be so dense as to mimic a lymphoma. The most recent study reports a majority of the LEL-HCCs arising in non-cirrhotic livers with no evidence of underlying liver disease [10]. Association with Epstein-Barr virus (EBV) has only been shown in one reported case [10, 11]. Little is known about the prognostic significance of this variant due to its rarity.

2.3.5   Sarcomatoid HCC

Sarcomatoid HCC is partially or completely composed of malignant spindle cells with or without heterologous differentiation [12]. Sarcomatoid changes are seen in 1.1–5.9% of HCCs and are associated with an aggressive clinical course, regardless of the initial stage [9]. Sarcomatoid changes can be seen in tumors after locoregional therapy and in tumors with no prior therapy. The sarcomatous component can be discrete or intimately admixed with classic HCC. Immunophenotypically, the sarcomatous component may stain similar to various sarcomas including fibrosarcoma, leiomyosarcoma, or rhabdomyosarcoma, or it may be undifferentiated [9].

2.3.6   Undifferentiated Carcinoma

Undifferentiated carcinoma is a rare neoplasm defined as a primary hepatic malignancy that can only be diagnosed as carcinoma with the use of immunohistochemistry and cannot be further subclassified. These tumors are thought to have a worse prognosis than conventional HCC [5, 12].

2.3.7   Diffuse Cirrhosis-Like HCC (CL-HCC)

CL-HCC is a rare variant with only ten cases reported. Clinically, these tumors are undetectable using standard imaging protocols for HCC and instead are identified at the grossing bench after transplant. These occur in a background of cirrhosis and are composed of innumerable pale and/or cholestatic small nodules of HCC which have thin sclerotic rims. Reportedly, these have a propensity to invade small vessels and lack large vessel invasion of classic HCC. Histologically, these tumors are easily differentiated from the nonneoplastic nodules of cirrhosis and frequently display cholestasis and ballooning with Mallory-Denk bodies. The immunohistochemical profile is the same as expected in classic HCC. The Ki-67 proliferation index tends to be low, but prognostic information is currently lacking due to this tumor's rarity [13].

2.3.8   Combined Hepatocellular-Cholangiocarcinoma

Combined hepatocellular-cholangiocarcinomas (HCC-CC) comprise less than 1% of all primary hepatic carcinomas. The World Health Organization (WHO) in their most recent classification has accepted the concept that HCC-CC arise from hepatic progenitor cells (HPCs). HPCs (also called oval cells) reside in the adult liver and harbor facultative bipotential and can give rise to both hepatocytes and cholangiocytes [14]. Terminology of the WHO embraces this concept and divides HCC-CC into classic type and those with stem cell features. The classic type has unequivocal areas of both HCC and CC (Fig. 2.6). The stem cell type is further subdivided into three subtypes: typical, intermediate, and cholangiolocellular [14].

The typical subtype is characterized by nests of mature hepatocytes with peripheral clusters of small cells that are positive for CK7 and CK19, nuclear cell adhesion molecule (NCAM1/CD56), KIT, and/or epithelial cell adhesion molecule (EpCAM). Intermediate type has features intermediate between hepatocytes and cholangiocytes, characterized by oval cells in trabeculae, nests, or strands within fibrous stroma, that have positivity for both hepatocellular and cholangiocyte markers. Cholangiolocellular type is characterized by small cells with high nuclear-cytoplasmic ratio growing in tubular, cord-like, anastomosing architecture within fibrous stroma and can be positive for CK19, KIT, NCAM, and EpCAM [14].

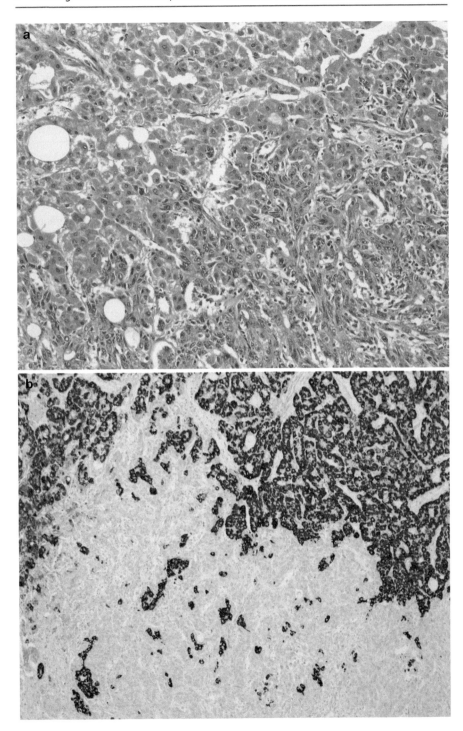

Fig. 2.6 Mixed HCC with both hepatocellular differentiation and cholangiolocellular differentiation. (**a**) H&E stain; (**b**) Immunohistochemical stain for CD19 showing cholangiolocellular differentiation

Differentiating CC, HCC, and HCC-CC does have clinical implications. Serum CA19-9 and/or carcinoembryonic antigen (CEA) may be elevated in patients presumed to have HCC, and serum AFP may be elevated in patients presumed to have CC. Overall HCC-CC has a worse prognosis than classic HCC with more frequent lymph node metastasis, but the prognosis of each HCC-CC subtype remains unknown. In addition, a diagnosis of HCC-CC can preclude a patient from transplant consideration [12].

2.4   Grading and Staging

2.4.1   Grading HCC

Several grading systems have been proposed. Generally, the higher the grade, the less the resemblance of the tumor to the "normal" liver. Both the College of American Pathologists (CAP) and the *AJCC Cancer Staging Manual* recommend using the Edmondson-Steiner grading system although the correlation between this grading system and prognosis has been disputed [2]. The Edmondson-Steiner system grades HCC on a scale from I to IV based on nuclear irregularity, hyperchromasia, and increasing N:C ratio with the greatest emphasis placed on the amount of cytoplasm and the N:C ratio (Table 2.1). The AFIP uses a modified four-category grading system based primarily on nuclear features alone, and this staging system has been reported to correlate survival with tumor grade (Table 2.2). The WHO recognizes four types: well-differentiated, moderately differentiated, poorly differentiated, and undifferentiated [5]. While histologic grade has been shown to have a relationship to tumor size, tumor presentation, and metastatic rate, it is not evident that in individual cases, the grade is clinically relevant [2]. In many cases, you can find a mixture of grades throughout a tumor.

Table 2.1 Edmondson-Steiner grading system (adapted from [15])

Grade I	Reserved for hepatocellular carcinomas where the difference between the tumor cells and hyperplastic liver cells is so minor that a diagnosis of carcinoma rests upon the demonstration of more aggressive growths in other parts of the neoplasm. Grade is assigned based upon the highest grade present. In fact grade I is rarely used for overall tumor grade designation
Grade II	Cells show marked resemblance to normal hepatic cells. Nuclei are larger and more hyperchromatic than in normal cells. The cytoplasm is abundant and acidophilic. Cell borders are sharp and clear-cut. Acini are frequent and variable in size. Lumina are often filled with bile or protein precipitate
Grade III	Nuclei are larger and more hyperchromatic than in grade II cells. The nuclei occupy a relatively greater proportion of the cell (high nuclear to cytoplasmic [N:C] ratio). The cytoplasm is granular and acidophilic but less so than grade II tumors. Acini are less frequent and not as often filled with bile or protein precipitate. More single-cell growth in vascular channels is seen than in grade II
Grade IV	Nuclei are intensely hyperchromatic and occupy a high percentage of the cell. The cytoplasm is variable in amount and often scanty and contains fewer granules. The growth pattern is medullary in character, trabeculae are difficult to find, and cell masses seem to lie loosely without cohesion in vascular channels. Only rare acini are seen. Spindle cell areas have been seen in some tumors. Short plump cell forms, resembling "small-cell" carcinoma of the lung, are seen in some grade IV tumors

Table 2.2 AFIP grading system (adapted from [2])

Grade 1	Nearly indistinguishable from hepatocellular adenomas with cells with abundant cytoplasm and minimal nuclear pleomorphism
Grade 2	Nuclei have prominent nucleoli, hyperchromasia, and mild nuclear pleomorphism
Grade 3	Tumors have even more nuclear pleomorphism and angulated nuclei
Grade 4	Tumors have marked nuclear pleomorphism and typically have anaplastic giant cells

2.4.2 Staging HCC

The majority of hepatocellular carcinomas occur with a background of chronic liver disease, which has a significant impact on prognosis irrespective of tumor stage [16]. This is the reason staging systems that only include the anatomic characterization of the tumor do not necessarily have good predictive value. These staging systems include the American Joint Committee on Cancer (AJCC)/Union for International Cancer Control (UICC) staging systems.

Other staging systems provide a clinical classification of HCC that incorporates the tumor characteristics (tumor size, number, and vascular invasion), the degree of liver function (Child-Pugh score), and the general health of the patient (ECOG classification). Of these available systems, the Barcelona Clinic Liver Cancer (BCLC) staging system is recommended for prognostic prediction and treatment allocation [17].

References

1. Krings G, Ramachandran R, Jain D, Wu TT, Yeh MM, Torbenson M, et al. Immunohistochemical pitfalls and the importance of glypican 3 and arginase in the diagnosis of scirrhous hepatocellular carcinoma. Mod Pathol. 2013;26(6):782–91.
2. MacSween RNM, Burt AD, Portmann B, Ferrell LD. MacSween's pathology of the liver. 6th ed. Edinburgh, New York: Churchill Livingstone/Elsevier; 2012. xiii, 1020 p.
3. Shafizadeh N, Kakar S. Diagnosis of well-differentiated hepatocellular lesions: role of immunohistochemistry and other ancillary techniques. Adv Anat Pathol. 2011;18(6):438–45.
4. International Consensus Group for Hepatocellular Neoplasia. The International Consensus Group for Hepatocellular Neoplasia. Pathologic diagnosis of early hepatocellular carcinoma: a report of the international consensus group for hepatocellular neoplasia. Hepatology. 2009;49(2):658–64.
5. WHO classification of tumours of the digestive system. IARC Press; 2010.
6. Lim II, Farber BA, LaQuaglia MP. Advances in fibrolamellar hepatocellular carcinoma: a review. Eur J Pediatr Surg. 2014;24(6):461–6.
7. Salomao M, Yu WM, Brown RS, Emond JC, Lefkowitch JH. Steatohepatitic hepatocellular carcinoma (SH-HCC): a distinctive histological variant of HCC in hepatitis C virus-related cirrhosis with associated NAFLD/NASH. Am J Surg Pathol. 2010;34(11):1630–6.
8. Yeh MM, Liu Y, Torbenson M. Steatohepatitic variant of hepatocellular carcinoma in the absence of metabolic syndrome or background steatosis: a clinical, pathological, and genetic study. Hum Pathol. 2015;46(11):1769–75.
9. Mitchell KA. Hepatocellular carcinoma: histologic considerations: pure, mixed, and motley. J Clin Gastroenterol. 2013;47(Suppl):S20–6.
10. Patel KR, Liu TC, Vaccharajani N, Chapman WC, Brunt EM. Characterization of inflammatory (lymphoepithelioma-like) hepatocellular carcinoma: a study of 8 cases. Arch Pathol Lab Med. 2014;138(9):1193–202.

11. Si MW, Thorson JA, Lauwers GY, DalCin P, Furman J. Hepatocellular lymphoepithelioma-like carcinoma associated with Epstein Barr virus: a hitherto unrecognized entity. Diagn Mol Pathol. 2004;13(3):183–9.
12. Shafizadeh N, Kakar S. Hepatocellular carcinoma: histologic subtypes. Surg Pathol Clin. 2013;6(2):367–84.
13. Jakate S, Yabes A, Giusto D, Naini B, Lassman C, Yeh MM, et al. Diffuse cirrhosis-like hepatocellular carcinoma: a clinically and radiographically undetected variant mimicking cirrhosis. Am J Surg Pathol. 2010;34(7):935–41.
14. Akiba J, Nakashima O, Hattori S, Tanikawa K, Takenaka M, Nakayama M, et al. Clinicopathologic analysis of combined hepatocellular-cholangiocarcinoma according to the latest WHO classification. Am J Surg Pathol. 2013;37(4):496–505.
15. Schlageter M, Terracciano LM, D'Angelo S, Sorrentino P. Histopathology of hepatocellular carcinoma. World J Gastroenterol. 2014;20(43):15955–64.
16. Maida M, Orlando E, Cammà C, Cabibbo G. Staging systems of hepatocellular carcinoma: a review of literature. World J Gastroenterol. 2014;20(15):4141–50.
17. Duseja A. Staging of hepatocellular carcinoma. J Clin Exp Hepatol. 2014;4(Suppl 3):S74–9.

Molecular Classification of Hepatocellular Carcinoma and Precision Medicine

3

Michael Feely

3.1 Introduction

The incidence of hepatocellular carcinoma in increasing globally and malignant liver tumors now represents the second leading cause of cancer-related mortality worldwide [1–3]. In the United States, the incidence of hepatocellular carcinoma has tripled over the past 30 years where it has become the fastest rising cause of cancer-related deaths [4]. With this emergence has come an increased effort, largely within the preceding decade, to better appreciate the molecular pathogenesis of this disease. As with other malignancies that have been examined in this way, the eventual goal of these investigations is to identify potential targets for therapy and to correlate these molecular mechanisms with patient prognosis. Here a summary of many of the molecular mechanisms identified in hepatocellular carcinoma is provided as well as outline of the current attempts at a molecular classification system of these tumors.

3.2 Molecular Alterations

3.2.1 TERT

Alterations in telomerase reverse transcriptase (*TERT*) expression, mainly through promoter mutation, have been identified in a diverse group of malignancies including melanoma, urothelial carcinoma of the bladder, anaplastic thyroid carcinoma, malignant glioma, and hepatocellular carcinoma [5, 6]. These alterations lead to increased levels of telomerase, a protein complex that is responsible for telomere maintenance

M. Feely, M.D.
Department of Pathology, Immunology, and Laboratory Medicine, College of Medicine, University of Florida, 1600 SW Archer Road, Gainesville, FL 32610-0275, USA
e-mail: mfeely@ufl.edu

© Springer International Publishing AG 2018
C. Liu (ed.), *Precision Molecular Pathology of Liver Cancer*,
Molecular Pathology Library, https://doi.org/10.1007/978-3-319-68082-8_3

and elongation during normal cell division [7]. These telomeres, which consist of short repeats of DNA, are essential for the protection of chromosomes during this process [8]. While telomerase remains functioning during development, this complex is relatively inactive during adulthood which contributes to the shortening of telomeres and the subsequent normal process of cell senescence and apoptosis [8].

Despite the vast diversity of molecular pathways and etiologies which contribute to hepatocellular carcinogenesis, *TERT* upregulation with telomerase reactivation is commonly appreciated in hepatocellular carcinomas. In fact, alterations in *TERT* expression have been demonstrated in greater than 90% of these malignancies, which makes these changes the most common alterations in hepatocellular carcinoma [9]. This prevalence is likely why telomere maintenance through increased levels of telomerase is considered to play a key role in tumor initiation [10]. In addition, while alterations in *TERT* expression appear quite common in hepatocellular carcinoma, other primary liver malignancies such as intrahepatic cholangiocarcinomas and classic pediatric hepatoblastomas have not been shown to have similar changes [11, 12].

While telomerase is not typically found to any significant level in normal human hepatocytes, reactivation of this complex is frequent in the early stages of hepatocellular carcinoma development [13]. Indeed, studies have shown an increased frequency of *TERT* alterations in premalignant lesions arising in cirrhotic livers including dysplastic nodules and early hepatocellular carcinomas [14]. Additionally, *TERT* promoter alterations have also been implicated in the progression of hepatocellular adenomas to their malignant counterparts [15]. Just as the molecular underpinnings of hepatocellular carcinogenesis are quite varied, the means by which telomerase reactivation occurs is also diverse and includes *TERT* promoter mutations (54–60%) [9, 16], *TERT* amplification (5–6%) [9], and HBV insertion in the *TERT* promoter (10–15%) [17–19]. Of these, *TERT* promoter mutations are associated with hepatocellular carcinomas developing through the β-catenin pathway, and these mutations are frequently located 124 base pairs upstream of the start codon [16].

3.2.2   Wnt/β-Catenin

β-catenin functions in normal cells as a mediator of cell adhesion as well as an activator of the Wnt signaling pathway. Alterations in this protein, or those responsible for regulating levels of β-catenin, contribute to elevated cytoplasmic and nuclear accumulation which activates the transcription of Wnt target genes [20]. This intimate association between β-catenin and the Wnt ligands has been termed the canonical Wnt pathway. This differs from the non-canonical Wnt pathway which is largely independent of β-catenin [21]. In normal human hepatocytes, the Wnt/β-catenin pathway plays a crucial role in a number of processes including liver growth and regeneration, metabolic zonation, and biliary homeostasis [22].

While normal development requires activation of this pathway, aberrant stimulation is implicated in a significant percentage of hepatocellular carcinomas through a number of alterations including activating mutations of *CTNNB1* (β-catenin) (11–37%) and less frequently inactivating mutations of *AXIN1* (5–15%) or *APC* [23–25]. The most common defect leading to activation of the Wnt signaling pathway in hepatocellular carcinoma, *CTNNB1* mutations, typically consists of in-frame deletions or substitutions in a hotspot on exon 3. These mutations affect the domain of β-catenin which is the target of the APC/AXIN1/GSK3B inhibitory complex [23]. Tumors with these mutations have been shown to have a specific gene expression profile with overexpression of classic Wnt pathway targets such as *LGR5* and *GLUL* [26].

While Wnt signaling activation, involving β-catenin, has been associated with well-differentiated hepatocellular carcinomas, upregulation of the canonical Wnt signaling pathway has been more closely associated with poorly differentiated aggressive tumors [27]. Corroborating this dichotomy is the finding that hepatocellular carcinomas harboring mutations in *CTNNB1* have been noted to have an increased incidence of specific histologic findings including microtrabecular and pseudoglandular architecture, well-differentiated cytology, and bile accumulation within the tumor [28]. This latter finding is thought to be directly related to β-catenin's role in bile homeostasis within normal liver tissue. Given these findings, it has been suggested that while Wnt signaling is a common theme across hepatocellular carcinomas, the specific pathways and affected cellular processes are different for tumor initiation than they are for tumor progression [28].

3.2.3 p53

p53, encoded by *TP53*, is a well-known tumor suppressor which functions as a transcription factor involved in many cellular processes including cell cycle regulation and cellular development and differentiation. While the role of this protein has traditionally concentrated on its function as a tumor suppressor, it is now understood that p53 is also involved in seemingly contrary processes such as supporting cell survival [29]. Given its integral role in crucial cellular activities, it is not surprising that *TP53* is the most frequently altered gene in human malignancies [30]. This finding is exemplified by hepatocellular carcinoma where alterations in p53 pathways have been found to be involved in the development of at least half of these tumors [31].

Alterations in p53 expression have been associated with a number of hepatocellular carcinoma etiologies including metabolic derangements, toxin exposure, and involvement of HBV or HCV [32]. In the multifaceted network of hepatocellular carcinoma molecular alterations, it should come as no surprise that changes in this pathway do not occur as singular events, and other genetic findings such as chromosomal instability are commonly found in *TP53*-mutated tumors [33].

While mutations in *TP53* do not appear to characteristically occur in specific hotspots in hepatocellular carcinoma, there is a single exception [34]. Tumors that develop in the setting of aflatoxin B1 exposure have been shown to have recurrent *TP53* mutations involving codon 249 [35]. This toxin, which is produced by several

Aspergillus species, is a common contaminate of a variety of food products includ-ing corn and other grains. Exposure is most common in developing countries of Southeast Asia, South America, and sub-Saharan Africa [36]. Consequently, hepa-tocellular carcinomas that develop in these regions often contain *TP53* R249S muta-tions, the hallmark of aflatoxin B1 exposure [35].

Just as in other malignancies, *TP53* mutations in hepatocellular carcinomas have been known to be characterized by poor differentiation [37]. Indeed recent studies comparing the histologic features of tumors with specific genetic alterations have shown hepatocellular carcinomas with *TP53* alterations to frequently harbor a mac-rotrabecular architecture, compact growth pattern, and nuclear pleomorphism. Additionally, in contrast to *CTNNB1*-mutated tumors, these lesions are not associ-ated with intratumoral cholestasis [38]. Beyond the correlations to aggressive histo-logic features, hepatocellular carcinomas with *TP53* mutations are also associated with a worse patient prognosis [39–41].

3.2.4   CDKN2A (p16)

Cyclin-dependent kinase inhibitor 2A, also referred to as p16, is regarded as a tumor suppressor protein and acts as a potent negative modulator of cell cycle progression at G_1. Alterations in p16 expression and loss of function are therefore commonly associated with uncontrolled cellular proliferation [42]. While decreased expression of p16 has been reported in hepatocellular carcinomas for some time, it was origi-nally believed that this alteration was largely mediated by homozygous deletions in chromosome 9 or mutations in *CDKN2A* [43, 44]. It has now been recognized that the absence of p16 expression in hepatocellular carcinoma is more often due to methylation of the *CDKN2A* promoter, which has been documented in 30–70% of tumors [31, 45]. The significance of this finding is difficult to ascertain however since methylation of *CDKN2A* has also been documented to occur in chronic liver disease in the absence of tumor [46].

3.2.5   AXIN1 and 2

Axis inhibition proteins 1 and 2 (Axin1 and 2) are tumor suppressors whose roles are intimately associated with β-catenin and the Wnt signaling pathway. Mutations of the *AXIN1* gene prevent the phosphorylation of β-catenin, thereby contributing to its accumulation by preventing its degradation [47]. While the percentage of hepa-tocellular carcinomas exhibiting accumulation of β-catenin is relatively high, this phenomenon appears more frequently than the reported rate of *CTNNB1* mutations in these tumors. Given this finding it was presumed that other mechanisms existed for this increase and contributing alterations in *AXIN1* and *AXIN2* were encountered [24]. While the overall prevalence of mutations in these genes in hepatocellular carcinoma is relatively low, of those tumors exhibiting activation of the Wnt signal-ing pathway, alterations in *AXIN1* and *AXIN2* have been reported in 54% and 38% of those lesions, respectively [48]. Given that overexpression of *AXIN1* has been shown to downregulate β-catenin and lead to cycle inhibition and tumor cell apoptosis, it has been suggested that this pathway may be a potential target for future therapy [49].

3.2.6 RAS

The *RAS* family of proto-oncogenes consists of three highly homologous genes consisting of *HRAS*, *NRAS*, and *KRAS*. The Ras proteins function in signaling pathways which when activated contribute to cell growth, differentiation, and survival [50]. While alterations in this pathway play a significant role in the development of other malignancies such as pancreatic and colon cancers, only a small percentage of hepatocellular carcinomas have been identified as having mutations within the *RAS* family of genes [51]. The exception to this finding is hepatocellular carcinoma arising in the setting of vinyl chloride exposure. This carcinogen, which is more often implicated in the development of angiosarcomas of the liver, has been strongly associated with *KRAS2* mutations [52]. Beyond this exceptional occurrence, it has been suggested that persistent activation of the Ras pathway may be one mechanism by which tumors resist the multikinase inhibitor sorafenib, the only approved systemic therapy for advanced hepatocellular carcinomas [53, 54].

3.2.7 MET

The *MET* proto-oncogene encodes for the receptor of the ligand hepatocyte growth factor (Hgf) [55]. In this signaling pathway, these proteins contribute to liver development and regeneration through activation of cell proliferation, survival, and angiogenesis [56]. Given its function in normal liver tissue, multiple investigations have looked into the role *MET* plays in the development of hepatocellular carcinoma. While Hgf appears to play no direct role in carcinogenesis, increased expression of *MET* has been well documented in hepatocellular carcinoma [57]. In fact, increased concentrations of the Met protein have been observed in up to 70% of tumors [58]. This is typically secondary to activation elsewhere as somatic mutations in *MET* occur in less than 5% of tumors [59]. While transcriptome-based studies have suggested that *MET* overexpression is not an oncogenic driver in hepatocellular carcinomas, increased activation of this pathway has been associated with metastases, tumor recurrence, and poor overall survival [60]. Recent investigations in the use of the oral Met inhibitor tivantinib have shown some benefit in patients with tumor found to have high *MET* expression [61].

3.2.8 TGFβ

The cytokine transforming growth factor β (TGFβ) is involved in a number of essential biologic processes such as cellular proliferation, differentiation, migration, and adhesion [62]. This pathway exerts its influence through a number of mediators including the small mothers against decapentaplegic (SMAD) family of transcriptional regulators [63]. The role of this pathway in neoplasia is complex as TGFβ has been found to act as both a tumor suppressor in the early stages of carcinogenesis and as a promoter of tumor progression later on in this process [64]. It has also been regarded as a driver of epithelial-mesenchymal transitions [65]. In terms of hepatocellular carcinoma development, the dichotomous activity of the TGFβ pathway has been documented [66]. Furthermore, it has been suggested that activation of the TGFβ pathway may represent an alternative method of Wnt signaling stimulation, independent of β-catenin [67, 68]. In fact, TGFβ stimulation in hepatocellular carcinoma cell lines has resulted in induced expression of Wnt target genes. Interestingly, this activation has also been associated with suppressed expression of AFP protein [68]. Manipulation of the TGFβ pathway is being investigated as a potential therapeutic target in hepatocellular carcinomas through the use of a small-molecular inhibitor [69].

3.2.9 VEGFA

Vascular endothelial growth factor A (VEGFA) is a potent angiogenesis regulator with significant impacts on tumor progression by promoting endothelial growth and migration [70]. Given the vascular nature of hepatocellular carcinomas, it has been postulated that VEGFA may play a role in the carcinogenesis of these liver tumors.

Indeed, overexpression of the *VEGFA* gene has been shown to occur in a subset of hepatocellular carcinomas through focal gains in chromosome 6p21 [71]. There also appears to be an association of increased expression of VEGFA protein with vascular density and tumor size on hepatocellular carcinomas [70].

3.2.10 EpCAM

The glycoprotein epithelial cell adhesion molecule (EpCAM) has been recognized for some time for its role in the growth and differentiation of epithelial cells. While EpCAM mediates cell-to-cell adhesions, this action appears to restrict the development of such junctions formed through classic cadherins [72]. Additionally, increased expression of EpCAM has also been associated with epithelial proliferation and decreased cellular differentiation [73]. Just as in other epithelial malignancies, hepatocellular carcinomas with increased expression of EpCAM often demonstrate stem cell-like features such as the ability to self-renew and differentiate [74]. Furthermore, hepatocellular carcinomas with increased expression of the *EpCAM* gene or its protein product have been shown to overexpress other stemness markers such as *KRT19* and *AFP* as well as FGF19 [75, 76]. Tumors found to have this set of gene expression have been associated with an overall poor patient prognosis [68].

3.2.11 PTEN

Phosphatase and tensin homolog (PTEN) is a tumor suppressor which oversees a variety of cellular processes such as proliferation, metabolism, and survival by downregulating the PI3K/AKT/mTOR pathway [77]. Somatic alterations in the expression of *PTEN* have been linked to a number of malignancies including prostate cancer and glioblastoma, while germline mutations are associated with the development of Cowden syndrome. Given the number and variety of malignancies affected by PTEN, it should come as no surprise that PTEN also appears to play a role in the development and progression of hepatocellular carcinomas. While mutations in the *PTEN* gene have only been identified in 5% of these tumors, loss of PTEN expression has been documented in up to 40% of hepatocellular carcinomas [78–80]. Reduced expression has also been associated with higher recurrence rates and shorter overall patient survival [78]. Not only is PTEN expression altered within neoplastic lesions of the liver, it has also been found to be dysregulated in liver diseases associated with obesity, viral infections, and alcohol abuse [81].

3.2.12 Epigenetic Alterations

While the role of genetic modifications through the process of mutations in the development of neoplasia has been recognized for some time, there is increasing evidence that epigenetic alterations also play a critical role in this process. Through aberrant hypermethylation of gene promoters or global genomic hypomethylation, the expression of particular genes can be manipulated in the absence of direct sequence changes [82]. In hepatocellular carcinoma, the relative frequency of genetic alterations through mutations is relatively low and limited to a small subset of tumor suppressor and proto-oncogenes [31]. In contrast, epigenetic modifications occur far more frequently in these tumors and are responsible for many of the altered gene expressions that are observed over the course of their development [83].

The understanding of the mechanisms by which the methylation process is altered in hepatocellular carcinogenesis is still being explored. However, several important insights have been uncovered. It has been shown that the process of epigenetic modification through hypermethylation can be detected in diseased livers in the absence of tumor [84]. Similarly, hepatitis B and C proteins have been shown to alter the expression of DNA methyltransferase, an enzyme responsible for epigenetic changes [85, 86]. These findings suggest that viral hepatitis and other chronic liver diseases may be laying the groundwork for carcinogenesis by intervening through aberrant methylation. Indeed it has also been shown that hepatocellular carcinomas associated with viral hepatitis have a tendency to harbor more frequent epigenetic alterations than tumors unassociated with these infections [87].

The expression of miRNAs is intimately associated with epigenetic mechanisms and has been increasingly recognized as a potent disease modifier through posttranscriptional gene regulation. In liver disease and carcinogenesis, increased and reduced expression of various miRNAs has been associated not only with specific disease etiologies but also with tumor progression. For example, decreased expression of miR-26 within tumor cells has been linked to poor patient survival but increased susceptibility to adjuvant therapy with interferon alfa [88]. Potential therapeutic targets have also been identified among miRNAs, including miR-122, whose expression is significantly reduced in hepatocellular carcinomas despite it being the most abundant miRNA in the liver, constituting up to 72% of the total liver miRNA [89]. Restoration of miR-122 has been shown to significantly inhibit hepatocellular carcinoma growth and increase tumor sensitivity to sorafenib [90, 91].

3.2.13 Chromosome Instability

While genetic alterations within tumors can occur at the level of methylation or individual gene mutation, genetic instability can also occur in the setting of large gains or losses of whole or parts of chromosomes. These changes, which contribute to tumor aneuploidy and intratumoral heterogeneity, have been termed chromosomal instability. Evaluations of chromosomal changes in hepatocellular carcinoma have revealed chromosomal instability in approximately half of these tumors. These lesions demonstrated loss of heterozygosity at chromosomes 1p, 4q, 13q, and 16 and mutations of *TP53* and *AXIN1*. In contrast, tumors which were found to be chromosome stable were closely associated with alterations in chromosome 8p and *CTNNB1* mutations [33].

While the circumstances contributing to chromosomal instability in hepatocellular carcinoma are likely multifactorial, the presence of this genomic volatility appears more closely related to HBV infection than other chronic liver disease etiologies. This is supported by the fact that HBV infection can promote carcinogenesis by integrating viral DNA in the host genome inducing a chromosomal unstable state [92].

Furthermore, although there is a suggestion in some tumor types that increased epigenetic dysfunction or instability contributes to chromosomal instability through genome-wide hypomethylation, these two processes appear to be largely independent of one another in hepatocellular carcinoma [87].

While the relationship of chromosomal instability in hepatocellular carcinomas to other molecular alterations remains complicated, liver tumors demonstrating chromosomal instability are associated with a poor prognosis, a finding which is echoed in other malignancies [33, 93–95]. The degree of chromosomal changes is also reflected in the histologic findings of such tumors with the level of chromosomal instability paralleling the degree of tumor differentiation [96].

3.3 Molecular Classification

3.3.1 Overview

As our understanding of the molecular and genetic processes involved in carcinogenesis has advanced, the study of some tumor types such as colorectal and breast

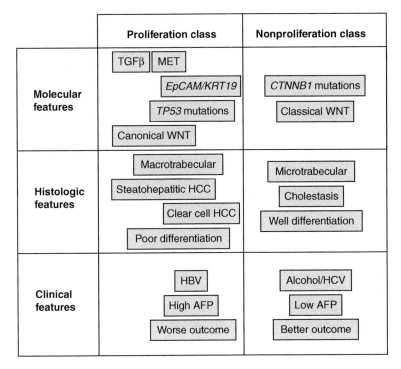

Fig. 3.1 Summary of the basic dichotomous classification of hepatocellular carcinomas and the associated clinical, histopathologic, and molecular themes common to those groups

carcinomas has resulted in widely accepted classification schemes which have both prognostic and therapeutic implications. Although much work has been done exploring the molecular underpinnings of hepatocellular carcinomas, and many investigators have proposed various classification schemes, no single system has gained wide adoption [33, 68, 71, 97]. Despite arriving at diverse final classifications based on the epigenetic alterations, somatic mutations, chromosomal stability, and gene expression profiling revealed in these studies, several general themes have been observed. So while investigators may have described various groups of hepatocellular carcinomas in several terms, the groupings themselves are remarkably similar. With that in mind, hepatocellular carcinomas can be broadly classified into two major subgroups, described by many as the proliferation and nonproliferation subclasses (Fig. 3.1).

3.3.2   Proliferation Class

The proliferation class of hepatocellular carcinomas, which represents approximately 55% of tumors, is characterized by lesions which harbor molecular features associated with cellular propagation and activation of prosurvival pathways such as MET and TGFβ [75, 98]. This group of tumors is also enriched for lesions with impaired expression of the tumor suppressor *TP53* [38]. These tumors tend to be large, less differentiated, and aggressive with lower survival rates and a higher risk of recurrence following surgery [68, 99, 100].

The proliferation class of lesions has been further divided into two groups based on a meta-analysis of the gene expression data from multiple previously published patient cohorts [68]. Following this scheme, the first subclass of this aggressive group is characterized by relatively higher activation of the TGFβ pathway with subsequent upregulation of the Wnt/β-catenin pathway and target genes such as *CCND1* and *MYC* [101]. This is accomplished in the absence of actual *CTNNB1* (β-catenin) mutations, which are more strongly associated with the nonproliferation class of hepatocellular carcinomas. These tumors, like all those in the proliferation class, tend to be less differentiated and may appear histologically as the so-called steatohepatitic variant of hepatocellular carcinoma [75, 102].

The second subclass within the proliferation group is characterized by increased expression of stemness markers such as *EpCAM* and *KRT19*. Increased protein expression and serum levels of GPC3 and AFP are also hallmarks of this group. This latter finding has noteworthy clinical consequences as serum AFP levels have been criticized as lacking sufficient sensitivity for hepatocellular carcinoma detection when in fact increased serum levels may be an indication of this particularly aggressive subclass of tumors [103]. While the predisposing etiologies of this subclass and the others are not strictly delineated among the groups, HBV infection is more strongly correlated with this subset of lesions [68, 75]. Histologically, these carcinomas appear as poorly differentiated tumors with a macrotrabecular or compact architecture. This subclass has also been associated with the clear cell variant of hepatocellular carcinoma [75].

3.3.3 Nonproliferation Class

The final class of hepatocellular carcinomas consists of tumors which are characterized by overexpression of liver-specific *WNT* targets such as *GLUL* and *LGR5* [26]. While *CTNNB1* mutations and activation of the Wnt/β-catenin pathway are common in this group, these changes do not appear to regulate the canonical Wnt targets associated with the proliferation class such as cyclin D1 and MYC [68]. *TP53* alterations are not a feature of this group and have been found to be mutually exclusive with *CTNNB1* mutations [38]. Furthermore, these lesions tend to be characterized by chromosome stability, as opposed to the proliferation class which often exhibits chromosomal instability [33]. While the etiologic factors vary, tumors in the nonproliferation class are more strongly correlated to alcohol-related liver disease and HCV [98]. Histologically, these lesions tend to be well differentiated, demonstrating a microtrabecular growth pattern and more often harboring a pseudoglandular architecture and intratumoral cholestasis than the proliferation class [28, 75]. Clinically, tumors with features of this class tend to be less aggressive with better patient outcomes [102].

References

1. Mittal S, El-Serag HB. Epidemiology of hepatocellular carcinoma: consider the population. J Clin Gastroenterol. 2013;47(Suppl):S2–6.
2. Bosch FX, Ribes J, Cleries R, Diaz M. Epidemiology of hepatocellular carcinoma. Clin Liver Dis. 2005;9(2):191–211, v.
3. Forner A, Llovet JM, Bruix J. Hepatocellular carcinoma. Lancet. 2012;379(9822):1245–55.
4. El-Serag HB. Hepatocellular carcinoma. N Engl J Med. 2011;365(12):1118–27.
5. Vinagre J, Almeida A, Populo H, et al. Frequency of TERT promoter mutations in human cancers. Nat Commun. 2013;4:2185.
6. Huang DS, Wang Z, He XJ, et al. Recurrent TERT promoter mutations identified in a large-scale study of multiple tumour types are associated with increased TERT expression and telomerase activation. Eur J Cancer. 2015;51(8):969–76.
7. Gunes C, Rudolph KL. The role of telomeres in stem cells and cancer. Cell. 2013;152(3):390–3.
8. Artandi SE. Telomeres, telomerase, and human disease. N Engl J Med. 2006;355(12):1195–7.
9. Totoki Y, Tatsuno K, Covington KR, et al. Trans-ancestry mutational landscape of hepatocellular carcinoma genomes. Nat Genet. 2014;46(12):1267–73.
10. Satyanarayana A, Manns MP, Rudolph KL. Telomeres and telomerase: a dual role in hepatocarcinogenesis. Hepatology. 2004;40(2):276–83.
11. Quaas A, Oldopp T, Tharun L, et al. Frequency of TERT promoter mutations in primary tumors of the liver. Virchows Arch. 2014;465(6):673–7.
12. Eichenmuller M, Trippel F, Kreuder M, et al. The genomic landscape of hepatoblastoma and their progenies with HCC-like features. J Hepatol. 2014;61(6):1312–20.
13. Farazi PA, Glickman J, Jiang S, Yu A, Rudolph KL, DePinho RA. Differential impact of telomere dysfunction on initiation and progression of hepatocellular carcinoma. Cancer Res. 2003;63(16):5021–7.
14. Nault JC, Calderaro J, Di Tommaso L, et al. Telomerase reverse transcriptase promoter mutation is an early somatic genetic alteration in the transformation of premalignant nodules in hepatocellular carcinoma on cirrhosis. Hepatology. 2014;60(6):1983–92.
15. Pilati C, Letouze E, Nault JC, et al. Genomic profiling of hepatocellular adenomas reveals recurrent FRK-activating mutations and the mechanisms of malignant transformation. Cancer Cell. 2014;25(4):428–41.
16. Nault JC, Mallet M, Pilati C, et al. High frequency of telomerase reverse-transcriptase promoter somatic mutations in hepatocellular carcinoma and preneoplastic lesions. Nat Commun. 2013;4:2218.
17. Sung WK, Zheng H, Li S, et al. Genome-wide survey of recurrent HBV integration in hepatocellular carcinoma. Nat Genet. 2012;44(7):765–9.
18. Minami M, Daimon Y, Mori K, et al. Hepatitis B virus-related insertional mutagenesis in chronic hepatitis B patients as an early drastic genetic change leading to hepatocarcinogenesis. Oncogene. 2005;24(27):4340–8.
19. Ferber MJ, Montoya DP, Yu C, et al. Integrations of the hepatitis B virus (HBV) and human papillomavirus (HPV) into the human telomerase reverse transcriptase (hTERT) gene in liver and cervical cancers. Oncogene. 2003;22(24):3813–20.
20. Behari J. The Wnt/beta-catenin signaling pathway in liver biology and disease. Expert Rev Gastroenterol Hepatol. 2010;4(6):745–56.
21. Takigawa Y, Brown AM. Wnt signaling in liver cancer. Curr Drug Targets. 2008;9(11):1013–24.
22. Cavard C, Colnot S, Audard V, et al. Wnt/beta-catenin pathway in hepatocellular carcinoma pathogenesis and liver physiology. Future Oncol. 2008;4(5):647–60.
23. de La Coste A, Romagnolo B, Billuart P, et al. Somatic mutations of the beta-catenin gene are frequent in mouse and human hepatocellular carcinomas. Proc Natl Acad Sci U S A. 1998;95(15):8847–51.
24. Satoh S, Daigo Y, Furukawa Y, et al. AXIN1 mutations in hepatocellular carcinomas, and growth suppression in cancer cells by virus-mediated transfer of AXIN1. Nat Genet. 2000;24(3):245–50.

25. Su LK, Abdalla EK, Law CH, Kohlmann W, Rashid A, Vauthey JN. Biallelic inactivation of the APC gene is associated with hepatocellular carcinoma in familial adenomatous polyposis coli. Cancer. 2001;92(2):332–9.
26. Boyault S, Rickman DS, de Reynies A, et al. Transcriptome classification of HCC is related to gene alterations and to new therapeutic targets. Hepatology. 2007;45(1):42–52.
27. Yuzugullu H, Benhaj K, Ozturk N, et al. Canonical Wnt signaling is antagonized by noncanonical Wnt5a in hepatocellular carcinoma cells. Mol Cancer. 2009;8:90.
28. Audard V, Grimber G, Elie C, et al. Cholestasis is a marker for hepatocellular carcinomas displaying beta-catenin mutations. J Pathol. 2007;212(3):345–52.
29. Kruiswijk F, Labuschagne CF, Vousden KH. p53 in survival, death and metabolic health: a lifeguard with a licence to kill. Nat Rev Mol Cell Biol. 2015;16(7):393–405.
30. Hollstein M, Sidransky D, Vogelstein B, Harris CC. p53 mutations in human cancers. Science. 1991;253(5015):49–53.
31. Laurent-Puig P, Zucman-Rossi J. Genetics of hepatocellular tumors. Oncogene. 2006;25(27): 3778–86.
32. Hussain SP, Schwank J, Staib F, Wang XW, Harris CC. TP53 mutations and hepatocellular carcinoma: insights into the etiology and pathogenesis of liver cancer. Oncogene. 2007;26(15):2166–76.
33. Laurent-Puig P, Legoix P, Bluteau O, et al. Genetic alterations associated with hepatocellular carcinomas define distinct pathways of hepatocarcinogenesis. Gastroenterology. 2001;120(7):1763–73.
34. Fujimoto A, Totoki Y, Abe T, et al. Whole-genome sequencing of liver cancers identifies etiological influences on mutation patterns and recurrent mutations in chromatin regulators. Nat Genet. 2012;44(7):760–4.
35. Bressac B, Kew M, Wands J, Ozturk M. Selective G to T mutations of p53 gene in hepatocellular carcinoma from southern Africa. Nature. 1991;350(6317):429–31.
36. Kew MC. Aflatoxins as a cause of hepatocellular carcinoma. J Gastrointestin Liver Dis. 2013;22(3):305–10.
37. Teramoto T, Satonaka K, Kitazawa S, Fujimori T, Hayashi K, Maeda S. p53 gene abnormalities are closely related to hepatoviral infections and occur at a late stage of hepatocarcinogenesis. Cancer Res. 1994;54(1):231–5.
38. Calderaro J, Couchy G, Imbeaud S, et al. Histological subtypes of hepatocellular carcinoma are related to gene mutations and molecular tumour classification. J Hepatol. 2017;67(4):727–38.
39. Hsu H, Peng S, Lai P, Chu J, Lee P. Mutations of p53 gene in hepatocellular-carcinoma (hcc) correlate with tumor progression and patient prognosis—a study of 138 patients with unifocal hcc. Int J Oncol. 1994;4(6):1341–7.
40. Yano M, Hamatani K, Eguchi H, et al. Prognosis in patients with hepatocellular carcinoma correlates to mutations of p53 and/or hMSH2 genes. Eur J Cancer. 2007;43(6):1092–100.
41. Hayashi H, Sugio K, Matsumata T, Adachi E, Takenaka K, Sugimachi K. The clinical significance of p53 gene mutation in hepatocellular carcinomas from Japan. Hepatology. 1995;22(6):1702–7.
42. Serrano M, Hannon GJ, Beach D. A new regulatory motif in cell-cycle control causing specific inhibition of cyclin D/CDK4. Nature. 1993;366(6456):704–7.
43. Hui AM, Sakamoto M, Kanai Y, et al. Inactivation of p16INK4 in hepatocellular carcinoma. Hepatology. 1996;24(3):575–9.
44. Jin M, Piao Z, Kim NG, et al. p16 is a major inactivation target in hepatocellular carcinoma. Cancer. 2000;89(1):60–8.
45. Csepregi A, Ebert MP, Rocken C, et al. Promoter methylation of CDKN2A and lack of p16 expression characterize patients with hepatocellular carcinoma. BMC Cancer. 2010;10:317.
46. Kaneto H, Sasaki S, Yamamoto H, et al. Detection of hypermethylation of the p16(INK4A) gene promoter in chronic hepatitis and cirrhosis associated with hepatitis B or C virus. Gut. 2001;48(3):372–7.
47. Song X, Wang S, Li L. New insights into the regulation of Axin function in canonical Wnt signaling pathway. Protein Cell. 2014;5(3):186–93.
48. Ishizaki Y, Ikeda S, Fujimori M, et al. Immunohistochemical analysis and mutational analyses of beta-catenin, Axin family and APC genes in hepatocellular carcinomas. Int J Oncol. 2004;24(5):1077–83.

49. Li J, Quan H, Liu Q, Si Z, He Z, Qi H. Alterations of axis inhibition protein 1 (AXIN1) in hepatitis B virus-related hepatocellular carcinoma and overexpression of AXIN1 induces apoptosis in hepatocellular cancer cells. Oncol Res. 2013;20(7):281–8.
50. Pylayeva-Gupta Y, Grabocka E, Bar-Sagi D. RAS oncogenes: weaving a tumorigenic web. Nat Rev Cancer. 2011;11(11):761–74.
51. Challen C, Guo K, Collier JD, Cavanagh D, Bassendine MF. Infrequent point mutations in codons 12 and 61 of ras oncogenes in human hepatocellular carcinomas. J Hepatol. 1992;14(2–3):342–6.
52. Weihrauch M, Benick M, Lehner G, et al. High prevalence of K-ras-2 mutations in hepatocellular carcinomas in workers exposed to vinyl chloride. Int Arch Occup Environ Health. 2001;74(6):405–10.
53. Rudalska R, Dauch D, Longerich T, et al. In vivo RNAi screening identifies a mechanism of sorafenib resistance in liver cancer. Nat Med. 2014;20(10):1138–46.
54. Llovet JM, Ricci S, Mazzaferro V, et al. Sorafenib in advanced hepatocellular carcinoma. N Engl J Med. 2008;359(4):378–90.
55. Bottaro DP, Rubin JS, Faletto DL, et al. Identification of the hepatocyte growth factor receptor as the c-met proto-oncogene product. Science. 1991;251(4995):802–4.
56. Goyal L, Muzumdar MD, Zhu AX. Targeting the HGF/c-MET pathway in hepatocellular carcinoma. Clin Cancer Res. 2013;19(9):2310–8.
57. Noguchi O, Enomoto N, Ikeda T, Kobayashi F, Marumo F, Sato C. Gene expressions of c-met and hepatocyte growth factor in chronic liver disease and hepatocellular carcinoma. J Hepatol. 1996;24(3):286–92.
58. Suzuki K, Hayashi N, Yamada Y, et al. Expression of the c-met protooncogene in human hepatocellular carcinoma. Hepatology. 1994;20(5):1231–6.
59. Park WS, Dong SM, Kim SY, et al. Somatic mutations in the kinase domain of the Met/hepatocyte growth factor receptor gene in childhood hepatocellular carcinomas. Cancer Res. 1999;59(2):307–10.
60. Kondo S, Ojima H, Tsuda H, et al. Clinical impact of c-Met expression and its gene amplification in hepatocellular carcinoma. Int J Clin Oncol. 2013;18(2):207–13.
61. Santoro A, Rimassa L, Borbath I, et al. Tivantinib for second-line treatment of advanced hepatocellular carcinoma: a randomised, placebo-controlled phase 2 study. Lancet Oncol. 2013;14(1):55–63.
62. Shi Y, Massague J. Mechanisms of TGF-beta signaling from cell membrane to the nucleus. Cell. 2003;113(6):685–700.
63. Massague J. How cells read TGF-beta signals. Nat Rev Mol Cell Biol. 2000;1(3):169–78.
64. Derynck R, Akhurst RJ, Balmain A. TGF-beta signaling in tumor suppression and cancer progression. Nat Genet. 2001;29(2):117–29.
65. Thiery JP, Sleeman JP. Complex networks orchestrate epithelial-mesenchymal transitions. Nat Rev Mol Cell Biol. 2006;7(2):131–42.
66. Coulouarn C, Factor VM, Thorgeirsson SS. Transforming growth factor-beta gene expression signature in mouse hepatocytes predicts clinical outcome in human cancer. Hepatology. 2008;47(6):2059–67.
67. Fischer AN, Fuchs E, Mikula M, Huber H, Beug H, Mikulits W. PDGF essentially links TGF-beta signaling to nuclear beta-catenin accumulation in hepatocellular carcinoma progression. Oncogene. 2007;26(23):3395–405.
68. Hoshida Y, Nijman SM, Kobayashi M, et al. Integrative transcriptome analysis reveals common molecular subclasses of human hepatocellular carcinoma. Cancer Res. 2009;69(18):7385–92.
69. Giannelli G, Villa E, Lahn M. Transforming growth factor-beta as a therapeutic target in hepatocellular carcinoma. Cancer Res. 2014;74(7):1890–4.
70. Simons M, Gordon E, Claesson-Welsh L. Mechanisms and regulation of endothelial VEGF receptor signalling. Nat Rev Mol Cell Biol. 2016;17(10):611–25.
71. Chiang DY, Villanueva A, Hoshida Y, et al. Focal gains of VEGFA and molecular classification of hepatocellular carcinoma. Cancer Res. 2008;68(16):6779–88.
72. Litvinov SV, Bakker HA, Gourevitch MM, Velders MP, Warnaar SO. Evidence for a role of the epithelial glycoprotein 40 (Ep-CAM) in epithelial cell-cell adhesion. Cell Adhes Commun. 1994;2(5):417–28.

73. Balzar M, Winter MJ, de Boer CJ, Litvinov SV. The biology of the 17-1A antigen (Ep-CAM). J Mol Med (Berl). 1999;77(10):699–712.
74. Yamashita T, Ji J, Budhu A, et al. EpCAM-positive hepatocellular carcinoma cells are tumor-initiating cells with stem/progenitor cell features. Gastroenterology. 2009;136(3):1012–24.
75. Tan PS, Nakagawa S, Goossens N, et al. Clinicopathological indices to predict hepatocellular carcinoma molecular classification. Liver Int. 2016;36(1):108–18.
76. Li Y, Zhang W, Doughtie A, et al. Up-regulation of fibroblast growth factor 19 and its receptor associates with progression from fatty liver to hepatocellular carcinoma. Oncotarget. 2016;7(32):52329–39.
77. Song MS, Salmena L, Pandolfi PP. The functions and regulation of the PTEN tumour suppressor. Nat Rev Mol Cell Biol. 2012;13(5):283–96.
78. Hu TH, Huang CC, Lin PR, et al. Expression and prognostic role of tumor suppressor gene PTEN/MMAC1/TEP1 in hepatocellular carcinoma. Cancer. 2003;97(8):1929–40.
79. Hu TH, Wang CC, Huang CC, et al. Down-regulation of tumor suppressor gene PTEN, overexpression of p53, plus high proliferating cell nuclear antigen index predict poor patient outcome of hepatocellular carcinoma after resection. Oncol Rep. 2007;18(6):1417–26.
80. Kawamura N, Nagai H, Bando K, et al. PTEN/MMAC1 mutations in hepatocellular carcinomas: somatic inactivation of both alleles in tumors. Jpn J Cancer Res. 1999;90(4):413–8.
81. Peyrou M, Bourgoin L, Foti M. PTEN in liver diseases and cancer. World J Gastroenterol. 2010;16(37):4627–33.
82. Allis CD, Jenuwein T. The molecular hallmarks of epigenetic control. Nat Rev Genet. 2016;17(8):487–500.
83. Nishida N, Goel A. Genetic and epigenetic signatures in human hepatocellular carcinoma: a systematic review. Curr Genomics. 2011;12(2):130–7.
84. Kondo Y, Kanai Y, Sakamoto M, Mizokami M, Ueda R, Hirohashi S. Genetic instability and aberrant DNA methylation in chronic hepatitis and cirrhosis—a comprehensive study of loss of heterozygosity and microsatellite instability at 39 loci and DNA hypermethylation on 8 CpG islands in microdissected specimens from patients with hepatocellular carcinoma. Hepatology. 2000;32(5):970–9.
85. Jung JK, Arora P, Pagano JS, Jang KL. Expression of DNA methyltransferase 1 is activated by hepatitis B virus X protein via a regulatory circuit involving the p16INK4a-cyclin D1-CDK 4/6-pRb-E2F1 pathway. Cancer Res. 2007;67(12):5771–8.
86. Arora P, Kim EO, Jung JK, Jang KL. Hepatitis C virus core protein downregulates E-cadherin expression via activation of DNA methyltransferase 1 and 3b. Cancer Lett. 2008;261(2):244–52.
87. Katoh H, Shibata T, Kokubu A, et al. Epigenetic instability and chromosomal instability in hepatocellular carcinoma. Am J Pathol. 2006;168(4):1375–84.
88. Ji J, Shi J, Budhu A, et al. MicroRNA expression, survival, and response to interferon in liver cancer. N Engl J Med. 2009;361(15):1437–47.
89. Lagos-Quintana M, Rauhut R, Yalcin A, Meyer J, Lendeckel W, Tuschl T. Identification of tissue-specific microRNAs from mouse. Curr Biol. 2002;12(9):735–9.
90. Nassirpour R, Mehta PP, Yin MJ. miR-122 regulates tumorigenesis in hepatocellular carcinoma by targeting AKT3. PLoS One. 2013;8(11):e79655.
91. Bai S, Nasser MW, Wang B, et al. MicroRNA-122 inhibits tumorigenic properties of hepatocellular carcinoma cells and sensitizes these cells to sorafenib. J Biol Chem. 2009;284(46):32015–27.
92. Aoki H, Kajino K, Arakawa Y, Hino O. Molecular cloning of a rat chromosome putative recombinogenic sequence homologous to the hepatitis B virus encapsidation signal. Proc Natl Acad Sci U S A. 1996;93(14):7300–4.
93. Walther A, Houlston R, Tomlinson I. Association between chromosomal instability and prognosis in colorectal cancer: a meta-analysis. Gut. 2008;57(7):941–50.
94. Bakhoum SF, Danilova OV, Kaur P, Levy NB, Compton DA. Chromosomal instability substantiates poor prognosis in patients with diffuse large B-cell lymphoma. Clin Cancer Res. 2011;17(24):7704–11.

95. How C, Bruce J, So J, et al. Chromosomal instability as a prognostic marker in cervical cancer. BMC Cancer. 2015;15:361.
96. Wilkens L, Flemming P, Gebel M, et al. Induction of aneuploidy by increasing chromosomal instability during dedifferentiation of hepatocellular carcinoma. Proc Natl Acad Sci U S A. 2004;101(5):1309–14.
97. Katoh H, Ojima H, Kokubu A, et al. Genetically distinct and clinically relevant classification of hepatocellular carcinoma: putative therapeutic targets. Gastroenterology. 2007;133(5):1475–86.
98. Zucman-Rossi J, Villanueva A, Nault JC, Llovet JM. Genetic landscape and biomarkers of hepatocellular carcinoma. Gastroenterology. 2015;149(5):1226–39.e24.
99. Kaposi-Novak P, Lee JS, Gomez-Quiroz L, Coulouarn C, Factor VM, Thorgeirsson SS. Met-regulated expression signature defines a subset of human hepatocellular carcinomas with poor prognosis and aggressive phenotype. J Clin Invest. 2006;116(6):1582–95.
100. Villanueva A, Hoshida Y, Battiston C, et al. Combining clinical, pathology, and gene expression data to predict recurrence of hepatocellular carcinoma. Gastroenterology. 2011;140(5):1501–12.e02.
101. Zucman-Rossi J, Benhamouche S, Godard C, et al. Differential effects of inactivated Axin1 and activated beta-catenin mutations in human hepatocellular carcinomas. Oncogene. 2007;26(5):774–80.
102. Goossens N, Sun X, Hoshida Y. Molecular classification of hepatocellular carcinoma: potential therapeutic implications. Hepat Oncol. 2015;2(4):371–9.
103. Toyoda H, Kumada T, Tada T, Sone Y, Kaneoka Y, Maeda A. Tumor markers for hepatocellular carcinoma: simple and significant predictors of outcome in patients with HCC. Liver Cancer. 2015;4(2):126–36.

Genomics Studies in Hepatocellular Carcinoma via Next-Generation Sequencing

4

Xiyang Wei, Niya Liu, Xin Wei Wang, and Junfang Ji

4.1 Hepatocellular Carcinoma and Its Heterogeneity

Hepatocellular carcinoma (HCC) accounts for 80% of all primary liver cancers worldwide and is a clinically and biologically heterogeneous disease. It ranks at the fifth most prevalent cancer and the third most deadly malignancy globally. Although most HCC patients are resided in eastern Asia and sub-Saharan Africa, it is along the way to be more prevalent in Western countries [1–5].

4.1.1 HCC Heterogeneity in Etiology

Various risk factors give rise to HCC, and the tumorigenesis of HCC exerts distinct regional differences [5]. Hepatitis B virus (HBV) infection and hepatitis C virus (HCV) infection are the two major risk factors of HCC, accounting for about 80% of HCC tumorigenesis globally. HBV infection is the dominant risk factor in eastern Asia and sub-Saharan Africa. While in Europe and North America, more than half of HCC are due to HCV infection [6–8]. Analysis of HBV genome sequencing data identifies eight distinct genotypes (A–H), which also exert obvious geographical and ethnic distributions [7]. HBV infection generally gives rise to the integration of viral DNA into the host genome, especially in hosts with attenuated immunity. While as a RNA virus, HCV is not able to integrate into host genome. HCV tends to escape from host's immune responses, implicates in chronic infection, and gives rise to liver cirrhosis. HCV proteins seem to change many potentially oncogenic

X. Wei, Ph.D. • N. Liu, Ph.D. • J. Ji, Ph.D. (✉)
Life Sciences Institute, Zhejiang University, Hangzhou 310058, China
e-mail: junfangji@zju.edu.cn

X.W. Wang, M.D., Ph.D.
Liver Carcinogenesis Section, Laboratory of Human Carcinogenesis, Center for Cancer Research, National Cancer Institute, Bethesda, MD 20892, USA

© Springer International Publishing AG 2018
C. Liu (ed.), *Precision Molecular Pathology of Liver Cancer*,
Molecular Pathology Library, https://doi.org/10.1007/978-3-319-68082-8_4

pathways and promote the malignant transformation of hepatocytes [1, 9]. In addition, hepatitis delta virus (HDV) is a defective RNA virus, which could also contribute to hepatic carcinogenesis [10, 11].

Many metabolic-related diseases also contribute to HCC development, which includes alcoholic fatty liver disease (AFLD), non-AFLD (NAFLD), diabetes, obesity, etc. Alcohol consumption and alcoholism is prevalent worldwide. Excessive alcohol consumption may cause AFLD, which ultimately gives rise to HCC [12–14]. NAFLD is one of the prevalent clinicopathological syndromes associated with insulin resistance and dyslipidemia. Synergistically with chronic HCV infection, alcoholic liver injury, or risk factors, NAFLD evolves into cirrhosis and HCC ultimately. As the prevalence of obesity in the industrialized countries, NAFLD has been a dominant element for chronic liver disease [15, 16]. Obesity itself is also proposed to relate with increased risk of HCC. In patients with chronic viral infection, obesity synergistically increases the risk of HCC by 100 folds [17, 18]. Meanwhile, diabetes is an independent risk factor for the development of HCC and ranks second of the most prevalent cause for HCC in the USA after viral infection [19–21].

In addition, HCC has been also associated with the increased exposure to aflatoxin B1, which mainly happened in Africa and Asia. Other HCC risk factors include neonatal hepatitis, autoimmune hepatitis, hereditary diseases (hemochromatosis, a-1AT deficiency, tyrosinemia, and Wilson's disease), other immune disorders, etc. [2, 22, 23].

4.1.2   HCC Heterogeneity in Clinical Presentation

HCC develops generally in a previously diseased liver that is related to various HCC risk factors as above. Either HCC tumor or previously diseased liver can be at different disease-progressing stage at the time of diagnosis and has diverse therapeutic perspectives. HCC population is therefore very heterogeneous. According to tumor size, differentiation grate, and nodular type, HCC could be presumably divided into early HCC and progressed HCC [24, 25]. The global HCC BRIDGE study scientifically documents various therapeutic approaches across regions and/or countries [26]. Tumor classification can help us identify the difference between various subtypes of HCC with comparable criteria and possibly provide specific subgroup candidate patients with appropriate therapeutic interventions [27].

A number of HCC staging systems and related treatment algorithms have been developed, which facilitate prognosis and guide clinical practice, prolonging survival of HCC patients eventually. These systems include Barcelona-Clinic Liver Cancer (BCLC) staging system, the Cancer of the Liver Italian Program (CLIP) score system, Okuda system, the Hong Kong Liver Cancer (HKLC) classification system, etc. [28–31]. Among them, HCC BCLC staging and treatment algorithm has been widely applied. At early stage, HCC patients with carcinoma in situ can be reliably curable. Curative therapies include liver transplantation, tumor resection, and local ablation. However, the number of nodules is relevant to resectability, and post-resection survival rates are variant [32]. Most HCC patients are diagnosed at intermediate stage and even advanced stage. In this case, trans-arterial chemoembolization (TACE) is the first-line option to extend live-life expectancy, but the overall survival is variable and limited. For those failed by TACE, sorafenib (a multityrosine kinase inhibitor) and radioembolization merit consideration [32]. Sorafenib currently is the only FDA-approved systemic therapy for advanced HCC. However, it only has a modest 2-month survival benefit for HCC patients without any preselection in several clinical trials.

4.1.3 HCC Heterogeneity at the Biological Level

Multiple array technologies including expression examination methods (cDNA/oligo/noncoding RNA arrays) and genetic assays (CGH/methylation arrays) have provided powerful tools to amend our understanding on the tumorigenesis, progression, and metastasis of HCC and hold potential of improving HCC therapeutic efficacy [33–44]. The accumulated studies have revealed that diverse changes in HCCs were associated with different viral backgrounds as well as different HCC subtypes.

Chronic HBV and HCV hepatic lesions present differential gene expression profiles. Genes being affected by HBV were related to inflammation, while HCV-associated genes were involved into the anti-inflammatory process [45]. Studies have also revealed increases of DNA copy number at 10p and decreases at 10q in HCV-HCCs [46], while gains on 1q, 6p, 8q, 9p, and losses at 1p, 16q, and 19p in many HBV-HCCs [47].

Several array studies have compared numerous HCC tumors to distinguish HCC subtypes. Via the combination of genomic and transcriptomic analysis, researchers have identified six robust HCC subclasses with distinct activation of biological pathways and therapeutic implications [48, 49]. Primary HCC tissues with a propensity for metastasis had a significantly different cDNA and microRNA expression profiles compared to profiles of relapse-free HCC tissues [40, 41, 43]. A 20-miRNA metastasis signature was significantly associated with recurrence in HCC at early stage [34].

In our group, we have found that a subgroup of HCCs with EpCAM and alpha-fetoprotein (AFP) high expression displayed a high rate of metastasis and poor outcome and were biologically different from other HCCs based on their stem cell-related gene expression profiles and singling pathway analysis [37, 42, 50]. Stem cell-related signaling pathways were highly active in these HCC cases, and isolated EpCAM + AFP + HCC cells were enriched hepatic cancer stem cells. In addition, our studies also revealed that HCC patients with low level of microRNA-26 had a significant prolonged survival after adjuvant interferon alpha (IFNα) therapy compared to the control treatment group. However, HCC patients with high level of microRNA-26 did not have survival benefit from adjuvant IFNα therapy [51, 52].

In this vein, HCC is a heterogeneous disease. It is thus important to identify the HCC tumor subtypes, in-depth study of each subtype using an unbiased high-throughput method to explore the potential early diagnostic, prognostic, as well as therapeutic biomarkers. The array technologies have been well established and widely used. However, they mainly focus on gene expression, only to detect known genes, and are at one genomic level per technology at a time. Recent advances in massively parallel nucleotide sequencing technologies allow for simultaneous identification of genetic substitutions, insertion/deletions, expression changes, and structural alterations with high accuracy and sensitivity. It is so-called next-generation sequencing (NGS) technology.

4.2 Next-Generation Sequencing System

NGS is now known as high-throughput parallel nucleotide sequencing. In 2005, a new massively parallel sequencing technique emerged and sequenced over 20 megabase data in a single run, which eventually launched the "next-generation" of genomic science [53]. Since that, NGS has largely revolutionized omics study in this decade. Now, the wide application of NGS has transformed the way scientists think about genetic information. Currently there are a number of different modern sequencing technologies including three dominate commercial platforms, i.e., Roche Genome Sequencer, Illumina Genome Analyzer, and Life Technologies Sequencing by Oligo Ligation Detection (SOLiD) System (Table 4.1).

4.2.1 Roche 454 Sequencing

In 2005, 454 Life Sciences (now Roche) developed the first commercially available NGS platform. Now the 454 family of platforms has been utilized for many

Table 4.1 Summary of major NGS technologies

Technology	Sequencing method (type, amplification, chemistry)	Reads/run (length, reads #)	Time/run	Advantages
Roche 454	Seq-by-synthesis, emulsion PCR, pyrosequencing	700 bp, 1 million reads	~24 h	Long reads, fast
Illumina	Seq-by-synthesis, bridge amplification, reversible dye terminator	50–300 bp, up to 6 million reads	1–10 days	High yield, cost-effective
SOLiD	Seq-by-ligation, emulsion PCR, 8-mer oligo chained ligation	35–75 bp, 1 billion reads	1–2 weeks	High accuracy, high yield, cost-effective
Ion Torrent	Seq-by-synthesis, emulsion PCR, proton detection	up to 400 bp, up to 80 million reads	~2 h	High yield, fast, portable equipment
The third generation (PacBio)	Seq-by-synthesis, N/A, phosphor-linked fluorescent bases	>1000 bp, up to 1 million bases	0.5–4 h	Longest read length, fast

applications due to its long reads. The overall approach for 454 is pyrosequencing based. It depends on the detection of pyrophosphate release on nucleotide incorporation [54]. The library DNAs with adapters are prepared using PCR primers or by ligation. These DNAs are then fixed to amplification beads followed by emulsion PCR. An emulsion PCR step produces a set of beads, and each set contains many cloned copies from the same DNA. The beads are loaded into PicoTiterPlate with one bead per well, and the sequencing by synthesis begins in a system with a group of enzymes and the substrates. The four DNA nucleotides are added sequentially in a fixed order. A nucleotide complementary to the template strand triggers pyrophosphate release, which generates a signal being recorded to infer the sequence of the DNA fragments as each base type is added. During the nucleotide flow, millions of copies of DNA are sequenced in parallel.

Currently Roche sequencing platforms are mainly GS-FLX and GS Junior Systems, which may be a good choice for certain applications where long read lengths are needed [55]. GS-FLX Titanium could generate about one million reads with the length of 700 bp per run within 24 h [53], while GS Junior Systems simplifies the library preparation and data processing.

The advantages of Roche sequencing are long read length (which generally offering higher accuracy) and sequencing speed (about 10 h). One shortcoming for this approach is the misidentification of homopolymers length [56]. In addition, 454 is relatively cost-ineffective compared to other sequencing platforms such as Illumina and SOLiD [57]. For downstream analysis, the GS Data analysis software packages are also available.

4.2.2 Illumina Sequencing

Illumina sequencing, Solexa platform, was first introduced in 2006. Now Illumina produces the most widely used platforms and have been used by numerous researchers due to its production of a large amount of data in a cost-effective manner. Similar to 454 technology, Illumina sequencing also uses a sequencing-by-synthesis method [58–60]. There are two major differences of Illumina technology from 454 sequencing. One is that Illumina uses a flow cell with coated oligoes instead of microwells with beads. As the DNA enters the flow cell, one of the adapters attaches to a complementary oligo. The other is that Illumina sequencing uses fluorescent reversible termination approach instead of pyrosequencing. A reversible terminator is on every nucleotide to prevent multiple additions in one round, one base per round and one unique emission for each of the four bases. After each round, the added base is recorded.

Now Illumina has many different sequencing platforms on the market including Genome Analyzer, HiSeq, MiSeq, and NextSeq [58, 59]. Each one has several different versions. Among them, MiSeq could produce the longest reads, about 300 bp and use the minimum sequencing time. It could sequence one sample in 10 h including sample and library preparation. MiSeqDx platform is the only one approved by the FDA for in vitro diagnostics. HiSeq could produce the greatest output amount. For example, HiSeq 2500 could generate four billion reads with 125 bp/read in a single run.

The superiorities of the Illumina system include small sample requirements, simple process, short run time, and high-quality data [58, 59]. It also has the proper data analysis flow and tools developed by Illumina so that the researchers can easily analyze and manage genome data. The major flaw is false positive when identifying sequence variations [60]. At this stage, more than 90% of sequencing data have been produced via Illumina technology.

4.2.3　SOLiD Sequencing

SOLiD system is appeared in 2006 and commercialized in 2009. This technology uses a sequencing-by-ligation method. After adaptor ligation and emulsion PCR, the library DNAs are sequenced in an entirely different method compared to 454 and Illumina. In SOLiD there are a set of four fluorescently labeled di-base probes and four di-base probes per dye. It uses DNA ligase for di-base incorporation, which makes a "sequencing by ligation" approach. Following each ligation cycle, the system removes the extension product and resets DNA template with a primer complementary to the $n - 1$ position for the next round ligation. There are several rounds of reset, by which each base is interrogated in two independent ligation reactions. Due to two-base probing and two-color encoding per base, the sequencing accuracy is very high (about 99.99%), and the systemic noise is very low [61, 62].

Now the updated version of SOLiD system can produce a mass of data, and the cost is substantially low. Since its read has relatively short length (up to 75 bp) but high accuracy, SOLiD technology has some advantages in detecting single-nucleotide polymorphism (SNP), small RNA sequencing, and ChIP-seq over other sequencers [55].

4.2.4　Ion Personal Genome Machine

Ion Torrent entered the sequencing market in 2010. The first semiconductor sequencing device was Ion Personal Genome Machine. This technology is mainly used for small genome sequencing and exome sequencing. It begins with a similar method with 454, which uses a chip of microwells containing beads being fixed with DNA fragments [63]. However, this chip is a semiconductor chip with micro-detectors sensitive to pH. As a base incorporation, a proton is released and alters the surrounding pH, and micro-detector could record the change. As each base type is added in turn and washed sequentially, the sequence is informed. Now, the accuracy rate of this instrument on a per read basis averages approximately 99%.

Ion Torrent Personal Genome Machine technology does not require fluorescence and camera recording, which leads to a higher speed, smaller instrument size, and lower cost. It now produces the highest output. Ion Torrent Sequencer can complete a DNA sequencing workflow in just 1 day. Since Ion AmpliSeq being launched in

2012, this technology has seen broad global adoption. However, similar to 454, Ion Torrent suffers homopolymer-related errors.

4.2.5 The Third-Generation Sequencers

Above NGS technologies start by fragmenting and amplifying DNA, which often sacrifices vital long-range connectivity. The third-generation sequencing is then developed to possibly overcome such defects. It has two major characteristics differing from the above sequencing technologies. One is that amplification of DNA fragments is not needed before sequencing. The other is that the base signal is obtained in real time during the enzyme reaction of adding nucleotide. Thus, the third-generation sequencing gains the advantages of high speed and long read length. Currently it mainly concentrates in the optical or electrical signal detection at single molecular level, such as single-molecule real-time (SMRT) and MinION system [64].

SMRT was developed by Pacific Biosciences, which uses nanotechnology (zero-mode waveguide, ZMW) [54]. The ZMW is a structure that is small enough to observe only a dye-labeled single nucleotide of DNA being incorporated by DNA polymerase. Four different fluorescent dyes are attached to A, T, C, and G. The sequencing is performed on a chip containing numerous ZMW detectors. As DNA strands are synthesized, the dye-labeled nucleotide incorporation is imaged in real time. SMRT completely depends on the role of DNA polymerase that enabled the length of sequencing.

The MinION system was released by Oxford Nanopore Technologies in 2014, which delivered long read real-time sequencing of individual molecules. It is the first commercial nanopore-based sequencer, small and portable. Nanopore is a tiny biopore with diameter in nanoscale and can facilitate ion exchange. Current MinION nanopore sequencing methods rely on the measurement of changes in ionic current at the time of a DNA molecule translocating through a protein nanopore. Biological nanopores aim at single nucleotide, so that this technique has good continuity and accuracy. Moreover, there is no need DNA polymerase ligase or dNTPs or complex optical detection system. It could potentially reach long read at length over 5 kb.

Fluorescence resonance energy transfer (FRET) is another third-generation sequencing technology, which is developed by VisiGen (now Life Tech). It uses a four-color set of FRET dideoxy nucleotide terminators. The fluorescence is cleaved off during the base incorporation and generates an optical signal to achieve the purpose of testing the sequence of DNA bases. The obvious advantages of FRET sequencing are simple and straightforward; the speed can reach one million bases per second.

Now sequencing technologies are widely utilized for mutation profiles, gene expression analysis, methylation analysis, metagenomics, disease-related gene identification, etc. [65]. It has also started to provide service of establishing personal genome information as well as noninvasive prenatal testing [66]. Since these, NGS has accelerated biological research by providing researchers a better understanding of the biology of diseases including carcinogenesis.

4.3   HCC Genomics Studies via NGS Technology

NGS has provided a sensitive, accurate, and cost-effective method to uncover the genetic basis of human disease including cancer at a single-nucleotide resolution [67, 68]. The tumorigenesis and progression of HCC are accompanied by the accumulation of somatic genetic variations. Previous microarray-based technologies have analyzed variations of HCC genome, transcriptome, epigenome, etc., which improved our understanding on HCC tumorigenesis, progression, and inter-/intra-heterogeneity as well as promoted HCC translational research. Here we summarized the original NGS studies in HCC as well as its potential clinical utilization, with an emphasis on understanding HCC heterogeneity (Table 4.2).

4.3.1   HCC Viral Risk Factors in Viral-Related HCCs

HBV Integration in HBV-Related HCCs
HBV is the most prevalent risk factor of HCC and the integration of HBV DNA into the host genome has been reported in 1980s [69]. Now, deep sequencing has been successfully applied to the study of HBV genome integration.

Whole-genome sequencing of 11 HBV-related HCC samples has revealed the HBV genome integration to the telomerase reverse transcriptase (*TERT*) locus [70], which is consistent with previous reports [71]. After that, a study of whole-genome sequencing using 88 HCC patients (81 HBV+ and 7 HBV−) further noted that HBV integration was more significantly frequent in tumors compared to control liver tissues and that about 40% of HBV breakpoints were around the HBV X and core genes [72]. Moreover, via a comparison of gene expression array data between tumors with and without HBV integration, the authors reported that five genes (*TERT*, *MLL4*, *CCNE1*, *SENP5*, and *ROCK1*) were recurrently affected by HBV integration. HCC patients with several HBV integration sites had shorter overall survival time [72].

One group recently reported that HBV was apt to integrate into promoters of genes, and recurrent integration into the promoter of *TERT* seemed to increase the expression level of *TERT*. HBx 3′-end was preferred to involve into integration, resulting into the expression of HBV-human chimeric proteins [73]. Li et al. developed high-throughput viral integration detection method to enrich and sequence HBV fragments. They identified 246 integration breakpoints in the gene *TERT*, *MLL4*, and *CCNE1* [74]. Meanwhile, the whole-exome sequencing and oncovirome sequencing in 68 HBV positive HCC cases have also revealed a group of genes close to the recurrent HBV integrations, including *TERT*, *MLL4*, *ALOX5*, etc. [75].

HCV Quasispecies Diversity in Chronic Liver Disease and HCC
In human, HCV presents as a group of genetic variants, which is known as "quasispecies." HCV quasispecies has been revealed to act as an important factor in HCC pathogenesis [76]. Park et al. performed pyrosequencing to compare the structural protein-coding genes of HCV genome between patients with chronic hepatitis C

Table 4.2 Summary of original NGS studies in HCC

Ref	Study design	Summary of two major results for each study
Genome and/or exome sequencing		
[109]	WGS of a HCV-HCC tumor and lymphocytes from a male	>11,000 somatic substitutions in HCC with less in genic region, 81/90 somatic variants in protein-coding regions was validated
[72]	WGS of 88 HCC tumor/non-tumor pairs (81 HBV, 7 HBV)	HBV integration was more frequent in tumors; ~40% of HBV breakpoints were around the X and core genes
[70]	WGS of 27 HCC tumors (11 HBV, 14 HCV)	Multiple chromatin regulators were mutated in ~50% of the tumors; HBV integration was found in the *TERT* locus
[110]	HBV integrates Seq of 40 HCC tumor/non-tumor pairs (40HBV)	HBV integration favored chromosome 17; 8 genes were recurrent target genes by HBV integration including *TERT1*
[111]	WES of 10 HBV-HCCs with portal vein tumor thromboses	475 candidate somatic substitutions were identified; genetic lesions in *ARID1A* contribute to high metastatic potential
[92]	WES of 3 matched HBV-HCC tumors and normal tissues	59 genes had mutations in HBV-related HCCs; variants of *ZNF717* and *PARP4* were detected in >10% HCCs from a validation cohort
[85]	WES of 87 HCC tumor/normal tissue pairs (38HBV; 19HCV)	Recurrent mutations in some key genes, such as *TP53* and *CTNNB1*. Some gene families were affected such as calcium channel subunits
[88]	WGS of 88 HCC tumor/normal pairs (81 HBV)	*CTNNB1* was the most frequently mutated oncogene (15.9%); *TP53* was the most frequently mutated tumor suppressor (35.2%)
[73]	HBV Seq of 48 matched HCC tumor/normal pairs	HBV integration favored chromosome 10; HBV recurrent integration was found in the promoter of *TERT*
[74]	HBV integrates sequencing of 28 HBV-HCC tumors	High-throughput viral integration detection method; HBV integration in *TERT*, *MLL4*, and *CCNE1* genes
[75]	WES and oncovirome Seq of 503 liver tumor/normal pairs (488HCC, 117HBV, 212HCV)	Reveal 30 candidate driver genes and 11 core pathway modules in HCC. Multiple types of *TERT* genetic alteration in HCC
[81]	WGS and RNA Seq of 12 HCC tumor/normal pairs; WES of 30 HCC tumor/normal pairs	Frequent mutations in *TP53*, *CTNNB1*, and *AXIN1*, *LAMA2* had multiple high-allelic frequency mutations and related to HCC prognosis
[102]	Targeted DNA Seq of 14 HCC tumors (3HBV, 5HCV)	Find mutations in Wnt, mTOR, etc. pathway; 2 out of 3 cases with mutations in mTOR pathway benefited from mTOR inhibitor therapy
[104]	WGS of 4 matched HCC/normal/lung metastatic tissues (4HBV)	Similar genetic variations in primary and metastatic tumors, a few somatic mutations (such as *ZNF*) were only in metastatic tumors
[90]	WGS of 88 matched HCC tumors/normal tissues (81HBV)	4314 genomic rearrangements in HCCs, Chromothripsis in 5 HCC genomes recurrently affecting chromosomal arms 1q and 8q
[103]	WGS of CTC/HCCs/PBMC from 20 HCCs and 10 controls	Characteristic gene mutations in CTC DNAs could stratify HCC metastasis patients; low frequency variants were higher in CTCs

(continued)

Table 4.2 (continued)

Ref	Study design	Summary of two major results for each study
[82]	WES of 243 tumors/normal tissue pairs (34HBV; 63HCV)	161 HCC driver genes associated with 11 recurrently altered pathways. Many alterations were potentially targetable by FDA-approved drugs
[91]	NGS of plasma DNAs from 31 HCCs and 8 controls	Visual CNV were identified in 13 HCCs at 150 kb per bin CNV plots; develop a CNV scoring method to evaluate the risk of HCC
RNA transcriptome sequencing		
[78]	HCV viral Seq of 79 HCV patients (25HCCs)	HCV isolates differed genetically based on the mutation status at HCV core aa 70; a ratio of mutant Q/H vs. wild R was increased in HCC
[98]	RNA Seq of 4 AFB1-treated rat livers and 4 control rat livers	Gene profiling differed between AFB1 treatment and controls Several low copy and novel transcripts were found in AFB1 group
[87]	RNA Seq of 1 matched HCC tumor/normal liver pairs	Identify a novel gene with coding regions, termed *DUNQU1*. The abundance of *FGFR2-IIIc* is associated with HCC prognosis
[89]	RNA Seq of normal, low-/high-grade dysplastic lesion, early/progressed HCC of 8 HBV-HCCs	Transcriptome changes in early lesions were modest and homogenous. Extensive alterations happened in progressed HCCs and changes were mainly on TGF-beta, WNT, NOTCH, and EMT-associated genes
[93]	RNA Seq of 3 HCC tumor/normal liver pairs (2HCV)	Gene expression differed between HCCs and normal controls; five non-synonymously mutational genes were related to metabolic diseases
[77]	HCV RNA Seq of 49 HCV patients (23 HCCs)	Quasispecies diversity of HCV E1 was low in HCCs. 14 amino acid positions differed in HCC patients compared to chronic HCV patients
Small RNA deep sequencing		
[96]	2 HCC cell lines and 1 immortalized hepatocyte lines	piR-Hep1, a new PIWI-interacting RNA was identified and involved in liver carcinogenesis. Show the abundance of miR-1323 in HCC
[94]	14 HCCs and 6 matched non-tumor livers (3HBV, 10HCV)	NGS was comparable to microarray; several novel microRNAs were identified
[99]	1 pooled liver from AFB1-treated rat and 1 from control rat	HCC-associated microRNAs were abnormally expressed in rats under AFB1 stress; 16 novel microRNAs were identified
[95]	24 matched HCC tumors and non-tumor tissues	MiR-122-5p was the most abundant microRNA of the hepatic miRnome. Almost every microRNA gene produced isomiRNAs
[39]	2 paired of EpCAM+/− primary HCC cells, 2 hepatic stem cells and 2 hepatoblasts, 3 hepatocytes and 1 pooled human ESC, etc.	Ten microRNAs were specifically altered in EpCAM+ primary HCC cells. MiR-155, one of these microRNAs, was validated at the expression level and functionally related to HCC malignant feature
[97]	12 matched HCC tumors and non-tumor pairs (4HBV, 4HCV)	5′ tRNA-halves were abundant in nonmalignant liver; 5′ tRNA-halves abundance was increased under chronic hepatitis but reduced in HCC

Table 4.2 (continued)

Ref	Study design	Summary of two major results for each study
Bisulfite DNA sequencing		
[100]	Plasma DNAs of 26 HCCs/32 controls; 15 matched HCC tumor DNAs and buffy coat DNAs	Significant hypomethylation in the plasma DNAs of HCC patients, genome-wide methylation and CNV analysis could be detected at the same time and likely be used synergistically to predict cancer
[101]	Targeted Seq of 28 genes in 24 paired tumor/non-tumor DNAs	Methylation status of all 28 amplicons were significant different between tumor and non-tumors. Preform the correlation of methylation status and expression of these amplicons

Notes: Illumina sequencing platforms were used in majority of above HCC NGS studies. A few of studies have used Roche technology [73, 77, 78], SOLiD technology [39, 111], and Personal Genome Machine technology [103]. *Abbreviations*: *CNV* copy number variation, *CTC* circulating tumor cell, *hESC* human embryonic stem cells, *PBMC* peripheral blood mononuclear cell, *WES* whole-exome sequencing, *WGS* whole-genome sequencing

($n = 26$) and HCC patients ($n = 23$) [77]. Data analysis revealed that quasispecies diversity in HCV E1 was significantly lower in HCC patients compared to patients chronic HCV, and 14 amino acid positions significantly differed between two groups. Miura et al. also conducted deep sequencing of serum samples from 79 HCV-infected patients (25 of chronic hepatitis, 29 of liver cirrhosis, 25 HCCs) to examine the association of HCV quasispecies with HCC [78]. They have found the HCV core amino acid that 70 residue sequencing data could reflect the status of liver disease. The ratio of mutant residue to wild-type one in HCV core was increased as liver disease advanced to liver cirrhosis and HCC.

4.3.2   Mutational Landscapes in HCC

NGS technologies have discovered many known and novel genetic alterations in numerous cancers including HCC. Recently, accumulated NGS studies in HCC have suggested that some genetic alterations being grouped in several important HCC oncogenic pathways are likely to be oncogenic driver mutations [70, 75, 79–82].

WNT/Beta-Catenin Pathway and P53 Pathway

It has been known that *CTNNB1* (encoding protein beta-catenin) and *TP53* are two frequently mutated genes in HCC [83, 84]. Many recent NGS studies in HCCs have confirmed *CTNNB1* as the most frequently mutated oncogene while *TP53* as the most frequently mutated tumor suppressor [74, 75, 80–82, 85]. These studies have also consistently revealed that *CTNNB1* mutation was more frequent in HCV and non-viral-related HCC cases (20–40%) but less frequent in HBV-related HCC cases (~10%). In a recent study, Schulze et al. performed a large scale of whole-exome sequencing in 243 HCCs with different etiologic background [82]. In their study,

CTNNB1 mutation was associated with alcohol-related HCCs, while *Tp53* mutation was related with HBV-HCCs. Further, two studies reported that *AXIN1*, one of WNT pathway regulators, had a high mutation rate in HCCs [75, 81]. Its mutation was more frequent in HBV-HCCs compared to HCV-HCCs and non-viral-related HCCs [75]. These results indicate that different viral etiologies might activate WNT pathways in distinct ways. Strikingly, about 66% of HCCs presented WNT pathway-related genetic alterations [75]. In P53 pathway, besides *TP53* mutation, *CDKN2A/CDKN2B*, *MDM2*, and *IRF2* mutation have also been noticed in a rate of over 1% in HCC, respectively. Together, about 49% of HCCs presented P53 pathway-related genetic alterations [75, 82].

Chromatin Regulators

Using exome sequencing of 24 HCC samples, researchers demonstrated that chromatin regulation pathway was commonly altered by genetic alterations including somatic mutations and gene deletions [80]. They noticed the frequent mutation of *ARID1A*, a chromatin-remodeling gene, in alcohol-related HCC. This study was further confirmed by Huang and his colleagues [47]. *ARID1A* mutations were found in 13% of HBV-related HCCs, and mutated *ARID1A* played an important role in HCC invasion and migration [47]. Interestingly, *ARID2* mutation was also identified in HCCs, and its mutation was significantly enriched in HCV-HCC cases compared to HBV-HCCs (14% vs. 2%) [86]. Furthermore, using whole-genome sequencing of HCC samples, Fujimoto et al. found recurrent somatic mutations in a group of chromatin regulation-related genes [70]. These genes were *ARID1A*, *ARID1B*, *ARID2*, *MLL*, *MLL3*, etc. In more than 50% of HCC tissues, they noticed mutations in at least one of these chromatin regulator genes. Therefore, dysregulated chromatin remodeling might play a key role in HCC.

Several studies have also revealed that genetic alterations of transcription modulators. Cleary et al. performed whole-exome sequencing for 87 pairs of HCC tumors and adjacent normal tissues and identified several significantly mutated transcription modulators, including genes in NFE2L2-KEAP1 pathways [85]. Totoki's study has also revealed the frequent alterations in *NFE2L2* [75].

PI3K/Akt/mTOR-Pathway and MAPK Pathway

Two groups have consistently reported that about 50% of HCC cases have genetic alterations in mTOR/PI3K pathway [75, 82]. They have noticed recurrent inactivating mutations in tuberous sclerosis 1 (*TSC1*) (3%) and *TSC2* (5%), activating mutations and copy again in *PIK3CA* (2%), and mutations in other modulators including *RPS6KA3* (7%), *PTEN* (3%), *DAPK1* (3%), *MTOR* (2%), etc. In MAPK pathway, a group of growth factors and their receptors have shown mutations in HCCs, including *FGF3* (4%), *FGF4* (5%), *FGF19* (19%), *HGF* (3%), *PDGFRs* (3%), *IGF1R* (2%), etc. Meanwhile, Lin et al. have also detected three cancer-related alternative splicing events including *FGFR2*, *ADAM15*, and abundance of *FGFR2-IIIc* (one of *FGFR2* isoform) that were associated with tumor recurrence [87]. Mutations of *IGFALS* and *JAK1* have also been found as key genetic determinants in HCC [88, 89].

Others

Fernandez-Banet et al. provided a comprehensive set of somatic genomic rearrangement and gene fusion predictions in HCCs by performing whole-genome sequencing with 88 pairs of primary HCC tumor and non-tumor tissues [90]. They predicted 4314 genomic rearrangements and 260 gene fusions that frequently result in aberrant overexpression of the 3′ genes in tumors. Further, 18 gene fusions, including recurrent fusion (2/88) of *ABCB11-LRP2*, were validated in HCCs. Xu et al. analyzed copy number variations using DNA sequencing in plasma samples from 31 HCC patients and 8 patients with chronic hepatitis or cirrhosis [91]. They found that copy number variations were recognizable in the majority of HCC plasma samples with large tumor size, and in few HCCs with small tumor size, but not in samples from chronic hepatitis/cirrhosis-related patients. Chen et al. sequenced the exomes of three pairs of HBV-HCC tumor and normal tissues and identified 59 original genes mutated in HBV-associated HCCs [92]. In combination with whole-genome sequencing data from the European Genome-phenome Archive database, 33 of these 59 genes were confirmed, and variants of two mutated genes, *ZNF717* and *PARP4*, were detected in more than 10% of samples from this database. In addition, high-proportion mutations of *LAMA2* (encoding an extracellular matrix protein), *BAP1*, and *IDH1* in HCCs have also been reported [81]. The sequencing in three HCCs and adjacent tissue pairs revealed five non-synonymously mutational genes (*IRS1*, *HMGCS1*, *ATP8B1*, *PRMT6*, and *CLU*), which were associated with metabolic diseases diabetes and obesity [93].

4.3.3 Expression Profiles of HCC

Besides the genetic changes, whole transcriptome sequencing also reveals gene expression levels from mapped RNA-seq reads. Compared to microarray, RNA sequencing could identify low copy and novel transcripts and is affected at a minimum level by probe efficacy and hybridization condition. Murakami et al. have performed both small RNA sequencing and microarray in 11 HCCs and found that microRNA profiling from sequencing is comparable and reproducible to that from microarray. Moreover, RNA sequencing discovered novel microRNAs (such as miR-9985 and miR-1843) that were otherwise undetectable by array [94]. Wojcicka et al. performed microRNA transcriptome sequencing on total RNAs from 24 paired HCC tumors and adjacent non-tumor tissues [95]. Among all 374 detected microRNAs, miR-122-5p was the most abundant, 64 miRNAs were differentially expressed, and almost every microRNA generated isomiRNAs. Among the most deregulated miRNAs, miR-199a-3p/miR-199b-3p was significantly downregulated in HCCs compared to adjacent non-tumor tissues, expressed in nine isoforms with three different seeds, dramatically activated TGF-β signaling pathway [95].

We have also performed small RNA deep sequencing using isolated EpCAM+ cancer cells with stem cell features and EpCAM− cancer cells with mature hepatocyte features, as well as EpCAM+ normal hepatic stem cells and EpCAM− hepatocytes from health liver donors [39]. Through the comprehensive comparison, we have discovered a group of microRNAs with a specific altered level in purified EpCAM+ hepatic cancer stem cells but not in other cells. The expression of miR-155 in EpCAM+ hepatic cancer stem cells was further validated, and the putative miR-155 targets were correlated with overall survival or time to recurrence [39]. Other groups have revealed the upregulation of a new PIWI-interacting RNA (piR-Hep1) via small RNA deep sequencing using RNAs from an immortalized hepatocyte and two HCC cell lines [96]. The functional study has also discovered that piR-Hep1 was involved in the regulation of HCC cell viability, proliferation, and invasiveness. Selitsky et al. performed small RNA sequencing on liver samples from advanced hepatitis B or C and HCC patients [97]. Compared to microRNAs, small RNAs derived from tRNAs, specifically 5′ tRNA-halves (5′ tRHs), were more abundant in nonmalignant liver. However, 5′ tRH abundance was reduced in matched cancer tissue.

As the development and progression of HCC is a multistage process, Thorgeirsson's group has performed sequential transcriptome analysis with liver samples in various HCC stages [89]. These samples include tumor-free surrounding liver ($n = 7$), low ($n = 4$)- and high ($n = 9$)-grade dysplastic lesions, early HCCs ($n = 5$), and progressed HCC ($n = 3$) from a total of eight HBV-HCC patients. They further integrated genetic and transcriptomic changes during hepatic carcinogenesis to characterize the genomic alteration. In their study, transcriptomes changes of early lesions (from low-grade dysplastic lesion to early HCC) were modest and homogenous. Extensive genetic and transcriptomic alterations occurred at late stage during hepatic carcinogenesis. The deregulated pathways were centered on TGF-beta, WNT, NOTCH, MYC, and EMT-related genes highlighting HCC molecular diversity. Meanwhile, other researchers reported that Aurora B signaling, Wnt pathways, and FOXM1 transcription factor network were altered in HCC via transcriptome sequencing [93]. In addition, two groups have performed transcriptome sequencing on RNAs obtained from rats with or without Aflatoxin B1 (a potent HCC carcinogen) treatment. A group of known and novel transcripts were identified to be differentially expressed under Aflatoxin B1 stress [98, 99].

4.3.4 Epigenetic Alterations in HCC

It has been shown that HCC has large panels of genes with aberrant DNA methylation. Whole-genome bisulfite sequencing could provide a comprehensive view of methylation patterns at single-base resolution across the genome. Chan et al. first explored the detection of genome-wide methylation in plasma from HCC patients using shotgun bisulfite sequencing [100]. Plasma DNAs from 26 HCC patients and 32 non-tumor control subjects were submitted to bisulfite conversion and then massively parallel sequencing. Meanwhile, available tumor DNAs and buffy coat DNAs from 15 HCC cases were also subjected to massively parallel bisulfite sequencing. Analysis of sequencing data revealed hypomethylation was pervasive across the genome. The hypomethylation pattern has high sensitivity and specificity for HCC diagnosis. They further applied the same analysis using copy number variation.

However, the diagnostic role of tumor-associated copy number variation is much more dependent on the depth of sequencing. Meanwhile, Shen et al. performed targeted bisulfite sequencing with 24 pairs of HCC tumor and adjacent non-tumor tissues, to investigate associations of DNA methylation and mRNA expression in HCC [101]. In this study, they reported that downregulation of *GRASP* and *TSPYL5* in HCC were regulated by DNA hypermethylation.

4.3.5 Potential Clinical Utilization in HCC

Inter- and intra-tumor heterogeneity has been observed in HCC tumors from both array-based technology and NGS-based technology. Thus HCC patient stratification is important for the introduction of precision medicine for clinical cancer care. Large-scale NGS mutational screening approaches have revealed some key driving signaling pathways in HCC based on the most frequent mutation profiles. Since these, HCC might be subjected to different subgroups based on their genetic alterations in TP53 pathway, WNT pathway, chromatin-remodeling regulation, PI3K/mTOR signaling, MAPK pathway, etc. [75, 82, 89]. For patients who have distinct genetic profiles, different treatment might be required for the best care. It is expected that patient survival will be largely improved with molecular-targeted therapies directed against these pathways. Encouraging data have been shown in a small-scale study. Two HCC patients at advanced stage had genetic alteration in PI3K/AKT/mTOR pathway being identified via targeted NGS and benefited from the treatment of an mTOR inhibitor, everolimus [102]. Schulze et al. reported that 28% of HCC patients harbored at least one damaging genetic alteration potentially targetable by one FDA-approved drug [82]. Meanwhile, some genetic alterations might be potentially related to the drug sensitivity in HCC cells such as *NQO1* mutation increasing the sensitivity of HCC cell growth inhibition with HSP90 inhibitor treatment.

In addition, Kelley et al. performed Personal Genome Machine sequencing using DNAs from circulating HCC cells and showed that analysis of genomic interrogation of circulating tumor cells could provide precise information for stratifying patients with metastatic HCC [103]. Ouyang et al. performed whole-genome sequencing with primary HCC and paired lung metastases samples and identified very similar genomic variations including genetic mutations and copy number alterations between primary and metastatic pairs [104]. These indicate the possibility of using the genomic variations to identify the primary tumor site for patients having cancer in multiorgans.

4.4   Conclusion and Prospective

NGS analysis for identifying genetic profiles in human malignancies has become a research priority. It has enabled the identification of new cancer drivers in several solid tumors including lung and melanoma. Molecular-targeted cancer therapies against genetic alterations in oncogenic genes have prolonged patient survival, such as vemurafenib treatment in BRAF-mutated melanoma [105, 106], crizotinib in lung cancer with ALK rearrangements [107]. Unfortunately, the molecular-based HCC treatment stratification has not been fulfilled reached for HCC. Now, sorafenib is the only FDA-approved molecular drug in HCC and could only moderately improve survival of patients with advanced HCC [108]. It might be valuable to test whether HCC patients with genetic alterations in PI3K and MAPK signaling could gain significant survival benefit from sorafenib instead of nonselected HCC populations.

A group of NGS data have shown HCC heterogeneity and identified several possible drivers that might be useful for sub-classifying HCC populations. However, such subgrouping should be further confirmed through basic and clinical investigation. Meanwhile, therapies targeting the most prevalent genetic alterations including *TERT*, *CTNNB1*, and *TP53* in HCC have not been clinically applied. It is also necessary to discover new therapeutic targets that come from genomic studies assessing chromosomal amplifications or deletions. Overall, HCC NGS studies have improved our understanding on HCC biological features and would eventually contribute to the treatment selection for heterogeneous HCC populations. Further efforts are needed to investigate the application the genomic information in patient decision-making and the utilization of molecular-targeted therapies against genetic alternations in some key signaling pathways.

References

1. Farazi PA, DePinho RA. Hepatocellular carcinoma pathogenesis: from genes to environment. Nat Rev Cancer. 2006;6:674–87.
2. Thorgeirsson SS, Grisham JW. Molecular pathogenesis of human hepatocellular carcinoma. Nat Genet. 2002;31:339–46.
3. Llovet JM, et al. Hepatocellular carcinoma. Lancet. 2003;362:1907–17.
4. Lozano R, et al. Global and regional mortality from 235 causes of death for 20 age groups in 1990 and 2010: a systematic analysis for the Global Burden of Disease Study 2010. Lancet. 2012;380:2095–128.
5. El-Serag HB. Epidemiology of viral hepatitis and hepatocellular carcinoma. Gastroenterology. 2012;142:1264–73.e1.
6. Arzumanyan A, et al. Pathogenic mechanisms in HBV- and HCV-associated hepatocellular carcinoma. Nat Rev Cancer. 2013;13:123–35.
7. Pujol FH, et al. Worldwide genetic diversity of HBV genotypes and risk of hepatocellular carcinoma. Cancer Lett. 2009;286:80–8.
8. Forner A, et al. Hepatocellular carcinoma. Lancet. 2012;379:1245–55.
9. Levrero M. Viral hepatitis and liver cancer: the case of hepatitis C. Oncogene. 2006;25:3834–47.
10. Fattovich G, et al. Hepatocellular carcinoma in cirrhosis: incidence and risk factors. Gastroenterology. 2004;127:S35–50.
11. Romeo R, et al. High serum levels of HDV RNA are predictors of cirrhosis and liver cancer in patients with chronic hepatitis delta. PLoS One. 2014;9:e92062.
12. Boffetta P, Hashibe M. Alcohol and cancer. Lancet Oncol. 2006;7:149–56.
13. El-Serag HB. Hepatocellular carcinoma. N Engl J Med. 2011;365:1118–27.
14. Hartling L, et al. Association between alcohol consumption and cancers in the Chinese population—a systematic review and meta-analysis. PLoS One. 2011;6:e18776.
15. Baffy G, et al. Hepatocellular carcinoma in non-alcoholic fatty liver disease: an emerging menace. J Hepatol. 2012;56:1384–91.

16. Nobili V, et al. A 360-degree overview of paediatric NAFLD: recent insights. J Hepatol. 2013;58:1218–29.
17. Calle EE, et al. Overweight, obesity, and mortality from cancer in a prospectively studied cohort of US adults. N Engl J Med. 2003;348:1625–38.
18. Larsson S, Wolk A. Overweight, obesity and risk of liver cancer: a meta-analysis of cohort studies. Br J Cancer. 2007;97:1005–8.
19. Arase Y, et al. Effect of type 2 diabetes on risk for malignancies includes hepatocellular carcinoma in chronic hepatitis C. Hepatology. 2013;57:964–73.
20. Hsiang JC, et al. Type 2 diabetes: a risk factor for liver mortality and complications in hepatitis B cirrhosis patients. J Gastroenterol Hepatol. 2015;30:591–9.
21. Lai MS, et al. Type 2 diabetes and hepatocellular carcinoma: a cohort study in high prevalence area of hepatitis virus infection. Hepatology. 2006;43:1295–302.
22. Feitelson MA, et al. Genetic mechanisms of hepatocarcinogenesis. Oncogene. 2002;21:2593–604.
23. Nault JC, Zucman-Rossi J. Genetics of hepatocellular carcinoma: the next generation. J Hepatol. 2014;60:224–6.
24. Roncalli M, et al. Histopathological classification of hepatocellular carcinoma. Dig Liver Dis. 2010;42(Suppl 3):S228–34.
25. Severi T, et al. Tumor initiation and progression in hepatocellular carcinoma: risk factors, classification, and therapeutic targets. Acta Pharmacol Sin. 2010;31:1409–20.
26. Park JW, et al. Global patterns of hepatocellular carcinoma management from diagnosis to death: the BRIDGE Study. Liver Int. 2015;35:2155–66.
27. Villanueva A, et al. Hepatocellular carcinoma: novel molecular approaches for diagnosis, prognosis, and therapy. Annu Rev Med. 2010;61:317–28.
28. Bruix J, et al. Focus on hepatocellular carcinoma. Cancer Cell. 2004;5:215–9.
29. Yau T, et al. Development of Hong Kong Liver Cancer staging system with treatment stratification for patients with hepatocellular carcinoma. Gastroenterology. 2014;146:1691–700.e3.
30. Kudo M, et al. Prognostic staging system for hepatocellular carcinoma (CLIP score): its value and limitations, and a proposal for a new staging system, the Japan Integrated Staging Score (JIS score). J Gastroenterol. 2003;38:207–15.
31. Okuda K, et al. Natural history of hepatocellular carcinoma and prognosis in relation to treatment. Study of 850 patients. Cancer. 1985;56:918–28.
32. Forner A, et al. Treatment of intermediate-stage hepatocellular carcinoma. Nat Rev Clin Oncol. 2014;11:525–35.
33. Quetglas IM, et al. Integration of genomic information in the clinical management of HCC. Best Pract Res Clin Gastroenterol. 2014;28:831–42.
34. Budhu A, et al. Identification of metastasis-related microRNAs in hepatocellular carcinoma. Hepatology. 2008;47:897–907.
35. Budhu A, et al. Integrated metabolite and gene expression profiles identify lipid biomarkers associated with progression of hepatocellular carcinoma and patient outcomes. Gastroenterology. 2013;144:1066–75.e1.
36. Ji J, Wang XW. New kids on the block: diagnostic and prognostic microRNAs in hepatocellular carcinoma. Cancer Biol Ther. 2009;8:1686–93.
37. Ji J, et al. Identification of microRNA-181 by genome-wide screening as a critical player in EpCAM-positive hepatic cancer stem cells. Hepatology. 2009;50:472–80.
38. Ji J, et al. Let-7g targets collagen type I alpha2 and inhibits cell migration in hepatocellular carcinoma. J Hepatol. 2010;52:690–7.
39. Ji J, et al. Identification of microRNAs specific for epithelial cell adhesion molecule-positive tumor cells in hepatocellular carcinoma. Hepatology. 2015;62:829–40.
40. Kim JW, et al. Cancer-associated molecular signature in the tissue samples of patients with cirrhosis. Hepatology. 2004;39:518–27.
41. Lee JS, et al. Classification and prediction of survival in hepatocellular carcinoma by gene expression profiling. Hepatology. 2004;40:667–76.
42. Yamashita T, et al. EpCAM-positive hepatocellular carcinoma cells are tumor-initiating cells with stem/progenitor cell features. Gastroenterology. 2009;136:1012–24.

43. Ye QH, et al. Predicting hepatitis B virus-positive metastatic hepatocellular carcinomas using gene expression profiling and supervised machine learning. Nat Med. 2003;9:416–23.
44. Parpart S, et al. Modulation of miR-29 expression by alpha-fetoprotein is linked to the hepatocellular carcinoma epigenome. Hepatology. 2014;60:872–83.
45. Honda M, et al. Differential gene expression between chronic hepatitis B and C hepatic lesion. Gastroenterology. 2001;120:955–66.
46. Hashimoto K, et al. Analysis of DNA copy number aberrations in hepatitis C virus-associated hepatocellular carcinomas by conventional CGH and array CGH. Mod Pathol. 2004;17:617–22.
47. Huang J, et al. Correlation between genomic DNA copy number alterations and transcriptional expression in hepatitis B virus-associated hepatocellular carcinoma. FEBS Lett. 2006;580:3571–81.
48. Boyault S, et al. Transcriptome classification of HCC is related to gene alterations and to new therapeutic targets. Hepatology. 2007;45:42–52.
49. Zucman-Rossi J, et al. Genetic landscape and biomarkers of hepatocellular carcinoma. Gastroenterology. 2015;149:1226–39.e4.
50. Yamashita T, et al. EpCAM and alpha-fetoprotein expression defines novel prognostic subtypes of hepatocellular carcinoma. Cancer Res. 2008;68:1451–61.
51. Ji J, et al. MicroRNA expression, survival, and response to interferon in liver cancer. N Engl J Med. 2009;361:1437–47.
52. Ji J, et al. Development of a miR-26 companion diagnostic test for adjuvant interferon-alpha therapy in hepatocellular carcinoma. Int J Biol Sci. 2013;9:303–12.
53. Margulies M, et al. Genome sequencing in microfabricated high-density picolitre reactors. Nature. 2005;437:376–80.
54. Eid J, et al. Real-time DNA sequencing from single polymerase molecules. Science. 2009;323:133–8.
55. Metzker ML. Sequencing technologies—the next generation. Nat Rev Genet. 2010;11:31–46.
56. Rothberg JM, Leamon JH. The development and impact of 454 sequencing. Nat Biotechnol. 2008;26:1117–24.
57. Ronaghi M, et al. Real-time DNA sequencing using detection of pyrophosphate release. Anal Biochem. 1996;242:84–9.
58. Feng YJ, et al. Parallel tagged amplicon sequencing of relatively long PCR products using the Illumina HiSeq platform and transcriptome assembly. Mol Ecol Resour. 2016;16:91–102.
59. Jeon YS, et al. Improved pipeline for reducing erroneous identification by 16S rRNA sequences using the Illumina MiSeq platform. J Microbiol. 2015;53:60–9.
60. Morozova O, Marra MA. Applications of next-generation sequencing technologies in functional genomics. Genomics. 2008;92:255–64.
61. Cloonan N, et al. Stem cell transcriptome profiling via massive-scale mRNA sequencing. Nat Methods. 2008;5:613–9.
62. Valouev A, et al. A high-resolution, nucleosome position map of C. elegans reveals a lack of universal sequence-dictated positioning. Genome Res. 2008;18:1051–63.
63. Quail MA, et al. A tale of three next generation sequencing platforms: comparison of Ion Torrent, Pacific Biosciences and Illumina MiSeq sequencers. BMC Genomics. 2012;13:341.
64. Schadt EE, et al. A window into third-generation sequencing. Hum Mol Genet. 2010;19:R227–40.
65. Buermans HP, den Dunnen JT. Next generation sequencing technology: advances and applications. Biochim Biophys Acta. 2014;1842:1932–41.
66. Wheeler DA, et al. The complete genome of an individual by massively parallel DNA sequencing. Nature. 2008;452:872–6.
67. Meyerson M, et al. Advances in understanding cancer genomes through second-generation sequencing. Nat Rev Genet. 2010;11:685–96.
68. Shendure J, Ji H. Next-generation DNA sequencing. Nat Biotechnol. 2008;26:1135–45.
69. Brechot C, et al. Presence of integrated hepatitis B virus DNA sequences in cellular DNA of human hepatocellular carcinoma. Nature. 1980;286:533–5.

70. Fujimoto A, et al. Whole-genome sequencing of liver cancers identifies etiological influences on mutation patterns and recurrent mutations in chromatin regulators. Nat Genet. 2012;44:760–4.
71. Paterlini-Brechot P, et al. Hepatitis B virus-related insertional mutagenesis occurs frequently in human liver cancers and recurrently targets human telomerase gene. Oncogene. 2003;22:3911–6.
72. Sung WK, et al. Genome-wide survey of recurrent HBV integration in hepatocellular carcinoma. Nat Genet. 2012;44:765–9.
73. Toh ST, et al. Deep sequencing of the hepatitis B virus in hepatocellular carcinoma patients reveals enriched integration events, structural alterations and sequence variations. Carcinogenesis. 2013;34:787–98.
74. Li W, et al. HIVID: an efficient method to detect HBV integration using low coverage sequencing. Genomics. 2013;102:338–44.
75. Totoki Y, et al. Trans-ancestry mutational landscape of hepatocellular carcinoma genomes. Nat Genet. 2014;46:1267–73.
76. Pawlotsky JM. Hepatitis C virus population dynamics during infection. Curr Top Microbiol Immunol. 2006;299:261–84.
77. Park CW, et al. Comparison of quasispecies diversity of HCV between chronic hepatitis c and hepatocellular carcinoma by Ultradeep pyrosequencing. Biomed Res Int. 2014;2014:853076.
78. Miura M, et al. Deep-sequencing analysis of the association between the quasispecies nature of the hepatitis C virus core region and disease progression. J Virol. 2013;87:12541–51.
79. Jiang JH, et al. Clinical significance of the ubiquitin ligase UBE3C in hepatocellular carcinoma revealed by exome sequencing. Hepatology. 2014;59:2216–27.
80. Guichard C, et al. Integrated analysis of somatic mutations and focal copy-number changes identifies key genes and pathways in hepatocellular carcinoma. Nat Genet. 2012;44:694–8.
81. Jhunjhunwala S, et al. Diverse modes of genomic alteration in hepatocellular carcinoma. Genome Biol. 2014;15:436.
82. Schulze K, et al. Exome sequencing of hepatocellular carcinomas identifies new mutational signatures and potential therapeutic targets. Nat Genet. 2015;47:505–11.
83. Forbes SA, et al. COSMIC: mining complete cancer genomes in the Catalogue of Somatic Mutations in Cancer. Nucleic Acids Res. 2011;39:D945–50.
84. Forbes SA, et al. COSMIC (the Catalogue of Somatic Mutations in Cancer): a resource to investigate acquired mutations in human cancer. Nucleic Acids Res. 2010;38:D652–7.
85. Cleary SP, et al. Identification of driver genes in hepatocellular carcinoma by exome sequencing. Hepatology. 2013;58:1693–702.
86. Li M, et al. Inactivating mutations of the chromatin remodeling gene ARID2 in hepatocellular carcinoma. Nat Genet. 2011;43:828–9.
87. Lin KT, et al. Identification of latent biomarkers in hepatocellular carcinoma by ultra-deep whole-transcriptome sequencing. Oncogene. 2014;33:4786–94.
88. Kan Z, et al. Whole-genome sequencing identifies recurrent mutations in hepatocellular carcinoma. Genome Res. 2013;23:1422–33.
89. Marquardt JU, et al. Sequential transcriptome analysis of human liver cancer indicates late stage acquisition of malignant traits. J Hepatol. 2014;60:346–53.
90. Fernandez-Banet J, et al. Decoding complex patterns of genomic rearrangement in hepatocellular carcinoma. Genomics. 2014;103:189–203.
91. Xu H, et al. Non-invasive analysis of genomic copy number variation in patients with hepatocellular carcinoma by next generation DNA sequencing. J Cancer. 2015;6:247–53.
92. Chen Y, et al. Exome capture sequencing reveals new insights into hepatitis B virus-induced hepatocellular carcinoma at the early stage of tumorigenesis. Oncol Rep. 2013;30:1906–12.
93. Meerzaman DM, et al. Genome-wide transcriptional sequencing identifies novel mutations in metabolic genes in human hepatocellular carcinoma. Cancer Genomics Proteomics. 2014;11:1–12.
94. Murakami Y, et al. Comparison of hepatocellular carcinoma miRNA expression profiling as evaluated by next generation sequencing and microarray. PLoS One. 2014;9:e106314.

95. Wojcicka A, et al. Next generation sequencing reveals microRNA isoforms in liver cirrhosis and hepatocellular carcinoma. Int J Biochem Cell Biol. 2014;53:208–17.
96. Law PT, et al. Deep sequencing of small RNA transcriptome reveals novel non-coding RNAs in hepatocellular carcinoma. J Hepatol. 2013;58:1165–73.
97. Selitsky SR, et al. Small tRNA-derived RNAs are increased and more abundant than microRNAs in chronic hepatitis B and C. Sci Rep. 2015;5:7675.
98. Merrick BA, et al. RNA-Seq profiling reveals novel hepatic gene expression pattern in aflatoxin B1 treated rats. PLoS One. 2013;8:e61768.
99. Yang W, et al. Genome-wide miRNA-profiling of aflatoxin B1-induced hepatic injury using deep sequencing. Toxicol Lett. 2014;226:140–9.
100. Chan KC, et al. Noninvasive detection of cancer-associated genome-wide hypomethylation and copy number aberrations by plasma DNA bisulfite sequencing. Proc Natl Acad Sci U S A. 2013;110:18761–8.
101. Shen J, et al. Integrative epigenomic and genomic filtering for methylation markers in hepatocellular carcinomas. BMC Med Genet. 2015;8:28.
102. Janku F, et al. Identification of novel therapeutic targets in the PI3K/AKT/mTOR pathway in hepatocellular carcinoma using targeted next generation sequencing. Oncotarget. 2014;5:3012–22.
103. Kelley RK, et al. Circulating tumor cells in hepatocellular carcinoma: a pilot study of detection, enumeration, and next-generation sequencing in cases and controls. BMC Cancer. 2015;15:206.
104. Ouyang L, et al. Whole-genome sequencing of matched primary and metastatic hepatocellular carcinomas. BMC Med Genet. 2014;7:2.
105. Chapman PB, et al. Improved survival with vemurafenib in melanoma with BRAF V600E mutation. N Engl J Med. 2011;364:2507–16.
106. Chapman PB, et al. Frontline approach to metastatic BRAF-mutant melanoma diagnosis, molecular evaluation, and treatment choice. Am Soc Clin Oncol Educ Book. 2014;34:e412–21.
107. Kwak EL, et al. Anaplastic lymphoma kinase inhibition in non-small-cell lung cancer. N Engl J Med. 2010;363:1693–703.
108. Llovet JM, et al. Sorafenib in advanced hepatocellular carcinoma. N Engl J Med. 2008;359:378–90.
109. Totoki Y, et al. High-resolution characterization of a hepatocellular carcinoma genome. Nat Genet. 2011;43:464–9.
110. Ding D, et al. Recurrent targeted genes of hepatitis B virus in the liver cancer genomes identified by a next-generation sequencing-based approach. PLoS Genet. 2012;8:e1003065.
111. Huang J, et al. Exome sequencing of hepatitis B virus-associated hepatocellular carcinoma. Nat Genet. 2012;44:1117–21.

Epigenetic Regulations in the Pathogenesis of HCC and the Clinical Application

5

Williams Puszyk, Keith Robertson, and Chen Liu

5.1 Introduction

Hepatocellular carcinoma (HCC) arises from hepatocytes, which constitute 70–80% of all liver cells, and is the most frequent liver malignancy, causing more than 80% of liver cancer cases globally. HCC is rarely associated with the inheritance of familial genetic mutations [73, 135]; this explains in part why pediatric HCC cases are so rare. In fact most HCC cases are diagnosed later in life and are caused by prolonged exposure to environmental factors known to damage the liver progressively over time. Two of the major risk factors associated with the development of HCC include chronic infection with hepatitis B virus (HBV) and chronic infection with hepatitis C virus (HCV); these viruses are detectable in approximately 80% of all HCC cases [113, 128, 138]. Another contributing factor driving the development of viral HCC is the accidental consumption of aflatoxin B_1 (AFB_1). The toxin is found in contaminated food stores containing *Aspergillus* fungal species. Heavy chronic cigarette smoking has also recently emerged as a contributory factor [21]. Apart from the hepatitis viruses, the other major independent risk factor for the development of HCC is chronic over consumption of alcohol [37, 95]. Another emerging risk factor is overnutrition. Consumption of excess calories routinely can lead to nonalcoholic fatty liver disease (NAFLD). NAFLD can progress to nonalcoholic steatohepatitis

W. Puszyk, Ph.D. (✉)
Department of Pathology, Immunology, and Laboratory Medicine, University of Florida, Gainesville, FL 32611, USA
e-mail: william_p100@hotmail.com

K. Robertson, Ph.D.
Department of Molecular Pharmacology and Experimental Therapeutics, Mayo Clinic Comprehensive Cancer Center, Mayo Clinic, Rochester, MN 85259, USA

C. Liu, M.D., Ph.D.
Department of Pathology and Laboratory Medicine, New Jersey Medical School, Rutgers, The State University of New Jersey, Newark, NJ 07103, USA
e-mail: Chen.liu@rutgers.edu

© Springer International Publishing AG 2018
C. Liu (ed.), *Precision Molecular Pathology of Liver Cancer*,
Molecular Pathology Library, https://doi.org/10.1007/978-3-319-68082-8_5

(NASH) which may then further develop into HCC. HCC caused by overnutrition is also linked to obesity and diabetes [125].

These environmental risk factors cause both genetic and epigenetic changes that have been shown to drive the progression of liver disease, leading to the development of HCC [103]. HCC is often identified by biopsy followed by the application of traditional immunohistochemical staining. Immunological markers can be informative and provide additional diagnostic features to traditional histological staining techniques. However, biopsies for liver cancer are often only obtained after the patient has presented with late stage disease. Over the past few decades, the fields of molecular genetics and epigenetics have emerged as an area of intense clinical translational research. Due to the complex nature and a lack of key-shared genetic mutations in HCC, the development of epigenetic molecular biomarkers may prove useful in the detection and characterization of HCC [62, 127, 154].

5.2 Epigenetics

In normal healthy cells, epigenetic pathways function to allow cells to follow programs of development and differentiation; when the epigenetic signature or profile of a cell becomes corrupted, this may lead to a loss of cell identity and function. This may eventually lead to the development of tumor cells. There are many different epigenetic mechanisms that enable the coordinate gene expression of healthy cells; these mechanisms may act independently or synergistically to maintain healthy cellular activity. In cancer cells epigenetic changes may initiate and drive tumor progression, by altering normal cellular gene expression without causing changes to the DNA sequence [103]. Epigenetic regulation occurs at the transcriptional, posttranscriptional, and posttranslational levels. Epigenetic mechanisms include DNA methylation, micro RNA (miR) expression, posttranslational modification of histone proteins, and structural chromatin changes [6, 48, 53, 78, 82, 144, 145, 152].

5.2.1 DNA Methylation

DNA methylation occurs predominantly in the mammalian genomes at CpG sites [32]. CpG sites are regions of DNA where a cytosine nucleotide is followed by a guanine nucleotide in the linear sequence of bases, that is to say that cytosine and guanine are separated by only one phosphate group on the same strand of DNA [32]. In this conformation the cytosine is capable of receiving a methyl group conferred by enzymes known as DNA methyl-transferase family, which is a family of enzymes that are able to regulate gene transcription by the addition of methyl groups at CpG sites located throughout the genome. The average frequency of occurrence of CpG sites across the human genome is approximately 1 in every 100 nucleotides; however, many genes have regions which are CpG enriched; these are known as CpG islands (CGIs) [4]. CpGs may occur as frequently as one in every ten nucleotides in CGIs. CGIs are predominantly located upstream of coding genes in a region that is termed the gene promoter. Many commonly transcribed genes including housekeeping genes have a CGI in the promoter [74]. Most transcriptionally active genes are relatively unmethylated at the gene promoter and methylated in transcribed gene body; therefore, the transcriptional effects conferred by DNA methylation are greatly dependent on the relative position of the methylated DNA [86].

DNA methylation changes that are known to occur in the development of liver cancer include hypermethylation of gene promoters and global hypomethylation of genomic DNA. While cumulative DNA methylation of gene promoters has been associated with loss of function of tumor suppressor genes in HCC, global DNA hypomethylation has been associated with genome instability and chromosomal rearrangement [18, 56]. This chapter will explore the role of DNA methylation changes in the development of HCC and also discuss the utility of DNA methylation biomarkers for the development of HCC diagnosis toward the goal of better personalized medicine.

5.2.2 Micro RNAs

Recently another epigenetic mechanism involving the transcription of short RNA molecules known as micro RNAs (miRs) has been identified. miRs are typically 21–23 nucleotides in length and have the capability to modify gene expression at the posttranscriptional level by binding to the 3′ untranslated region of target messenger RNA, preventing the translation of target mRNAs [52, 59]. Micro RNAs may be found within coding genes (intronic miRNAs) and act in cis to downregulate the coding gene they are located within. Micro RNAs may also be found either upstream of genes around enhancer sites or even gene deserts and may be trans-acting in their targeting of mRNAs [5, 14, 35, 102]. miRs are also highly evolutionarily conserved among species and relatively well conserved compared to other noncoding RNAs; this high level of evolutionary conservation indicates the importance of miRs in the epigenetic regulation of genes at the posttranslational level [139]. Micro RNAs may exert their effects by several alternative degradation pathways including; the cleavage of mRNA targets into two strands, the destabilization of mRNA through the shortening of the poly A tail, and the less efficient translation of the mRNA into proteins by ribosomes [9, 42]. Altered miR expression has been associated with metabolic and phenotypic changes in HCC. Alterations in miR expression have been shown to be tumor-specific, indicating the potential for the development of biomarkers based on miR expression profiles and the expression profile of miR target genes [16, 96, 114]. Aberrant miR expression has been linked to the repression of tumor suppressor genes and may also contribute to the overexpression of proto-oncogenes in HCC [88, 148, 156]. In this chapter we aim to discuss the role of miRs that are most frequently altered in HCC and represent significant putative biomarkers of HCC; we will also discuss how miR expression may also be used to indicate tumor stage and aggression.

5.2.3 Histone Modifications and Histone Variants

Histones are alkaline proteins which function to package and order genomic DNA into structures known as nucleosomes. Histones exist as dimers, with four dimer subunits coming together to form an octameric histone core. 147 bp of DNA wraps around each core approximately 1.65 times [87, 91]. The histone family is made up of a linker histone H1 and the core histones H2A, H2B, H3, and H4. Each family has several variants that may constitute part of the nucleosomal structure; these variants are also associated with altered transcriptional activity [111, 157]. The study of histone modifications has emerged as an area on intense scientific investigation in cancer research. Histone proteins can be modified at the N terminal tails, which protrude from the histone core and serve to act as binding sites for histone modification proteins. Histone modifiers may then confer chemical marks to the histone tails; these marks or histone modifications act as signals to recruit proteins that alter the structure of chromatin. These modification signals may act to recruit proteins that can then go on to open the chromatin into an accessible conformation (euchromatin). Chromatin modification signals may also act as repressive markers for the recruitment of chromatin modifiers which alter chromatin structure into a non-accessible conformation (heterochromatin). Histone modifications include methylation, acetylation, sumoylation, and ubiquitination. Amino acids frequently modified on the histone tails include lysine, arginine, serine, threonine, and glutamate. Histone modification nomenclature is summarized concisely in [130]. It is known that aberrant alterations to histone modifications and chromatin structure are associated with HCC, and histone-modifying proteins are druggable targets for the treatment of HCC [22, 26, 158]. Semiquantitative detection of histone modifications by immunohistochemistry may provide additional clinical information regarding the identification and stratification of diseased tissues, and some studies have shown the utility of this approach [54, 99]. Immunostaining for histone modifications and variants may potentially improve the diagnosis of HCC over currently available immunohistochemical approaches. However, due to the paucity of studies in this area of research, the utility of immunostaining of histones for the detection of HCC has yet to be verified. In this chapter we will not discuss histone modifications further as the molecular approaches for the identification of histone modifications remain technically challenging; this is due to the relatively larger amounts of tissue samples required compared with RNA and DNA techniques. Many archived tissue collections or biobanks maintained for clinical purposes store tissue as "formalin-fixed paraffin-embedded tissue" (ffpe). This is the standard method employed to preserve tissue samples in many pathology departments, this method enables samples to be stored for many years. Molecular markers based on DNA methylation and miRs also have a greater potential to be developed using ffpe tissue samples, as DNA and RNA can be extracted even from relatively small amounts obtained from just a few recut slides [93, 155]. DNA methylation markers and miR markers also have the possibility to be developed into minimally invasive diagnostic tests, using patient sera [38, 39]. Therefore the overall aim of this chapter is to summarize the current knowledge regarding the alterations to DNA methylation and aberrant miR expression in HCC and to comment on the future direction of these approaches for improving patient care through personalized medicine.

5.3   Hepatitis B Virus-Associated Hepatocellular Carcinoma

Hepatitis B virus (HBV) is a member of the small enveloped DNA virus family known as hepadnaviruses; these viruses preferentially infect human hepatocytes inducing minimal cytotoxicity. The HBV genome is a double-stranded circular DNA structure and is approximately 3.2 kb in length and consists of four overlapping reading frames, coding for five mRNA transcripts [1, 25]. The smallest transcript is just 0.8 kb in length and encodes the HBx protein; this protein is essential for viral replication [1, 25]. The precise mechanism of HBV entry into hepatocytes has yet to be fully elucidated. However, it is known that upon entry the virus nucleocapsid disintegrates and releases a relaxed form of viral circular DNA into the cytoplasm. The DNA is then quickly transported into the host cell nucleus and converted into a more rigid covalently closed circular DNA structure. Chronic infection with HBV is a major risk factor for the development of HCC. Currently there are more than 350 million individuals living with chronic HBV infection globally. Chronic HBV infection accounts for around 55% of HCC incidence, with increased prevalence in China and sub-Saharan Africa [116]. As a double-stranded DNA virus, HBV is able to integrate into the human genome. One of the proposed mechanisms by which HBV promotes disease progression to HCC is by integration into the host genome. Multiple integration sites have been identified. It is also possible for one or more copies to cocurrently infect each host cell. However, there is little evidence to suggest that HBV integration drives HCC by inserting into preferential sites to alter expression of specific genes. HBV integration is a stochastic process of random insertion, and the most likely contribution of these random insertions toward the development of HCC is the production of mutated HBx proteins that retain the ability to block P53 activity [138].

So far, tissue testing of HCC has revealed that the majority of HCC cases do not have a distinctive set of coding gene mutations that can account for all of the cases. P53 is the most frequently occurring coding mutation, with mutations of P53 detected in over 60% of cases (dependent on the cohort). The next most frequent coding gene mutation is beta-catenin, occurring in 20–40% cases [117, 134, 136]. During the development of HBV-related HCC, many epigenetic changes in DNA methylation have been observed. Both genome-wide DNA hypomethylation and promoter-specific DNA hypermethylation have been shown to occur. HBV-related HCC is characterized as a CpG island methylator phenotype positive (CIMP+) tumor type [140]. CIMP+ cancers progress by a process of cumulative hypermethylation of DNA at gene promoters, where both the number of methylated CpGs and methylated gene promoters increase over time [78, 82, 144, 145].

In cases of HBV-related HCC, the HBx protein induces increased expression of two proteins known to regulate the methylation of DNA. The HBx protein induces the expression of both DNA methyltransferase 1 (DNMT1) and DNA methyltransferase 3a (DNMT3a) [81]. DNMT1 is required for methylation of hemi-methylated DNA, acting as the maintenance methyltransferase, maintaining methylation levels during DNA replication. DNMT3a is a de novo methyltransferase conferring methylation marks to unmethylated DNA without the need for a hemi-methylated primer [65]. Studies have shown that the recruitment of these enzymes to specific gene promoters induces DNA methylation-mediated silencing [80, 112]. Perhaps counterintuitively HBx expression has also been shown to induce gene-specific DNA hypomethylation also. Recent studies have shown that HBx induces the expression of several genes by inducing DNA hypomethylation at the gene promoter [83]. The mechanism of this hypomethylation effect is unknown. However, it has been proposed that the effect may be caused by sequestration HBx binding to the promoter of DNMT3a [75]. Genes frequently aberrantly methylated in HBV-related HCC include GSTP1, XAF1, CAV1, APC, RASSF1A, SOCS1, p16, and COX2. GSTP1 downregulation exposes cells to oxidation damage by inhibiting the glutathione-mediated removal of endogenous and exogenous electrophiles. Notably both COX2 and p16 showed correlation between tumor progression and hypermethylation incidence. Loss of p16 function directly influences the p53 degradation pathway, and COX2 loss promotes a more pro-inflammatory state [132]. COX2 and p16 could be utilized and developed into epigenetic biomarker assays of HBV-related HCC; these assays may be informative of HCC recurrence risk when used to analyze biopsied tissue or patient sera. (See Table 5.1.)

Although HBV is a DNA virus, it may be targeted by host cell micro RNAs. HBV may also target transcripts in the host and alter normal host gene expression in order to promote viral replication. miRs overexpressed at different stages of liver disease induced by HBV have the potential to be utilized as markers of liver disease progression. Altered miR expression profiles may be useful for the stratification of HCC in order to determine aggression and risk of recurrence. miRs under expressed at different stages of liver disease may also be useful in treating HBV-HCC, as replacing these miRs may reduce the stability of viral products or inhibit viral replication.

miR-602 is upregulated in hepatitis, indicating an early role for miR-602 expression in liver disease; miR-602 downregulates RASSF1A gene, a gene known to be

Table 5.1 HBV-related HCC methylation markers

Gene	Gene function	Methylation	Effect
APC	Tumor suppressor protein antagonist of the WNT pathway	Hypermethylated in cirrhotic and HCC cases	WNT activation
RASSF1A	Tumor suppressor, inhibits accumulation of cyclin D and induces cell cycle arrest	Hypermethylated in cirrhotic and HCC cases	Loss of cell cycle inhibition
SOCS1	STAT-induced STAT inhibitor, suppresses cytokine signaling	Hypermethylated in cirrhotic and HCC cases	STAT activation
p16	Inhibitors of CDK4 Kinase, stabilizes P53 and sequesters MDM2. Highly important regulator of cell cycle	Hypermethylated in early and late HCC	Loss of cell cycle regulation, loss of tumor suppression of P53
COX2	Key enzyme in prostaglandin synthesis required in inflammation and mitogenesis	Hypermethylated in high-grade dysplasia and early and late HCC	Inhibition of AKT pathway

Table 5.2 HBV-related HCC miR markers

miR accession number	Gene target	miRNA expression	miRNA function
miR-199a5p	CHC	Upregulated	Promotes cell proliferation
miR-21	PDCD4	Upregulated	Promotes anti-apoptotic pathways
miR-29a	PTEN/PI3K/ Akt/MMP-2	Upregulated	Enhances cell migration
Let-7	STAT3	Upregulated	Enhances angiogenesis, cell proliferation and migration
miR-122	CCNG1	Downregulated	Promotes cell cycle progression
miR-145	MAP3K/CUL5	Downregulated	Enhances cell proliferation, promotes cell cycle progression and anti-apoptotic pathways
miR-222D	p27	Downregulated	Inhibition of cell cycle progression
miR-429	Rab18	Downregulated	Promoting dysregulation of lipogenesis and cell proliferation
miR-661	MTA1/NK-kB/ iNOS/NO	Downregulated	Enhances angiogenesis, cell proliferation and migration

frequently downregulated in cancer. RASSF1A has been classified as an important tumor suppressor gene, reduced expression or loss of expression appears to be an early stage hit in the development of HBV-related HCC. However, the expression of miR-602 is also consistently maintained in cirrhosis and HCC; therefore, it could not be used as a marker to distinguish between liver disease and cancer. In the cirrhotic liver, both miR-145 and miR-199 are frequently downregulated. In vitro studies restoring miR-145 in HepG2 cells indicate a tumor suppressor role for miR-145, and HepG2 cells treated to restore miR-145 showed inhibited cell proliferation and reduced invasion and migration [45]. Other changes in miR expression in HBV-related liver disease include the upregulation of miR-10B, miR-21, miR-224, miR-221, and miR34a; these increases in expression continue to persist through to HCC and may be used as biomarkers to monitor liver disease progression in HBV patients [70]. Expression of miR-96 in HBV patient serum has been observed; an assay for miR-96 could be an ideal marker for monitoring tumor progression in patients with chronic HBV infection [22, 26]. The HBx protein interacts with a number of miRs and affects a broad spectrum of pathways which act synergistically to promote HCC [153]. (See Table 5.2 for the list of miRs affected by HBV.) However, the expression of any given miR may also be further complicated by single nucleotide polymorphisms, which alter miR targets; therefore, assays developed must include a component of sequence information for the best results [69].

5.4   Hepatits C Virus-Associated Hepatocellular Carcinoma

The hepatitis C virus (HCV) is an enveloped positive-strand RNA virus, classified within the hepatic virus genus in the Flaviviridae family [29]. The viral genome encodes several proteins including structural proteins (Core, E21, E2, and P7) and nonstructural proteins (NS3 NS4A, NS4B, NS5A, and NS5B) [94]. Globally there are approximately 130 million people infected with HCV with around 80% of infected individuals progressing to develop persistent infection. Chronic HCV infection is a major risk factor for the development of hepatitis, liver cirrhosis, and hepatocellular carcinoma [119]. Despite the common pathophysiological aspects of hepatitis, fibrosis followed by cirrhosis, leading to the development of hepatocellular carcinoma, differences between HBV-related and HCV-related disease have become apparent [60]. HCV viral entry occurs when HCV particles present in the blood stream come into contact with hepatocytes after crossing the fenestrated endothelium of the liver sinusoids. This allows HCV particles and cell surface markers on hepatocytes to interact; although the precise mechanism for initial contact has yet to be fully elucidated, the LDL and ApoE receptors have been proposed to play a role in initiation of viral entry [34, 63]. Initial attachment of HCV particles onto the surface hepatocytes is mediated by several cell surface receptors including heparan sulfate proteoglycan, syndecan-1, syndecan-4, CD81, CLDN1, OCLN, and the scavenger receptor B1 (SRB1) [40, 76, 115, 120]. SRB1's role in HCV viral entry was first proposed when it was discovered that SRB1 binds to the HCV protein E2; the E2 protein contains a hyper variable region (HVR1) which is essential for binding to SRB1 [115]. However, this role in initiation has been contested since SRB1 is also able to bind to HCV-associated lipoproteins [34, 90]. An alternative interaction has also been proposed whereby SRB1 binding reveals the CD81 binding site, allowing E2 to bind to CD81. This interaction has been proposed as the mode of HCV viral entry, in studies using mutant HCV viruses where the HVR1 is deleted [8, 33, 49]. CD81 is another potential HCV entry factor. CD81 is a tetraspanin family member, which binds to the core amino acids in the HCV protein E2; this interaction primes the HCV envelope for low-pH-dependent fusion [118]. CD81 has also been associated with CLAUDIN (CLDN), which may act as a co-complex receptor to facilitate the internalization of the HCV particle [84]. In addition to CLDN, OCCLUDIN (OCLN) is another essential HCV entry factor [108]. The role of OCLN is poorly understood, and the evidence suggests that OCLN plays a role in the late stage of viral entry [11].

The HCV genome contains a single open reading frame encoding for all of the transcripts necessary for viral translation and replication. The 5′ non-translated region contains an internal ribosomal entry site (IRES) that initiates HCV translation into a polyprotein [85]. After initial translation HCV induces intracellular membrane rearrangement to create a structure known as the membranous web [85]. HCV protein NS4B is proposed to act as the scaffold of the membranous web with NS5A performing structural remodeling to form double-membrane vesicles [50]. In this way HCV and HBV have very different effects on the hepatocytes as they alter normal cellular activity by interfering with different cellular pathways. HCV is proposed to induce hepatocarcinogenesis via host and viral protein interactions and to cause effects in pathways including inhibition of apoptosis, oncogene activation, and increased production of reactive oxygen species [124].

Both HBV and HCV infection alter genomic DNA methylation patterns of infected cells. HCV infection of hepatocytes is known to increase the expression of DNA methyltransferases (DNMTs). It has also been shown that knockdown of DNMTs can inhibit sub-genomic replication of HCV. Experimental studies have previously shown that by reducing the amount of the functional DNA methyltransferases, DNMT1 and DNMT3B, by short hairpin RNA-mediated knockdown, the sub-genomic replication of HCV was severely inhibited, as detected by either the measurement of the HCV proteins NS3 and NS5A or the signal generated from HCV constructs tagged with green fluorescent protein [24]. It was also shown that the known DNA methylation inhibitors 5-Aza-cytidine and 5′-Aza-dCytidine reduced HCV viral replication by inhibition of DNA methyltransferases. The specific DNA methyltransferases affected by HCV infection are DNMT1 and DNMT3b [12]. The precise mechanism by which HCV induces overexpression of DNMTs is unknown. Evidence suggests a role for the HCV core protein, as virus subspecies with different core protein genotypes have been shown to induce variable expression of DNMT1 and DNMT3b [12]. The overexpression of DNMTs induced by HCV drives aberrant genomic DNA methylation, which in turn drives disease progression. Important genes shown to be hypermethylated in HCV-related HCC include the WNT inhibitors SFRP2 and DKK1, with hypermethylation of both gene promoters observed in early stage disease [133]. The methylation index of SFRP shows a clear increase in DNA methylation between cirrhotic liver tissues and HCC tissues [133]. SFRP is an example of a highly desirable epigenetic biomarker which could be developed as a test to detect HCC; other epigenetic markers are shown in Table 5.3. These markers show the potential of using DNA methylation biomarkers to detect HCC in cases complicated by liver cirrhosis, which may often confound tests [133, 151]. This opens up the possibility of DNA methylation biomarkers for the detection of HCC biomarkers in biopsied tissue and in the future could lead to the development of minimally invasive biomarkers of HCC by the detection of aberrantly methylated DNA of tumor origin circulating in the peripheral blood [110].

Table 5.3 HCV-related HCC methylation markers

Gene	Gene function	Methylation	Effect
SFRP2	WNT inhibitor	Promoter hypermethylation	WNT activation
DKK1	WNT inhibitor	Promoter hypermethylation	WNT activation
SPINT2/HAI2	HGF inhibitor	Hypermethylation in cirrhosis and HCC	HGF activation
p14	Tumor suppressor gene	Cumulative promoter hypermethylation in cirrhosis and HCC	Enhances cell cycle progression and anti-apoptotic pathways
p15	Tumor suppressor gene	Cumulative promoter hypermethylation in cirrhosis and HCC	Enhances cell cycle progression and anti-apoptotic pathways
p73	Tumor suppressor gene	Cumulative promoter hypermethylation in cirrhosis and HCC	Enhances cell cycle progression and anti-apoptotic pathways
06MGMT	DNA mismatch repair	Cumulative promoter hypermethylation in cirrhosis and HCC	Increases the effects of ROS damage

HCV like HBV interacts with a number of host cell miRs and may selectively induce either upregulation or downregulation of specific miRs. Because HCV is a single-stranded RNA genome, it may also be targeted by host miRs [66, 67]. Several important miRs have been shown to effect the progression of the HCV life cycle [79]. miR 122 is the single most abundant micro RNA expressed in the liver, accounting for more than 70% of the miR species present in the liver [77], and promotes HCV accumulation and retention by binding to the 5′ UTR of the HCV genome; this interaction increases HCV genome stability and also increases HCV translation [66, 67, 101, 121]. miR-122 anneals to the 5′ end of the HCV virus via adjacent binding motifs. miR-122 also binds to the 3′ untranslated region of HCV, an action which normally leads to degradation of mRNA but appears to have an opposing or protective effect on HCV. Both 5′ and 3′ UTR binding of HCV by miR-122 promote virus accumulation; it is proposed that miR-122 binding creates an overhang thereby preventing viral genome detection by antiviral restriction enzymes [89].

miR-196 b is another micro RNA expressed in the liver, it functions to suppress the translation of BACH1 mRNA, a known transcriptional repressor of the anti-inflammatory protein HMOX1. Infection with HCV has been shown to downregulate miR-196 b expression and cause a decrease in HMOX1 expression as the activity of BACH1 is no longer inhibited, reducing anti-inflammatory responses in the liver [68, 105]. HCV infection has also been shown to downregulate the expression of miR-29. miR-29 downregulates the translation of TGFβ meaning that HCV infection increases the expression of TGFβ; the increase in TGFβ has been linked to enhanced production of collagen and extracellular matrix; both are markers of liver fibrosis; TGFβ also acts as a mitogen in cancer [7]. miRs 192, 215, and 491 have also been identified as minor modifiers of HCV, with the expression of each miR increasing HCV expression between 1.5- and 2-fold [61]. Let-7a is another micro RNA which also has two binding sites in the HCV genome. Let-7a has been shown to reduce HCV replication in cell culture studies and is able to bind to different HCV genotypes [28]. Micro RNAs known to be altered in HCV-related HCC are summarized in Table 5.4. The detection and quantification of these markers could

Table 5.4 HCV-related miR markers

miR accession number	Gene target	Upregulated or downregulated	Effect
miR-122	HCV binding motifs	Competitive downregulation	Enhances HCV stabilization and viral persistence
miR-196b	BACH1	Downregulated	Causes inflammatory response, promotes viral replication and persistence
miR-155	PTEN	Upregulated	Causes inflammatory response, promotes viral replication and persistence, enhances hepatocyte proliferation
miR-29	TGFB	Downregulated	Promotes fibrosis and mitogenesis
miR-192	HCV	Upregulated	Enhances HCV expression and viral persistence
miR-215	HCV	Upregulated	Enhances HCV expression and viral persistence
miR-491	HCV	Upregulated	Enhances HCV expression and viral persistence
Let-7a	HCV	Downregulated	Enhances HCV expression and viral persistence

form the basis of an assay for minimally invasive diagnostic tests. These markers could also enhance current immunohistochemical pathology practices for the detection and stratification of HCC.

5.5   Alcohol-Associated Hepatocellular Carcinoma

Heavy alcohol consumption is a known independent risk factor for the development of HCC. In the United States, state reporting on the incidence of youth alcohol abuse has shown that the percentage of youths (under the age of 18) who admitted to previously binge-drinking alcohol increased from an average of 34% (from 1993 to 1999) to an average of 49% (2001–2005). This trend of increasing alcohol abuse correlates with a predicted increase in liver cancer-related deaths, with liver cancer deaths (including HCC) expected to surpass breast, colorectal, and prostate cancer by 2030.

Following ingestion alcohol is absorbed through the stomach and duodenum and enters the hepatic circulation where it is metabolized. The metabolism of ethanol alcohol forms by-products including acetaldehyde and acetic acid; further metabolism of these by-products requires the reduction of NAD+ to NADH. Acetic acid produced by the metabolism of alcohol also increases the labile pool of acetyl-CoA, driving among other processes an increase in genome-wide histone acetylation. Alcohol causes damage to the liver by multiple pathways including glutathione (GSH) depletion and the generation of reactive oxygen species (ROS). These pathways also affect epigenetic mechanistic pathways. Excessive production of ROS acutely depletes GSH promoting the transsulfuration pathway utilizing available homocysteine to generate new GSH. This reduction in the availability of homocysteine greatly reduces the production of S-adenosylmethionine (SAM). SAM is a methyl donor for the reactions of the DNA methyltransferase family [150]. ROS may also demethylate DNA by the direction oxidation of guanine to form 8-OHdG. The presence of 8-OHdG has been shown alter DNA methylation by blocking DNA methyltransferase binding and preventing local cytosine methylation [141].

Until recently not many studies have been performed specifically on the methylation of alcohol-related HCC; this is due to the paucity of patients presenting with chronic alcohol abuse but without either HCV or HBV. Previous studies have suggested the possibility of unique DNA methylation profiles in different HCC subtypes, as would be indicated by their divergent etiologies [57, 72]. In 2011 Lambert and colleagues published a study demonstrating that different subtypes of HCC had overlapping epigenetic changes, with many of the same genes sharing similar epigenetic alternations independent of viral etiology or alcohol involvement [72]. However, the study also showed that some genes were uniquely altered depending on whether the HCC was virally or alcohol-induced; this was an important step as it showed that each subtype of HCC can be considered as a separate disease and may have different putative pharmacological targets. In this study MGMT was shown to be hypermethylated in some alcohol-related HCC cases compared with HBV and HCV cases [72]. In 2014 we performed a study of genome-wide DNA methylation on a large cohort of HCC cancer patients and compared them to normal healthy liver samples. The groups we analyzed included HCV-related HCC, HBV-related HCC, alcohol-related HCC, and cryptogenic HCC cases. We employed the infinium bead array to obtain methylation information on approximately 473,000 CpGs across the genome (excluding sex chromosomes). While HBV and HCV had very similar methylation profiles (with notable differences), we found that alcohol-related HCC had a much different methylation profile [58]. We analyzed a subset of CpGs which had a minimum 25% change in DNA methylation, indicating that the changes were highly stringent (between tumor and normal liver tissue). We found that in this subset of 18,257 stringent CpGs there was a fair amount of overlap in methylation changes between HCV-related HCC and alcohol-related HCC tissues; the two groups shared 5732 methylation changes. However, we also found that while HCV-related HCC had fewer unique changes (1245), alcohol-related HCC had more than 10 times the number of unique methylation changes (16,574). We also observed that while HCV-related HCC has a steady number of changes between cirrhotic, T1-T2, and T3-T4 groups that alcohol-related HCC had a massive increase of DNA hypomethylation in late stage cancer [58]. We also found that in alcohol-related HCC there was an enrichment of hypomethylation of genes involved in alcoholism, alcohol dependence, alcohol abuse, heroin abuse, and schizophrenia [58]. Subsequent studies have validated these findings and have further elucidated some of the genes involved which may prove to be useful biomarkers of alcohol-related HCC. In 2015 a small study involving eight patients who had chronically consumed alcohol for a minimum of 20 years was undertaken. The patients were identified to be free from viral infection (HBV, HCV, HIV, Cytomegalovirus, EBV), and tumor tissues were compared with distal healthy liver tissue for analysis of genome-wide DNA methylation and gene expression [131]. This study built on ideas previously established and showed that DNA methylation could alter gene expression based on whether the gene promoter or gene body was altered. The study identified six genes involved in the retinol metabolism pathway (ADH1a, ADH1b, ADH6, CYP3A43, CYP4A22, and RDH16) and one gene in the carbon cycle (SHMT1); these genes were hypermethylated at the gene promoter and repressed in tumor tissue. Several other genes were found to hypomethylated at the gene promoter and induced in tumor tissue (NOX4, SPINK1, TAT1, and ESM 1) (Table 5.5). These markers could be used as biomarkers to detect the presence of alcohol-related HCC and could also be further developed into therapeutic targets for the targeted treatment of alcohol-related HCC. These biomarkers may also help pathologists to stratify between alcohol-related HCC and cryptogenic HCC cases where there is no viral involvement.

Alcohol has also been shown to alter the micro RNA expression of many cell types and tissues [46, 100] (Table 5.6). Although there have been few clinical studies to show the effects of alcohol on micro RNA expression, there have been some murine

Table 5.5 Alcohol-related HCC methylation markers

Gene	Gene function	Methylation	Effect
MGMT	DNA repair	Promoter hypermethylation in HCC	Increased frequency of DNA lesions and toxic effects on DNA
ADH1a	Alcohol dehydrogenase catalyzes the oxidation of alcohols and aldehydes	Promoter hypermethylation in HCC	Promotes hepatocyte growth and differentiation and anti-apoptotic pathways, promotes damage by alcohol metabolites
ADH1b	Alcohol dehydrogenase catalyzes the oxidation of ethanol and retinol alcohols, hydroxysteroids, and lipid peroxidation products	Promoter hypermethylation in HCC	Promotes hepatocyte growth and differentiation and anti-apoptotic pathways, promotes damage by alcohol metabolites
ADH6	Alcohol dehydrogenase catalyzes the oxidation of ethanol and retinol alcohols, hydroxysteroids, and lipid peroxidation products	Promoter hypermethylation in HCC	Promotes hepatocyte growth and differentiation and anti-apoptotic pathways, promotes damage by alcohol metabolites
CYP3A43	Cytochrome P450 member, metabolizing drugs, synthesis of cholesterol, steroids, and lipids	Promoter hypermethylation in HCC	Promotes hepatocyte growth and differentiation and anti-apoptotic pathways, promotes damage by alcohol metabolites
CYP4A22	Cytochrome P450 member, metabolizing drugs, synthesis of cholesterol, steroids, and lipids	Promoter hypermethylation in HCC	Promotes hepatocyte growth and differentiation and anti-apoptotic pathways, promotes damage by alcohol metabolites
RDH16	Retinol dehydrogenase, catalyzing retinol, and aldehyde metabolism	Promoter hypermethylation in HCC	Promotes hepatocyte growth and differentiation and anti-apoptotic pathways, promotes damage by alcohol metabolites
SHMT1	Serine hydroxymethyltransferase, synthesizes methionine and thymidylate and purines	Promoter hypermethylation in HCC	Promotes genomic hypomethylation by reducing the labile methionine pool
NOX4	Oxygen sensor catalyzing the reduction of molecular oxygen to various reactive oxygen species	Promoter hypomethylation	Promotes DNA damage
SPINK1	Trypsin inhibitor, prevents premature trypsin-catalyzed activation of zymogens, inhibits nitric oxide production	Promoter hypomethylation	Promotes inflammation and hepatocyte damage
ESM1	Endothelial cell-specific molecule	Promoter hypomethylation	Promotes angiogenesis and hepatocyte growth

Table 5.6 Alcohol-related miR markers

miR accession number	Gene target	Upregulated or downregulated	Effect
miR-34B/C	Promotes activity of P53	SNP polymorphism may upregulated transcription by formation of a GATA box	Polymorphism associated with increased RR of HCC in chronic alcohol abusers

studies indicating the role miR-122 in the activation of HIF-1α. Mice were induced to hepatitis using diethyl-nitrosamine (DEN) and then provided either saline or an alcohol substitute. The study showed that alcohol feeding had the effect of reducing miR-122 expression and also increased the expression of stemness markers [3]. Apart from altered expression, another mechanism by which micro RNAs may affect cancer development is through single nucleotide polymorphisms which prevent miRs from binding to mRNA targets. Some clinical studies have suggested that the existence of such micro RNA SNPs, rs4938723, has been associated with increased risk of HCC and has been shown to correlate with alcohol consumption in a cohort of Chinese patients studied (see Table 5.6) [149]. These studies point toward a putative mechanism of alcohol altering miR expression or inducing SNPs in micro RNAs to induce the progression of HCC; this area is currently under intense study, and the potential findings are tantalizing.

5.6   NAFLD-NASH-Associated Hepatocellular Carcinoma

Nonalcoholic fatty liver disease (NAFLD) is characterized by the accumulation of fat in the liver, in the absence of significant alcohol consumption, hereditary disease, or drug abuse [20]. NAFLD constitutes a clinicopathological disease comprising of broad-spectrum disease, ranging from simple steatosis (ss), which is usually benign, to nonalcoholic steatohepatitis (NASH), accompanied by inflammatory responses and hepatocellular damage [44]. NAFLD remains the most common cause of chronic liver disease in the United States with an estimated prevalence of 30–40% in the adult population [143]. With between 5 and 20% of NAFLD patients progressing to NASH, this translates to a national prevalence of 2–5% of the US adult population [15]. The pathogenesis of NAFLD is complex as the liver is the catalyst for many metabolic processes in the body; lipid and glucose metabolism are highly important processes disrupted in NAFLD; therefore, NAFLD is a disease representative of impaired homeostasis of metabolism in the liver [10]. In the well-established two-hit model of NAFLD, the primary insult is the accumulation of triglycerides in hepatocytes, which is followed by hepatocellular injury and fibrosis [43, 51, 126]. Obesity contributes to the risk of developing HCC with meta-analysis of cohort studies showing a 90% increased relative risk (RR) for the development of HCC in the obese [13, 31]. One cohort study showed that a body mass index of greater than 35 kg/m^2 increases the RR of developing HCC by 1.68 times in females and 4.52 in males [17]. Additional meta-analysis studies including data from

Table 5.7 NAFLD-NASH related HCC DNA methylation biomarkers

Gene	Gene function	Methylation	Effect
CASP1	Caspase 1 family, role in inducing apoptosis	Hypomethylation of promoter decreases with NAFLD severity	Promotes inflammation by driving interleukin activation
FGFR2	Fibroblast growth receptor 2	Hypomethylation of promoter decreases with NAFLD severity	Promotes mitogenesis and cell proliferation and anti-apoptotic pathways
MAT1A	Catalyzes the addition of adenosyl moiety to methionine in carbon cycle	Hypermethylation of promoter increases with NAFLD severity	Enhanced liver damage and drives genome-wide hypomethylation by abrogation of the carbon cycle
MT-ND6	NADH dehydrogenase, forms part of the electron transport chain	Promoter hypermethylation increases between NAFLD and with NASH severity	Putative accumulation of ROS in the mitochondria, putative anti-apoptotic effect

Greece, Sweden, and Denmark identify a similar increase in RR for the development of HCC in diabetic patients, with females having an increased RR of 1.86 and males an increased RR of 4.5 [2, 41, 71, 142]. Epigenetic changes during the development of HCC are well established [78, 82, 144, 145]. The difficulty in diagnosing HCC in patients with a background of NAFLD can be in detecting changes earlier that may distinguish simple steatosis from NASH or determining the severity of NASH. NASH has also been associated with changes in DNA methylation in hepatocyte cells. Several studies have been performed linking DNA methylation with NAFLD severity and progression to NASH [97]. Methylation of several genes was found to have gradually altered through NAFLD progression; both FGFR2 and CAPS1 were shown to lose methylation during NAFLD progression; MAT1A was shown to gain methylation during NAFLD progression [97]. Genes involved in lipid metabolism and vitamin D metabolism have also shown to be altered epigenetically in NAFLD [98]. Evidence has also shown that a DNA methyltransferase isoform DNMT1 is targeted to mitochondria in the cell for the purpose of maintaining the DNA methylation profile of mitochondrial genes [122]. Patient biopsies were used to assess the DNA methylation of several mitochondrial genes including MT-ND6, MT-CO1, and the D-loop control region. MT-ND6 or mitochondrial NADH dehydrogenase 6 was found to be associated with NAFLD and progression to NASH; patients with advanced fibrosis were also found to have increased DNA methylation and reduced expression of the MT-ND6 gene [107]. Aberrant DNA methylation of another mitochondrial gene NQ01 is also implicated in HBV virus-related HCC adding weight to the promising study of mitochondrial DNA methylation biomarkers of HCC progression [146]. See Table 5.7 for full list of methylation markers in NAFLD and NASH.

Micro RNAs are expressed in highly tissue-specific manner, and some miRs have been shown to regulate gene pathways involved in lipid metabolism, adipocyte differentiation, and glucose resistance [19, 23, 30, 92]. So far there have been few clinical studies on the altered micro RNA profiles of NAFLD and NASH patients.

Table 5.8 Putative NAFLD-NASH-related HCC miR markers from in vitro and in vivo experiments

miR accession number	Gene target	Upregulated or downregulated	Putative effect in NAFLD
miR-212	FGF21	Downregulated	Deregulated lipogenesis increased lipid peroxidation
miR-34a	PPAR/SIRT1	Upregulated	Drives lipid accumulation in hepatocytes
miR-146b	TRAF6/IRAK	Upregulated	Drives lipid accumulation and increase adipocyte proliferation

So far much of the data has been gathered from cell line and murine studies; these studies show that high-fat diet affects the expression of liver micro RNAs, and several miR biomarkers have emerged from experimental models and require further validation in a clinical setting [147, 36, 64]. See Table 5.8 for experimental micro RNA markers of NAFLD progression.

5.7   Future of Biomarkers for the early diagnosis of Hepatocellular Carcinoma

Both methylated DNA and micro RNA provide clinically accessible markers which can be developed into molecular tools for the early detection and diagnosis and classification of HCC. Both methylated DNA and micro RNAs can be detected in peripheral blood; methylated DNA has been shown to be stable and present in small subcellular vesicles, and micro RNAs have been shown to be attached to Ago proteins [47, 109, 129]. However, not all patients have the same quantities of cell-free circulating nucleic acids [55] with the micro RNAs also detectable at different levels in plasma and serum [137]. Often the low abundance of tumor nucleic acids present in the circulation limits the diagnostic potential of such biomarkers; contamination by non-tumor DNA and RNA can also make the analysis of such biomarkers technically challenging. The PDX model of tumor implantation in mice for the further development of heterogenic cell lines based on primary tumor offers a way of surmounting these limitations [104, 106] providing a virtually limitless amount of tumor genetic material for analysis of genetic and epigenetic markers and for the testing of putative chemotherapeutic treatments prior to patient treatment. However, we must also carefully evaluate the information arising from the PDX model as there is potential for the in vivo and ex vivo compartments to introduce cellular changes not present in the original tumor tissue [123]. Currently the most suitable methodology would be the development of clinical biomarker panels based on array data for HCC; these panels can be developed using technology that utilizes less genetic material such as digital droplet PCR (DDPCR) [27]. One thing is certain and that is whichever technological platform is eventually proven to be successful in the development of early patient diagnosis of HCC that it will in tandem with excellent histopathology. The epigenetic biomarkers presented in this chapter could point the way toward the development of epigenetic biomarker panels, for the development of better patient care and improved survival rates from HCC in the future.

References

1. Abu-Amara M, Feld JJ. Does antiviral therapy for chronic hepatitis B reduce the risk of hepatocellular carcinoma? Semin Liver Dis. 2013;33(2):157–66. https://doi.org/10.1055/s-0033-1345719.
2. Adami HO, Chow WH, Nyrén O, Berne C, Linet MS, Ekbom A, et al. Excess risk of primary liver cancer in patients with diabetes mellitus. J Natl Cancer Inst. 1996;88(20):1472–7.
3. Ambade A, Satishchandran A, Szabo G. Alcoholic hepatitis accelerates early hepatobiliary cancer by increasing stemness and miR-122-mediated HIF-1α activation. Sci Rep. 2016;6:21340. https://doi.org/10.1038/srep21340.
4. Antequera F, Bird A. CpG islands. EXS. 1993;64:169–85.
5. Arora A. MicroRNA targets: potential candidates for indirect regulation by drugs. Pharmacogenet Genomics. 2015;25(3):107–25. https://doi.org/10.1097/FPC.0000000000000111.
6. Augello C, Vaira V, Caruso L, Destro A, Maggioni M, Park YN, et al. MicroRNA profiling of hepatocarcinogenesis identifies C19MC cluster as a novel prognostic biomarker in hepatocellular carcinoma. Liver Int. 2012;32(5):772–82. https://doi.org/10.1111/j.1478-3231.2012.02795.x.
7. Bandyopadhyay S, Friedman RC, Marquez RT, Keck K, Kong B, Icardi MS, et al. Hepatitis C virus infection and hepatic stellate cell activation downregulate miR-29: miR-29 overexpression reduces hepatitis C viral abundance in culture. J Infect Dis. 2011;203(12):1753–62. https://doi.org/10.1093/infdis/jir186.
8. Bankwitz D, Steinmann E, Bitzegeio J, Ciesek S, Friesland M, Herrmann E, et al. Hepatitis C virus hypervariable region 1 modulates receptor interactions, conceals the CD81 binding site, and protects conserved neutralizing epitopes. J Virol. 2010;84(11):5751–63. https://doi.org/10.1128/JVI.02200-09.
9. Bartel DP. MicroRNAs: target recognition and regulatory functions. Cell. 2009;136(2):215–33. https://doi.org/10.1016/j.cell.2009.01.002.
10. Bechmann LP, Hannivoort RA, Gerken G, Hotamisligil GS, Trauner M, Canbay A. The interaction of hepatic lipid and glucose metabolism in liver diseases. J Hepatol. 2012;56(4):952–64. https://doi.org/10.1016/j.jhep.2011.08.025.
11. Benedicto I, Molina-Jiménez F, Bartosch B, Cosset FL, Lavillette D, Prieto J, et al. The tight junction-associated protein occludin is required for a postbinding step in hepatitis C virus entry and infection. J Virol. 2009;83(16):8012–20. https://doi.org/10.1128/JVI.00038-09.
12. Benegiamo G, Vinciguerra M, Mazzoccoli G, Piepoli A, Andriulli A, Pazienza V. DNA methyltransferases 1 and 3b expression in Huh-7 cells expressing HCV core protein of different genotypes. Dig Dis Sci. 2012;57(6):1598–603. https://doi.org/10.1007/s10620-012-2160-1.
13. Blonski W, Kotlyar DS, Forde KA. Non-viral causes of hepatocellular carcinoma. World J Gastroenterol. 2010;16(29):3603–15.
14. Bosia C, Osella M, Baroudi ME, Corà D, Caselle M. Gene autoregulation via intronic microRNAs and its functions. BMC Syst Biol. 2012;6:131. https://doi.org/10.1186/1752-0509-6-131.
15. Bruix J, Sherman M, Practice Guidelines Committee, American Association for the Study of Liver Diseases. Management of hepatocellular carcinoma. Hepatology. 2005;42(5):1208–36. https://doi.org/10.1002/hep.20933.
16. Burchard J, Zhang C, Liu AM, Poon RT, Lee NP, Wong KF, et al. microRNA-122 as a regulator of mitochondrial metabolic gene network in hepatocellular carcinoma. Mol Syst Biol. 2010;6:402. https://doi.org/10.1038/msb.2010.58.
17. Calle EE, Rodriguez C, Walker-Thurmond K, Thun MJ. Overweight, obesity, and mortality from cancer in a prospectively studied cohort of U.S. adults. N Engl J Med. 2003;348(17):1625–38. https://doi.org/10.1056/NEJMoa021423.
18. Calvisi DF, Simile MM, Ladu S, Pellegrino R, De Murtas V, Pinna F, et al. Altered methionine metabolism and global DNA methylation in liver cancer: relationship with genomic instability and prognosis. Int J Cancer. 2007;121(11):2410–20. https://doi.org/10.1002/ijc.22940.

19. Chakraborty C, Doss CG, Bandyopadhyay S, Agoramoorthy G. Influence of miRNA in insulin signaling pathway and insulin resistance: micro-molecules with a major role in type-2 diabetes. Wiley Interdiscip Rev RNA. 2014;5(5):697–712. https://doi.org/10.1002/wrna.1240.

20. Chalasani N, Younossi Z, Lavine JE, Diehl AM, Brunt EM, Cusi K, et al. The diagnosis and management of non-alcoholic fatty liver disease: practice guideline by the American Gastroenterological Association, American Association for the Study of Liver Diseases, and American College of Gastroenterology. Gastroenterology. 2012;142(7):1592–609. https://doi.org/10.1053/j.gastro.2012.04.001.

21. Chen CJ, Yu MW, Liaw YF. Epidemiological characteristics and risk factors of hepatocellular carcinoma. J Gastroenterol Hepatol. 1997;12(9–10):S294–308.

22. Chen HP, Zhao YT, Zhao TC. Histone deacetylases and mechanisms of regulation of gene expression. Crit Rev Oncog. 2015b;20(1–2):35–47.

23. Chen L, Hou J, Ye L, Chen Y, Cui J, Tian W, et al. MicroRNA-143 regulates adipogenesis by modulating the MAP2K5-ERK5 signaling. Sci Rep. 2014;4:3819. https://doi.org/10.1038/srep03819.

24. Chen WC, Wang SY, Chiu CC, Tseng CK, Lin CK, Wang HC, Lee JC. Lucidone suppresses hepatitis C virus replication by Nrf2-mediated heme oxygenase-1 induction. Antimicrob Agents Chemother. 2013;57(3):1180–91. https://doi.org/10.1128/AAC.02053-12.

25. Chen WN, Chen JY, Lin WS, Lin JY, Lin X. Hepatitis B doubly spliced protein, generated by a 2.2 kb doubly spliced hepatitis B virus RNA, is a pleiotropic activator protein mediating its effects via activator protein-1- and CCAAT/enhancer-binding protein-binding sites. J Gen Virol. 2010;91(Pt 10):2592–600. https://doi.org/10.1099/vir.0.022517-0.

26. Chen Y, Dong X, Yu D, Wang X. Serum miR-96 is a promising biomarker for hepatocellular carcinoma in patients with chronic hepatitis B virus infection. Int J Clin Exp Med. 2015a;8(10):18462–8.

27. Cheng H, Liu C, Jiang J, Luo G, Lu Y, Jin K, et al. Analysis of ctDNA to predict prognosis and monitor treatment responses in metastatic pancreatic cancer patients. Int J Cancer. 2017;140(10):2344–50. https://doi.org/10.1002/ijc.30650.

28. Cheng M, Si Y, Niu Y, Liu X, Li X, Zhao J, et al. High-throughput profiling of alpha interferon- and interleukin-28B-regulated microRNAs and identification of let-7s with anti-hepatitis C virus activity by targeting IGF2BP1. J Virol. 2013;87(17):9707–18. https://doi.org/10.1128/JVI.00802-13.

29. Choo QL, Kuo G, Weiner AJ, Overby LR, Bradley DW, Houghton M. Isolation of a cDNA clone derived from a blood-borne non-A, non-B viral hepatitis genome. Science. 1989;244(4902):359–62.

30. Christian P, Su Q. MicroRNA regulation of mitochondrial and ER stress signaling pathways: implications for lipoprotein metabolism in metabolic syndrome. Am J Physiol Endocrinol Metab. 2014;307(9):E729–37. https://doi.org/10.1152/ajpendo.00194.2014.

31. Clark JM. The epidemiology of nonalcoholic fatty liver disease in adults. J Clin Gastroenterol. 2006;40(Suppl 1):S5–10. https://doi.org/10.1097/01.mcg.0000168638.84840.ff.

32. Clark SJ, Harrison J, Frommer M. CpNpG methylation in mammalian cells. Nat Genet. 1995;10(1):20–7. https://doi.org/10.1038/ng0595-20.

33. Dao Thi VL, Dreux M, Cosset FL. Scavenger receptor class B type I and the hypervariable region-1 of hepatitis C virus in cell entry and neutralisation. Expert Rev Mol Med. 2011;13:e13. https://doi.org/10.1017/S1462399411001785.

34. Dao Thi VL, Granier C, Zeisel MB, Guérin M, Mancip J, Granio O, et al. Characterization of hepatitis C virus particle subpopulations reveals multiple usage of the scavenger receptor BI for entry steps. J Biol Chem. 2012;287(37):31242–57. https://doi.org/10.1074/jbc.M112.365924.

35. Deng JH, Deng P, Lin SL, Ying SY. Gene silencing in vitro and in vivo using intronic microRNAs. Methods Mol Biol. 2015;1218:321–40. https://doi.org/10.1007/978-1-4939-1538-5_20.

36. Ding J, Li M, Wan X, Jin X, Chen S, Yu C, Li Y. Effect of miR-34a in regulating steatosis by targeting PPARα expression in nonalcoholic fatty liver disease. Sci Rep. 2015;5:13729. https://doi.org/10.1038/srep13729.

37. Donato F, Tagger A, Gelatti U, Parrinello G, Boffetta P, Albertini A, et al. Alcohol and hepatocellular carcinoma: the effect of lifetime intake and hepatitis virus infections in men and women. Am J Epidemiol. 2002;155(4):323–31.
38. Dong H, Wang C, Lu S, Yu C, Huang L, Feng W, et al. A panel of four decreased serum microRNAs as a novel biomarker for early Parkinson's disease. Biomarkers. 2016;21(2):129–37. https://doi.org/10.3109/1354750X.2015.1118544.
39. Dou CY, Fan YC, Cao CJ, Yang Y, Wang K. Sera DNA methylation of CDH1, DNMT3b and ESR1 promoters as biomarker for the early diagnosis of hepatitis B virus-related hepatocellular carcinoma. Dig Dis Sci. 2016;61(4):1130–8. https://doi.org/10.1007/s10620-015-3975-3.
40. Dreux M, Dao Thi VL, Fresquet J, Guérin M, Julia Z, Verney G, et al. Receptor complementation and mutagenesis reveal SR-BI as an essential HCV entry factor and functionally imply its intra- and extra-cellular domains. PLoS Pathog. 2009;5(2):e1000310. https://doi.org/10.1371/journal.ppat.1000310.
41. El-Serag HB, Hampel H, Javadi F. The association between diabetes and hepatocellular carcinoma: a systematic review of epidemiologic evidence. Clin Gastroenterol Hepatol. 2006;4(3):369–80. https://doi.org/10.1016/j.cgh.2005.12.007.
42. Fabian MR, Sundermeier TR, Sonenberg N. Understanding how miRNAs post-transcriptionally regulate gene expression. Prog Mol Subcell Biol. 2010;50:1–20. https://doi.org/10.1007/978-3-642-03103-8_1.
43. Farrell GC, Larter CZ. Nonalcoholic fatty liver disease: from steatosis to cirrhosis. Hepatology. 2006;43(2 Suppl 1):S99–S112. https://doi.org/10.1002/hep.20973.
44. Farrell GC, van Rooyen D, Gan L, Chitturi S. NASH is an inflammatory disorder: pathogenic, prognostic and therapeutic implications. Gut Liver. 2012;6(2):149–71. https://doi.org/10.5009/gnl.2012.6.2.149.
45. Gao P, Wong CC, Tung EK, Lee JM, Wong CM, Ng IO. Deregulation of microRNA expression occurs early and accumulates in early stages of HBV-associated multistep hepatocarcinogenesis. J Hepatol. 2011;54(6):1177–84. https://doi.org/10.1016/j.jhep.2010.09.023.
46. Gardiner AS, Gutierrez HL, Luo L, Davies S, Savage DD, Bakhireva LN, Perrone-Bizzozero NI. Alcohol use during pregnancy is associated with specific alterations in MicroRNA levels in maternal serum. Alcohol Clin Exp Res. 2016;40(4):826–37. https://doi.org/10.1111/acer.13026.
47. Giacona MB, Ruben GC, Iczkowski KA, Roos TB, Porter DM, Sorenson GD. Cell-free DNA in human blood plasma: length measurements in patients with pancreatic cancer and healthy controls. Pancreas. 1998;17(1):89–97.
48. Gottschalk AJ, Timinszky G, Kong SE, Jin J, Cai Y, Swanson SK, et al. Poly(ADP-ribosyl) ation directs recruitment and activation of an ATP-dependent chromatin remodeler. Proc Natl Acad Sci U S A. 2009;106(33):13770–4. https://doi.org/10.1073/pnas.0906920106.
49. Gottwein JM, Scheel TK, Jensen TB, Lademann JB, Prentoe JC, Knudsen ML, et al. Development and characterization of hepatitis C virus genotype 1-7 cell culture systems: role of CD81 and scavenger receptor class B type I and effect of antiviral drugs. Hepatology. 2009;49(2):364–77. https://doi.org/10.1002/hep.22673.
50. Gouttenoire J, Penin F, Moradpour D. Hepatitis C virus nonstructural protein 4B: a journey into unexplored territory. Rev Med Virol. 2010;20(2):117–29. https://doi.org/10.1002/rmv.640.
51. Haider DG, Schindler K, Schaller G, Prager G, Wolzt M, Ludvik B. Increased plasma visfatin concentrations in morbidly obese subjects are reduced after gastric banding. J Clin Endocrinol Metab. 2006;91(4):1578–81. https://doi.org/10.1210/jc.2005-2248.
52. Haybaeck J, Zeller N, Heikenwalder M. The parallel universe: microRNAs and their role in chronic hepatitis, liver tissue damage and hepatocarcinogenesis. Swiss Med Wkly. 2011;141:w13287. https://doi.org/10.4414/smw.2011.13287.
53. He C, Xu J, Zhang J, Xie D, Ye H, Xiao Z, Cai M, Xu K, Zeng Y, Li H, Wang J. High expression of trimethylated histone H3 lysine 4 is associated with poor prognosis in hepatocellular carcinoma. Hum. Pathol. 2012;43(9):1425–35. https://doi.org/10.1016/j.humpath.2011.11.003; Epub 2012 Mar 9.

54. Hechtman JF, Beasley MB, Kinoshita Y, Ko HM, Hao K, Burstein DE. Promyelocytic leukemia zinc finger and histone H1.5 differentially stain low- and high-grade pulmonary neuroendocrine tumors: a pilot immunohistochemical study. Hum Pathol. 2013;44(7):1400–5. https://doi.org/10.1016/j.humpath.2012.11.014.

55. Heidary M, Auer M, Ulz P, Heitzer E, Petru E, Gasch C, et al. The dynamic range of circulating tumor DNA in metastatic breast cancer. Breast Cancer Res. 2014;16(4):421. https://doi.org/10.1186/s13058-014-0421-y.

56. Herath NI, Leggett BA, MacDonald GA. Review of genetic and epigenetic alterations in hepatocarcinogenesis. J Gastroenterol Hepatol. 2006;21(1 Pt 1):15–21. https://doi.org/10.1111/j.1440-1746.2005.04043.x.

57. Hernandez-Vargas H, Lambert MP, Le Calvez-Kelm F, Gouysse G, McKay-Chopin S, Tavtigian SV, et al. Hepatocellular carcinoma displays distinct DNA methylation signatures with potential as clinical predictors. PLoS One. 2010;5(3):e9749. https://doi.org/10.1371/journal.pone.0009749.

58. Hlady RA, Tiedemann RL, Puszyk W, Zendejas I, Roberts LR, Choi JH, et al. Epigenetic signatures of alcohol abuse and hepatitis infection during human hepatocarcinogenesis. Oncotarget. 2014;5(19):9425–43. 10.18632/oncotarget.2444.

59. Huang S, He X. The role of microRNAs in liver cancer progression. Br J Cancer. 2011;104(2):235–40. https://doi.org/10.1038/sj.bjc.6606010.

60. Ikeda M, Zhang ZW, Srianujata S, Hussamin N, Banjong O, Chitchumroonchokchai C, et al. Prevalence of hepatitis B and C virus infection among working women in Bangkok. Southeast Asian J Trop Med Public Health. 1998;29(3):469–74.

61. Ishida H, Tatsumi T, Hosui A, Nawa T, Kodama T, Shimizu S, et al. Alterations in microRNA expression profile in HCV-infected hepatoma cells: involvement of miR-491 in regulation of HCV replication via the PI3 kinase/Akt pathway. Biochem Biophys Res Commun. 2011;412(1):92–7. https://doi.org/10.1016/j.bbrc.2011.07.049.

62. Itano O, Ueda M, Kikuchi K, Hashimoto O, Hayatsu S, Kawaguchi M, et al. Correlation of postoperative recurrence in hepatocellular carcinoma with demethylation of repetitive sequences. Oncogene. 2002;21(5):789–97. https://doi.org/10.1038/sj.onc.1205124.

63. Jiang J, Wu X, Tang H, Luo G. Apolipoprotein E mediates attachment of clinical hepatitis C virus to hepatocytes by binding to cell surface heparan sulfate proteoglycan receptors. PLoS One. 2013;8(7):e67982. https://doi.org/10.1371/journal.pone.0067982.

64. Jiang W, Liu J, Dai Y, Zhou N, Ji C, Li X. MiR-146b attenuates high-fat diet-induced nonalcoholic steatohepatitis in mice. J. Gastroenterol. Hepatol. 2015;30(5):933–43. https://doi.org/10.1111/jgh.12878.

65. Jin B, Robertson KD. DNA methyltransferases, DNA damage repair, and cancer. Adv Exp Med Biol. 2013;754:3–29. https://doi.org/10.1007/978-1-4419-9967-2_1.

66. Jopling CL. Regulation of hepatitis C virus by microRNA-122. Biochem Soc Trans. 2008;36(Pt 6):1220–3. https://doi.org/10.1042/BST0361220.

67. Jopling CL, Norman KL, Sarnow P. Positive and negative modulation of viral and cellular mRNAs by liver-specific microRNA miR-122. Cold Spring Harb Symp Quant Biol. 2006;71:369–76. https://doi.org/10.1101/sqb.2006.71.022.

68. Kałużna EM. MicroRNA-155 and microRNA-196b: promising biomarkers in hepatitis C virus infection? Rev Med Virol. 2014;24(3):169–85. https://doi.org/10.1002/rmv.1785.

69. Kim HY, Yoon JH, Lee HS, Cheong JY, Cho SW, Shin HD, Kim YJ. MicroRNA-196A-2 polymorphisms and hepatocellular carcinoma in patients with chronic hepatitis B. J Med Virol. 2014;86(3):446–53. https://doi.org/10.1002/jmv.23848.

70. Ladeiro Y, Couchy G, Balabaud C, Bioulac-Sage P, Pelletier L, Rebouissou S, Zucman-Rossi J. MicroRNA profiling in hepatocellular tumors is associated with clinical features and oncogene/tumor suppressor gene mutations. Hepatology. 2008;47(6):1955–63. https://doi.org/10.1002/hep.22256.

71. Lagiou P, Kuper H, Stuver SO, Tzonou A, Trichopoulos D, Adami HO. Role of diabetes mellitus in the etiology of hepatocellular carcinoma. J Natl Cancer Inst. 2000;92(13):1096–9.

72. Lambert MP, Paliwal A, Vaissière T, Chemin I, Zoulim F, Tommasino M, et al. Aberrant DNA methylation distinguishes hepatocellular carcinoma associated with HBV and HCV

infection and alcohol intake. J Hepatol. 2011;54(4):705–15. https://doi.org/10.1016/j.jhep.2010.07.027.

73. Lapunzina P, Badia I, Galoppo C, De Matteo E, Silberman P, Tello A, et al. A patient with Simpson-Golabi-Behmel syndrome and hepatocellular carcinoma. J Med Genet. 1998;35(2):153–6.

74. Larsen F, Gundersen G, Lopez R, Prydz H. CpG islands as gene markers in the human genome. Genomics. 1992;13(4):1095–107.

75. Lee SM, Lee YG, Bae JB, Choi JK, Tayama C, Hata K, et al. HBx induces hypomethylation of distal intragenic CpG islands required for active expression of developmental regulators. Proc Natl Acad Sci U S A. 2014;111(26):9555–60. https://doi.org/10.1073/pnas.1400604111.

76. Lefèvre M, Felmlee DJ, Parnot M, Baumert TF, Schuster C. Syndecan 4 is involved in mediating HCV entry through interaction with lipoviral particle-associated apolipoprotein E. PLoS One. 2014;9(4):e95550. https://doi.org/10.1371/journal.pone.0095550.

77. Lewis AP, Jopling CL. Regulation and biological function of the liver-specific miR-122. Biochem. Soc. Trans. 2010;38(6):1553–7. https://doi.org/10.1042/BST0381553.

78. Li B, Liu W, Wang L, Li M, Wang J, Huang L, et al. CpG island methylator phenotype associated with tumor recurrence in tumor-node-metastasis stage I hepatocellular carcinoma. Ann Surg Oncol. 2010a;17(7):1917–26. https://doi.org/10.1245/s10434-010-0921-7.

79. Li G, Cai G, Li D, Yin W. MicroRNAs and liver disease: viral hepatitis, liver fibrosis and hepatocellular carcinoma. Postgrad. Med. J. 2014;90(1060):106–12. https://doi.org/10.1136/postgradmedj-2013-131883; Epub 2013 Nov 15. Review.

80. Li H, Rauch T, Chen ZX, Szabó PE, Riggs AD, Pfeifer GP. The histone methyltransferase SETDB1 and the DNA methyltransferase DNMT3A interact directly and localize to promoters silenced in cancer cells. J Biol Chem. 2006;281(28):19489–500. https://doi.org/10.1074/jbc.M513249200.

81. Li H, Yang F, Gao B, Yu Z, Liu X, Xie F, Zhang J. Hepatitis B virus infection in hepatocellular carcinoma tissues upregulates expression of DNA methyltransferases. Int J Clin Exp Med. 2015;8(3):4175–85.

82. Li R, Qian N, Tao K, You N, Wang X, Dou K. MicroRNAs involved in neoplastic transformation of liver cancer stem cells. J Exp Clin Cancer Res. 2010b;29:169. https://doi.org/10.1186/1756-9966-29-169.

83. Liu XY, Tang SH, Wu SL, Luo YH, Cao MR, Zhou HK, et al. Epigenetic modulation of insulin-like growth factor-II overexpression by hepatitis B virus X protein in hepatocellular carcinoma. Am J Cancer Res. 2015;5(3):956–78.

84. Liu Z, Tian Y, Machida K, Lai MM, Luo G, Foung SK, Ou JH. Transient activation of the PI3K-AKT pathway by hepatitis C virus to enhance viral entry. J Biol Chem. 2012;287(50):41922–30.

85. Lohmann V. Hepatitis C virus RNA replication. Curr Top Microbiol Immunol. 2013;369:167–98. https://doi.org/10.1007/978-3-642-27340-7_7.

86. Lokk K, Modhukur V, Rajashekar B, Märtens K, Mägi R, Kolde R, et al. DNA methylome profiling of human tissues identifies global and tissue-specific methylation patterns. Genome Biol. 2014;15(4):r54. https://doi.org/10.1186/gb-2014-15-4-r54.

87. Luger K, Rechsteiner TJ, Flaus AJ, Waye MM, Richmond TJ. Characterization of nucleosome core particles containing histone proteins made in bacteria. J Mol Biol. 1997;272(3):301–11. https://doi.org/10.1006/jmbi.1997.1235.

88. Ma Y, She XG, Ming YZ, Wan QQ, Ye QF. MicroRNA-144 suppresses tumorigenesis of hepatocellular carcinoma by targeting AKT3. Mol Med Rep. 2015;11(2):1378–83. https://doi.org/10.3892/mmr.2014.2844.

89. Machlin ES, Sarnow P, Sagan SM. Masking the 5′ terminal nucleotides of the hepatitis C virus genome by an unconventional microRNA-target RNA complex. Proc Natl Acad Sci U S A. 2011;108(8):3193–8. https://doi.org/10.1073/pnas.1012464108.

90. Maillard P, Huby T, Andréo U, Moreau M, Chapman J, Budkowska A. The interaction of natural hepatitis C virus with human scavenger receptor SR-BI/Cla1 is mediated by ApoB-containing lipoproteins. FASEB J. 2006;20(6):735–7. https://doi.org/10.1096/fj.05-4728fje.

91. Mariño-Ramírez L, Kann MG, Shoemaker BA, Landsman D. Histone structure and nucleosome stability. Expert Rev Proteomics. 2005;2(5):719–29. https://doi.org/10.1586/14789450.2.5.719.
92. Mattis AN, Song G, Hitchner K, Kim RY, Lee AY, Sharma AD, et al. A screen in mice uncovers repression of lipoprotein lipase by microRNA-29a as a mechanism for lipid distribution away from the liver. Hepatology. 2015;61(1):141–52. https://doi.org/10.1002/hep.27379.
93. McKinney MD, Moon SJ, Kulesh DA, Larsen T, Schoepp RJ. Detection of viral RNA from paraffin-embedded tissues after prolonged formalin fixation. J Clin Virol. 2009;44(1):39–42. https://doi.org/10.1016/j.jcv.2008.09.003.
94. Moradpour D, Gosert R, Egger D, Penin F, Blum HE, Bienz K. Membrane association of hepatitis C virus nonstructural proteins and identification of the membrane alteration that harbors the viral replication complex. Antiviral Res. 2003;60(2):103–9.
95. Morgan TR, Mandayam S, Jamal MM. Alcohol and hepatocellular carcinoma. Gastroenterology. 2004;127(5 Suppl 1):S87–96.
96. Murakami Y, Yasuda T, Saigo K, Urashima T, Toyoda H, Okanoue T, Shimotohno K. Comprehensive analysis of microRNA expression patterns in hepatocellular carcinoma and non-tumorous tissues. Oncogene. 2006;25(17):2537–45. https://doi.org/10.1038/sj.onc.1209283.
97. Murphy SK, Yang H, Moylan CA, Pang H, Dellinger A, Abdelmalek MF, et al. Relationship between methylome and transcriptome in patients with nonalcoholic fatty liver disease. Gastroenterology. 2013;145(5):1076–87. https://doi.org/10.1053/j.gastro.2013.07.047.
98. Mwinyi J, Boström AE, Pisanu C, Murphy SK, Erhart W, Schafmayer C, et al. NAFLD is associated with methylation shifts with relevance for the expression of genes involved in lipoprotein particle composition. Biochim Biophys Acta. 2017;1862(3):314–23. https://doi.org/10.1016/j.bbalip.2016.12.005.
99. Narayan PJ, Lill C, Faull R, Curtis MA, Dragunow M. Increased acetyl and total histone levels in post-mortem Alzheimer's disease brain. Neurobiol Dis. 2015;74:281–94. https://doi.org/10.1016/j.nbd.2014.11.023.
100. Natarajan SK, Pachunka JM, Mott JL. Role of microRNAs in alcohol-induced multi-organ injury. Biomolecules. 2015;5(4):3309–38. https://doi.org/10.3390/biom5043309.
101. Niepmann M. Activation of hepatitis C virus translation by a liver-specific microRNA. Cell Cycle. 2009;8(10):1473–7. https://doi.org/10.4161/cc.8.10.8349.
102. Nishizawa M, Ikeya Y, Okumura T, Kimura T. Post-transcriptional inducible gene regulation by natural antisense RNA. Front Biosci (Landmark Ed). 2015;20:1–36.
103. Ozen C, Yildiz G, Dagcan AT, Cevik D, Ors A, Keles U, et al. Genetics and epigenetics of liver cancer. N Biotechnol. 2013;30(4):381–4. https://doi.org/10.1016/j.nbt.2013.01.007.
104. Park D, Wang D, Chen G, Deng X. Establishment of patient-derived xenografts in mice. Bio Protoc. 2016;6(22). doi:10.21769/BioProtoc.2008.
105. Pedersen IM, Cheng G, Wieland S, Volinia S, Croce CM, Chisari FV, David M. Interferon modulation of cellular microRNAs as an antiviral mechanism. Nature. 2007;449(7164):919–22. https://doi.org/10.1038/nature06205.
106. Pham K, Delitto D, Knowlton AE, Hartlage ER, Madhavan R, Gonzalo DH, et al. Isolation of pancreatic cancer cells from a patient-derived xenograft model allows for practical expansion and preserved heterogeneity in culture. Am J Pathol. 2016;186(6):1537–46. https://doi.org/10.1016/j.ajpath.2016.02.009.
107. Pirola CJ, Gianotti TF, Burgueño AL, Rey-Funes M, Loidl CF, Mallardi P, et al. Epigenetic modification of liver mitochondrial DNA is associated with histological severity of nonalcoholic fatty liver disease. Gut. 2013;62(9):1356–63. https://doi.org/10.1136/gutjnl-2012-302962.
108. Ploss A, Evans MJ, Gaysinskaya VA, Panis M, You H, de Jong YP, Rice CM. Human occludin is a hepatitis C virus entry factor required for infection of mouse cells. Nature. 2009;457(7231):882–6. https://doi.org/10.1038/nature07684.
109. Puszyk WM, Chatha K, Elsenheimer S, Crea F, Old RW. Methylation of the imprinted GNAS1 gene in cell-free plasma DNA: equal steady-state quantities of methylated and unmethylated DNA in plasma. Clin Chim Acta. 2009;400(1–2):107–10. https://doi.org/10.1016/j.cca.2008.10.018.

110. Ramadan RA, Zaki MA, Awad AM, El-Ghalid LA. Aberrant methylation of promoter region of SPINT2/HAI-2 gene: an epigenetic mechanism in hepatitis C virus-induced hepatocarcinogenesis. Genet Test Mol Biomarkers. 2015;19(7):399–404. https://doi.org/10.1089/gtmb.2015.0025.

111. Redon C, Pilch D, Rogakou E, Sedelnikova O, Newrock K, Bonner W. Histone H2A variants H2AX and H2AZ. Curr Opin Genet Dev. 2002;12(2):162–9.

112. Reid G, Métivier R, Lin CY, Denger S, Ibberson D, Ivacevic T, et al. Multiple mechanisms induce transcriptional silencing of a subset of genes, including oestrogen receptor alpha, in response to deacetylase inhibition by valproic acid and trichostatin A. Oncogene. 2005;24(31):4894–907. https://doi.org/10.1038/sj.onc.1208662.

113. Saito I, Miyamura T, Ohbayashi A, Harada H, Katayama T, Kikuchi S, et al. Hepatitis C virus infection is associated with the development of hepatocellular carcinoma. Proc Natl Acad Sci U S A. 1990;87(17):6547–9.

114. Sandoval J, Esteller M. Cancer epigenomics: beyond genomics. Curr Opin Genet Dev. 2012;22(1):50–5. https://doi.org/10.1016/j.gde.2012.02.008.

115. Scarselli E, Ansuini H, Cerino R, Roccasecca RM, Acali S, Filocamo G, et al. The human scavenger receptor class B type I is a novel candidate receptor for the hepatitis C virus. EMBO J. 2002;21(19):5017–25.

116. Schweitzer A, Horn J, Mikolajczyk RT, Krause G, Ott JJ. Estimations of worldwide prevalence of chronic hepatitis B virus infection: a systematic review of data published between 1965 and 2013. Lancet. 2015;386(10003):1546–55. https://doi.org/10.1016/S0140-6736(15)61412-X.

117. Shanbhogue AK, Prasad SR, Takahashi N, Vikram R, Sahani DV. Recent advances in cytogenetics and molecular biology of adult hepatocellular tumors: implications for imaging and management. Radiology. 2011;258(3):673–93. https://doi.org/10.1148/radiol.10100376.

118. Sharma NR, Mateu G, Dreux M, Grakoui A, Cosset FL, Melikyan GB. Hepatitis C virus is primed by CD81 protein for low pH-dependent fusion. J Biol Chem. 2011;286(35):30361–76. https://doi.org/10.1074/jbc.M111.263350.

119. Shepard CW, Finelli L, Alter MJ. Global epidemiology of hepatitis C virus infection. Lancet Infect Dis. 2005;5(9):558–67. https://doi.org/10.1016/S1473-3099(05)70216-4.

120. Shi Q, Jiang J, Luo G. Syndecan-1 serves as the major receptor for attachment of hepatitis C virus to the surfaces of hepatocytes. J Virol. 2013;87(12):6866–75. https://doi.org/10.1128/JVI.03475-12.

121. Shimakami T, Yamane D, Jangra RK, Kempf BJ, Spaniel C, Barton DJ, Lemon SM. Stabilization of hepatitis C virus RNA by an Ago2-miR-122 complex. Proc Natl Acad Sci U S A. 2012;109(3):941–6. https://doi.org/10.1073/pnas.1112263109.

122. Shock LS, Thakkar PV, Peterson EJ, Moran RG, Taylor SM. DNA methyltransferase 1, cytosine methylation, and cytosine hydroxymethylation in mammalian mitochondria. Proc Natl Acad Sci U S A. 2011;108(9):3630–5. https://doi.org/10.1073/pnas.1012311108.

123. Sia D, Moeini A, Labgaa I, Villanueva A. The future of patient-derived tumor xenografts in cancer treatment. Pharmacogenomics. 2015;16(14):1671–83. https://doi.org/10.2217/pgs.15.102.

124. Simmonds P. The origin of hepatitis C virus. Curr Top Microbiol Immunol. 2013;369:1–15. https://doi.org/10.1007/978-3-642-27340-7_1.

125. Starley BQ, Calcagno CJ, Harrison SA. Nonalcoholic fatty liver disease and hepatocellular carcinoma: a weighty connection. Hepatology. 2010;51(5):1820–32. https://doi.org/10.1002/hep.23594.

126. Tacke F, Luedde T, Trautwein C. Inflammatory pathways in liver homeostasis and liver injury. Clin Rev Allergy Immunol. 2009;36(1):4–12. https://doi.org/10.1007/s12016-008-8091-0.

127. Tiwari AK, Laird-Fick HS, Wali RK, Roy HK. Surveillance for gastrointestinal malignancies. World J Gastroenterol. 2012;18(33):4507–16. https://doi.org/10.3748/wjg.v18.i33.4507.

128. Torres HA, Nevah MI, Barnett BJ, Mahale P, Kontoyiannis DP, Hassan MM, Raad II. Hepatitis C virus genotype distribution varies by underlying disease status among patients in the same geographic region: a retrospective multicenter study. J Clin Virol. 2012;54(3):218–22. https://doi.org/10.1016/j.jcv.2012.03.002.

129. Turchinovich A, Weiz L, Langheinz A, Burwinkel B. Characterization of extracellular circulating microRNA. Nucleic Acids Res. 2011;39(16):7223–33. https://doi.org/10.1093/nar/gkr254.

130. Turner BM. Reading signals on the nucleosome with a new nomenclature for modified histones. Nat Struct Mol Biol. 2005;12(2):110–2. https://doi.org/10.1038/nsmb0205-110.

131. Udali S, Guarini P, Ruzzenente A, Ferrarini A, Guglielmi A, Lotto V, et al. DNA methylation and gene expression profiles show novel regulatory pathways in hepatocellular carcinoma. Clin Epigenetics. 2015;7:43. https://doi.org/10.1186/s13148-015-0077-1.

132. Um TH, Kim H, Oh BK, Kim MS, Kim KS, Jung G, Park YN. Aberrant CpG island hypermethylation in dysplastic nodules and early HCC of hepatitis B virus-related human multistep hepatocarcinogenesis. J Hepatol. 2011;54(5):939–47. https://doi.org/10.1016/j.jhep.2010.08.021.

133. Umer M, Qureshi SA, Hashmi ZY, Raza A, Ahmad J, Rahman M, Iqbal M. Promoter hypermethylation of Wnt pathway inhibitors in hepatitis C virus—induced multistep hepatocarcinogenesis. Virol. J. 2014;11:117. https://doi.org/10.1186/1743-422X-11-117.

134. van Malenstein H, van Pelt J, Verslype C. Molecular classification of hepatocellular carcinoma anno 2011. Eur J Cancer. 2011;47(12):1789–97. https://doi.org/10.1016/j.ejca.2011.04.027.

135. Vilarinho S, Erson-Omay EZ, Harmanci AS, Morotti R, Carrion-Grant G, Baranoski J, et al. Paediatric hepatocellular carcinoma due to somatic CTNNB1 and NFE2L2 mutations in the setting of inherited bi-allelic ABCB11 mutations. J Hepatol. 2014;61(5):1178–83. https://doi.org/10.1016/j.jhep.2014.07.003.

136. Villanueva A, Hoshida Y. Depicting the role of TP53 in hepatocellular carcinoma progression. J Hepatol. 2011;55(3):724–5. https://doi.org/10.1016/j.jhep.2011.03.018.

137. Wang K, Yuan Y, Cho JH, McClarty S, Baxter D, Galas DJ. Comparing the MicroRNA spectrum between serum and plasma. PLoS One. 2012;7(7):e41561. https://doi.org/10.1371/journal.pone.0041561.

138. Wang XW, Hussain SP, Huo TI, Wu CG, Forgues M, Hofseth LJ, et al. Molecular pathogenesis of human hepatocellular carcinoma. Toxicology. 2002;181–182:43–7.

139. Warnefors M, Liechti A, Halbert J, Valloton D, Kaessmann H. Conserved microRNA editing in mammalian evolution, development and disease. Genome Biol. 2014;15(6):R83. https://doi.org/10.1186/gb-2014-15-6-r83.

140. Wei X, Xiang T, Ren G, Tan C, Liu R, Xu X, Wu Z. miR-101 is down-regulated by the hepatitis B virus x protein and induces aberrant DNA methylation by targeting DNA methyltransferase 3A. Cell Signal. 2013;25(2):439–46. https://doi.org/10.1016/j.cellsig.2012.10.013.

141. Weitzman SA, Turk PW, Milkowski DH, Kozlowski K. Free radical adducts induce alterations in DNA cytosine methylation. Proc Natl Acad Sci U S A. 1994;91(4):1261–4.

142. Wideroff L, Gridley G, Mellemkjaer L, Chow WH, Linet M, Keehn S, et al. Cancer incidence in a population-based cohort of patients hospitalized with diabetes mellitus in Denmark. J Natl Cancer Inst. 1997;89(18):1360–5.

143. Williams CD, Stengel J, Asike MI, Torres DM, Shaw J, Contreras M, et al. Prevalence of nonalcoholic fatty liver disease and nonalcoholic steatohepatitis among a largely middle-aged population utilizing ultrasound and liver biopsy: a prospective study. Gastroenterology. 2011;140(1):124–31. https://doi.org/10.1053/j.gastro.2010.09.038.

144. Wu LM, Yang Z, Zhou L, Zhang F, Xie HY, Feng XW, et al. Identification of histone deacetylase 3 as a biomarker for tumor recurrence following liver transplantation in HBV-associated hepatocellular carcinoma. PLoS One. 2010a;5(12):e14460. https://doi.org/10.1371/journal.pone.0014460.

145. Wu LM, Zhang F, Zhou L, Yang Z, Xie HY, Zheng SS. Predictive value of CpG island methylator phenotype for tumor recurrence in hepatitis B virus-associated hepatocellular carcinoma following liver transplantation. BMC Cancer. 2010b;10:399. https://doi.org/10.1186/1471-2407-10-399.

146. Wu YL, Wang D, Peng XE, Chen YL, Zheng DL, Chen WN, Lin X. Epigenetic silencing of NAD(P)H:quinone oxidoreductase 1 by hepatitis B virus X protein increases mitochondrial

injury and cellular susceptibility to oxidative stress in hepatoma cells. Free Radic Biol Med. 2013;65:632–44. https://doi.org/10.1016/j.freeradbiomed.2013.07.037.

147. Xiao J, Bei Y, Liu J, Dimitrova-Shumkovska J, Kuang D, Zhou Q, Li J, Yang Y, Xiang Y, Wang F, Yang C, Yang W. miR-212 downregulation contributes to the protective effect of exercise against non-alcoholic fatty liver via targeting FGF-21. J. Cell. Mol. Med. 2016;20(2):204–16. https://doi.org/10.1111/jcmm.12733; Epub 2015 Dec 9.

148. Xu H, Hu YW, Zhao JY, Hu XM, Li SF, Wang YC, et al. MicroRNA-195-5p acts as an anti-oncogene by targeting PHF19 in hepatocellular carcinoma. Oncol Rep. 2015;34(1):175–82. https://doi.org/10.3892/or.2015.3957.

149. Xu Y, Liu L, Liu J, Zhang Y, Zhu J, Chen J, et al. A potentially functional polymorphism in the promoter region of miR-34b/c is associated with an increased risk for primary hepatocellular carcinoma. Int J Cancer. 2011;128(2):412–7. https://doi.org/10.1002/ijc.25342.

150. Zakhari S. Alcohol metabolism and epigenetics changes. Alcohol Res. 2013;35(1):6–16.

151. Zekri AR, Bahnasy AA, Shoeab FE, Mohamed WS, El-Dahshan DH, Ali FT, et al. Methylation of multiple genes in hepatitis C virus associated hepatocellular carcinoma. J Adv Res. 2014;5(1):27–40. https://doi.org/10.1016/j.jare.2012.11.002.

152. Zhang C, Guo X, Jiang G, Zhang L, Yang Y, Shen F, et al. CpG island methylator phenotype association with upregulated telomerase activity in hepatocellular carcinoma. Int J Cancer. 2008;123(5):998–1004. https://doi.org/10.1002/ijc.23650.

153. Zhang F, Sodroski C, Cha H, Li Q, Liang TJ. Infection of hepatocytes with HCV increases cell surface levels of heparan sulfate proteoglycans, uptake of cholesterol and lipoprotein, and virus entry by up-regulating SMAD6 and SMAD7. Gastroenterology. 2017;152(1):257–70.e7. https://doi.org/10.1053/j.gastro.2016.09.033.

154. Zhang JC, Gao B, Yu ZT, Liu XB, Lu J, Xie F, et al. Promoter hypermethylation of p14 (ARF), RB, and INK4 gene family in hepatocellular carcinoma with hepatitis B virus infection. Tumour Biol. 2014;35(3):2795–802. https://doi.org/10.1007/s13277-013-1372-0.

155. Zhang S, Tan IB, Sapari NS, Grabsch HI, Okines A, Smyth EC, et al. Technical reproducibility of single-nucleotide and size-based DNA biomarker assessment using DNA extracted from formalin-fixed, paraffin-embedded tissues. J Mol Diagn. 2015;17(3):242–50. https://doi.org/10.1016/j.jmoldx.2014.12.001.

156. Zheng C, Li J, Wang Q, Liu W, Zhou J, Liu R, et al. MicroRNA-195 functions as a tumor suppressor by inhibiting CBX4 in hepatocellular carcinoma. Oncol Rep. 2015;33(3):1115–22. https://doi.org/10.3892/or.2015.3734.

157. Zink LM, Hake SB. Histone variants: nuclear function and disease. Curr Opin Genet Dev. 2016;37:82–9. https://doi.org/10.1016/j.gde.2015.12.002.

158. Zopf S, Ocker M, Neureiter D, Alinger B, Gahr S, Neurath MF, Di Fazio P. Inhibition of DNA methyltransferase activity and expression by treatment with the pan-deacetylase inhibitor panobinostat in hepatocellular carcinoma cell lines. BMC Cancer. 2012;12:386. https://doi.org/10.1186/1471-2407-12-386.

Biomarker Discovery and Validation in HCC Diagnosis, Prognosis, and Therapy

6

Lanjing Zhang

6.1 Introduction

In the USA, liver cancers are one of the only three cancers with rising mortality rates, while a steady decrease in mortality has been observed in other cancers [1]. They are also the fourth most common cancer in China and the third most deadly cancer in China [2]. The most common liver cancer is hepatocellular carcinoma (HCC) [1] and is the main focus of liver cancer research and that of this chapter. Biomarkers are critical for the diagnosis, prognostication, and management of HCC and have been developed significantly in the past decade, in part due to the advancement in molecular diagnostic and precision medicine [3–7]. The recent updates, discovery, and validation of liver cancer biomarkers will be reviewed here, as well as the methodological considerations on cancer biomarker research.

6.2 Epidemiological Considerations on Cancer Biomarkers

6.2.1 The Definition of Cancer Biomarker

The definition of biomarkers significantly varies among scholars. One school of thought considers the markers that could predict patients' responses to treatments as

L. Zhang, M.D., M.S., F.C.A.P., F.A.C.G.
Department of Pathology, University Medical Center of Princeton, Plainsboro, NJ, USA

Rutgers Cancer Institute of New Jersey, New Brunswick, NJ, USA

Department of Chemical Biology, Ernest Mario School of Pharmacy, Rutgers University, Piscataway, NJ, USA

Department of Biological Sciences, Faculty of Arts and Sciences, Rutgers University, Newark, NJ, USA
e-mail: lanjing.zhang@rutgers.edu

© Springer International Publishing AG 2018
C. Liu (ed.), *Precision Molecular Pathology of Liver Cancer*,
Molecular Pathology Library, https://doi.org/10.1007/978-3-319-68082-8_6

biomarkers [8–10], while the other uses a much broader definition. For example, the biomarkers referred to in the National Cancer Care Network (NCCN) compendium for cancer biomarkers include "all tests measuring genes or gene products, which are used for diagnosis, screening, monitoring, surveillance, or for providing predictive or prognostic information" [5]. Consistent with the NCCN guidelines, the term "biomarkers" used in recent updates on the biomarkers of HCC also includes markers useful for cancer risk stratification, screening, diagnosis, prediction of drug responses, and prognostication [6, 7, 11]. Due to the wide use of College of American Pathologists (CAP) guidelines among pathologists in the USA and the rest of the world, it is recommended adopting the boarder definition of cancer biomarkers which is used by the CAP Cancer Biomarker Reporting Group. The group develops the templates for reporting results of biomarker testing of specimens for common cancers, if not all cancer types, with strong collaboration with sister professional societies such as the American Society of Clinical Oncology and Association for Molecular Pathology [12, 13]. Twelve templates for reporting biomarker testing in various cancers have been published, with the latest one on thyroid cancer specimens [14], but no templates for liver cancer are yet developed or published by the group.

6.2.2 Epidemiological Considerations of Biomarker Discovery and Validation

The characteristics and performance of a diagnostic test are best described with its sensitivity, specificity, positive predictive value (PPV), negative predictive value (NPV), and receiver-operator curve [8]. Formula 6.1–6.4 illustrates how these parameters are calculated. It is noteworthy that PPV and NPV are both test-population dependent; therefore, the tested or applicable population must be defined when reporting PPV and NPV (Table 6.1).

$$\text{Sensitivity} = \frac{TP}{TP + FN} = \frac{TP}{\text{Gold standard test positive cases}} \tag{6.1}$$

$$\text{Specificity} = \frac{TN}{TN + FP} = \frac{TN}{\text{Gold standard test negative cases}} \tag{6.2}$$

$$PPV = \frac{TP}{TP + FP} = \frac{TP}{\text{New biomarker positive cases}} \tag{6.3}$$

$$NPV = \frac{TN}{TN + FN} = \frac{TN}{\text{New test negative cases}} \tag{6.4}$$

PPV, positive predictive value; NPV, negative predictive value

Discovery and validation of diagnostic and prognostic tests are hurdled in part by the lack of related standards and guidelines [15, 16]. Recently, several guidelines

Table 6.1 The 2 × 2 table for describing the performance of diagnostic tests

New biomarker	Gold standard test	
	Negative	Positive
Negative	True negative (TN)	False negative (FN)
Positive	False positive (FP)	True positive (TP)

have been developed or updated to increase the transparency, reporting quality and reproducibility of the studies concerning diagnostic and prognostic tests [17–19]. The 2015 Standards for Reporting Diagnostic Accuracy (STARD) statement is the latest guidelines devoted into reporting diagnostic tests and includes a checklist of 30 items [18]. The 2015 Transparent Reporting of a multivariable prediction model for Individual Prognosis Or Diagnosis (TRIPOD) statement is a checklist of 22 items and should be used for reporting results of any prediction-model study, regardless of the study methods [17]. Both checklists are accepted by many medical journals and required for manuscript submission. However, their validity and effects on improving reporting quality remain unclear.

The European group on tumor biomarkers developed two documents on tumor biomarker development and validation [20, 21]. This group proposed a clinical trial-type four-phase model for biomarker monitoring studies [21]. They later also proposed a four-step method in advancing a biomarker candidate to clinical application, including analytical validation of the biomarker assay, clinical validation of the biomarker test, demonstration of clinical value of the biomarker test, and regulatory approval [20]. This statement also recommends registering all clinical-value demonstration studies of tumor markers prior to their initiation at a clinical trial registry such as clinicaltrials.gov. However, despite the emphasis on registering biomarker studies [21], the (tumor) biomarker studies are less often incorporated in the clinical trials than the interventional studies [unpublished data, Zhang L]. Therefore, some scholars urge stronger collaborations and establishment of cancer biomarker registries [22]. On the other hand, much is unknown or misunderstood regarding how to rigorously design studies for and to analyze the data concerning cancer biomarkers [15, 20, 23–31]. Investigators are strongly recommended to familiarize and adhere to the guidelines or consensuses on the study design and data interpretation for cancer biomarkers [19–21, 32, 33]. Epidemiology or biostatistics experts should be consulted in any cancer biomarker research. In the meantime, epidemiologists and biostatisticians may also seek better optimizing or simplifying the study designs and modeling for cancer biomarker identification and validation.

Validation of cancer biomarker requires prospective, blinded trials, while randomization is often difficult, if not impossible, for the studies on diagnostic tests [20]. Early involvement of epidemiologists or biostatisticians is strongly recommended so that one could reduce the errors or biases in the study design, data interpretation, and reporting and modeling of the data. These errors and biases, if not reduced or prevented, could cost significant time, efforts, and resources because of the introduction of confounders and misinterpretation of the data.

6.2.3 The FDA-Defined Companion Diagnostics and Complementary Diagnostics

Predictive biomarkers for drug administration include companion diagnostic and complementary diagnostic tests. According to the US Food and Drug Administration (US FDA), a companion diagnostic device can be an in vitro diagnostic device or an imaging tool that provides information that is essential for the safe and effective use of a corresponding therapeutic product [34]. Therefore, companion diagnostics are required for approval, co-approval, and labeling of associated drugs and devices and subsequently any clinical use of either approved drugs or devices except in the setting of off-label uses. As of November 2016, approximately 35 approvals for companion diagnostics have been issued by the US FDA. Most of them (32/35 approvals, 91.4%) are for oncology drugs. Definition of complementary diagnostics is not yet given by the US FDA despite being used for two of the approved oncology drugs.

Recently, three programmed cell death-1 (PD-1)/programmed cell death ligand-1 (PDL-1)-based immune checkpoint inhibitors (antibodies) were approved by the US FDA for patients with advanced melanoma, non-small cell lung cancer (NSCLC), head and neck squamous cell carcinoma, or urothelial carcinoma, including alphabetically listed atezolizumab (anti-PD-L1, brand name TECENTRIQ® by Genentech Oncology), nivolumab (anti-PD-1, brand name OPDIVO® by Bristol-Myers Squibb Company), and pembrolizumab (anti-PD-1, brand name KEYTRUDA® by Merck & Co., Inc.) [35–41]. They appeared to offer sustainable antitumor effects, a significant advantage over other classes of oncology drugs. A companion diagnostic test (PD-L1 IHC 22C3 pharmDx, formerly Dako North America, now part of Agilent Technologies, Santa Clara, CA, 95051) is required for pembrolizumab uses [36]. On the other hand, perhaps confusingly, the US FDA approved complementary diagnostics for atezolizumab (complementary test: Ventana PD-L1 [SP142], Ventana Medical Systems, based in Tucson, Arizona) and nivolumab (complementary test: PD-L1 IHC 28-8 pharmDx, formerly Dako North America, now part of Agilent Technologies, Santa Clara, CA, 95051), respectively [36, 42–44]. These complementary diagnostics are important to "help physicians determine which patients may benefit most from treatment with" associated drugs [45]. Some scholars consider that complementary diagnostics may be applicable not only with a specific drug but with a class of drugs [46], although the specific definition of complementary diagnostics remains to be further clarified or explained by the US FDA.

The scoring algorithms and positivity criteria for the complementary/companion diagnostics are different among these drugs [36, 42–44]. To help choose patients for atezolizumab use, the positive tumor-infiltrating immune cell staining in urothelial carcinoma using Ventana PD-L1 [SP142] IHC should show "presence of discernible PD-L1 staining of any intensity in tumor-infiltrating immune cells covering >5% of tumor area occupied by tumor cells, associated intratumoral, and contiguous peritumoral stroma" [47]. For guiding the use of nivolumab for NSCLC patients, the percentage of tumor cells should be determined by the membranous PD-L1 staining of any intensity in a minimum of 100 evaluable tumor cells using the Dako PD-L1 IHC 28-8 pharmDx [36, 42, 43]. For the approved use of pembrolizumab in NSCLC, the tumor proportion score (TPS), as determined by the percentage of viable tumor cells showing partial or complete membrane staining for PD-L1 IHC (22C3 pharmDx), should be assessed [48]. The specimen should be considered PD-L1 positive, if TPS ≥ 50% of the viable tumor cells exhibit membrane staining at any intensity, and administration of pembrolizumab may then be considered [48]. It must be stressed that *a positive TPS is required* before pembrolizumab could be given to a patient with advanced NSCLC. To increase test portability, improve concordance of the PD-L1 test results, and decrease the costs of having different test platforms, standardization or harmonization of these tests seems important and is being considered in recent years [49, 50].

Despite that increasingly more cancers are approved for the anti-PD-1/PD-L1 immunotherapy, none of these anti-PD-1/PD-L1 based immunotherapies is yet approved by the US FDA for treating any of the tumors of the GI tract, liver, and pancreatobiliary tract by December 2016 [35]. However, several trials are undergoing for HCC. Specifically, a search in the US clinical trial registry (clinicaltrials.gov) in early December 2016 shows that seven trials on pembrolizumab, five trials on nivolumab, and no trials on atezolizumab are recruiting patients for treating HCC. If searched by the immune checkpoint inhibitor types, 8 clinical trials on the safety or efficacy of PD-1 or PD1 in HCC patients are undergoing and 11 on that of PD-L1 or PDL1. Therefore, it is reasonable to speculate that these drugs and their associated biomarkers/diagnostic tests may be applicable to HCC patients in a near future. It is noteworthy that the prospective companion or complementary diagnostics for the use of these drugs in HCC patients may be different from the currently approved ones for other cancers, such as NSCLC. In May, 2017, the US FDA approved the first tissue/site agonistic indication to pembrolizumab (Keytruda®). The drug is indicated for the treatment of adult and pediatric patients with unresectable or metastatic solid tumors, including HCC, that have been identified as having a biomarker referred to as microsatellite instability-high (MSI-H) or mismatch repair deficient (dMMR).

6.3 Established Biomarkers for HCC Diagnosis, Prognosis, and Treatment

6.3.1 Introduction

It is agreed among the guidelines developed by various international and regional hepatology societies (often named as an association for the study of the liver), that at-risk population should be screened for early detection of liver cancers [4, 5, 51–60]. However, the use of and the choice of cancer biomarkers vary among these guidelines. Several recent, noteworthy reviews and updates highlight the major differences among the guidelines and may help the caring physicians manage liver cancer patients and better use cancer biomarkers [3, 61–64]. The guidelines of various hepatology societies concerning HCC biomarkers are here compared and discussed. It is hoped that this section may provide some evidence which physicians, surgeons, and pathologists could refer to in their daily practices. A noteworthy reference book for clinical pathology also briefly discusses the tumor markers of HCC and its mimickers [65].

6.3.2 Liver Cancer Biomarkers for Screening

Guidelines and consensus statements on liver cancer biomarkers have been developed and revised by many local and regional hepatological and oncological societies, including the American Association for the Study of Liver Diseases (AASLD), European Association for the Study of the Liver (EASL), Asia-Pacific Association for the Study of the Liver (APASL), European Society for Medical Oncology (ESMO), and Sociedad Española de Oncología Médica (SEOM) [55, 66–69]. With advancement in imaging technology, most of the traditional liver cancer biomarkers are no longer favored by recent or updated guidelines [55, 66–69], except the 2015 Japanese guidelines [52].

Alpha-Fetoprotein (AFP)

AFP is a major α-fetal serum protein isoform and a carcinoembryonic protein. Elevated AFP could be seen in patients with primary HCC or germ cell tumors, while transiently elevation of AFP is also seen during pregnancy and in many benign liver diseases [65]. Combination of AFP and ultrasound was the most commonly used screening tool for liver cancer. However, due to limited sensitivity and specificity, AFP was no longer recommended by AASLD, EASL, APASL, ESMO, and SEOM for liver cancer screening in *at-risk populations* [55, 66–69]. The same position is adopted by the NCCN in 2016 [5], while AFP was recommended for liver cancer screening in junction with ultrasound and posttreatment follow-up in the 2009 NCCN guidelines [60]. Interestingly, the latest NCCN guidelines also state that AFP may still be considered for liver cancer screening in the *no-risk population*. However, comparison of the guidelines showed the other professional societies (especially Eastern Asians) had different opinions regarding using AFP as a screening tool for the at-risk populations [3, 62–64]. Specifically, the Japanese, Korean, and Singaporean societies recommended using AFP as a screening tool for HCC early detection in at-risk populations [51, 70, 71], while the Latin America Association for the Study of the Liver (LAASL) recommended using AFP to surveil at-risk populations when quality ultrasound imaging studies are not available [72]. In addition, some scholars still appreciate the usefulness of AFP as a screening tool [73]. Therefore, one must consider the local and regional guidelines and personal experiences in deciding whether to use AFP as a biomarker for liver cancer screening.

Lens culinaris agglutinin-Reactive Glycoform of AFP (AFP-L3)

Compared with the AFP produced by normal hepatocytes, the AFP secreted by malignant hepatocytes contains unusual and complex sugar chains [65]. AFP-L3 is one of the AFP isoforms with unusual sugar chains and, as the name implies, is reactive to *Lens culinaris agglutinin* [74, 75]. In patients with a total AFP of 10–200 ng/mL, >10% of AFP-L3% had a sensitivity of 71% and a specificity of 63% for diagnosis of HCC, while >35% of AFP-L3% had a reduced sensitivity of 33% and a specificity of 100% [75]. At the cutoff of 10.9 ng/mL, AFP-L3 is more specific for detecting early HCC than APF (94% versus 82%) but less sensitive

(37% versus 65%) [7, 74]. Therefore, it is understandable that the Japanese guidelines still recommends using APF-L3 for screening early HCC in high-risk population, with a US study and an optional CT or MRI study [52, 62]. It is noteworthy that NCCN, EASL, ESMO, and AASLD do not support the use of AFP-L3 for screening early HCC [5, 55, 66–69].

Des-γ-Carboxy Prothrombin (DCP)

Plasma DCP, also known as proteins induced by vitamin K absence-II (PIVKA-II), is raised in most of the HCC patients [65]. A possible cause is an overproduction of prothrombin precursor with reduced gamma-carboxylation [76]. At the current clinical cutoff of 150 mAU/mL, DCP is more sensitive than APF and APF-L3 but less specific than APF and APF-L3 in HCC [74]. Similar findings are also present in the early-stage HCC [74]. Interestingly, combination of using DCP and AFP (either above the cutoffs) would reach the highest sensitivity of 86% in all HCC and 78% in early-stage HCC, as well as the largest area under the curve, while with the lowest septicity [74]. Therefore, it is reasonable that several recent or updated guidelines do not support the use of DCP for early HCC screening, including the NCCN, EASL, Singaporean, and Korean guidelines [5, 51, 67, 77]. This recommendation is indeed consistent with the FDA-approved use of DCP for risk stratification in chronic liver disease patients. However, the Japanese guidelines still recommend its use [52]. And two other guidelines did not comment on the use of DCP for screening HCC [55, 66].

6.3.3 Liver Cancer Biomarkers for Predicting Treatment Responses

It is agreed by various guidelines that no known biomarkers are useful for predicting treatment responses in the HCC patients with surgical treatment, radiotherapy, or chemotherapy [5, 55, 67, 71]. Specifically, there is a lack of (molecular) biomarkers for predicting responses to sorafenib, the mainstream treatment option for HCC patients with preserved liver functions (Child-Pugh A class) and advanced cancer stage (BCLC C) [5, 67].

Regarding overall prognosis, the NCCN guidelines mention that AFP ≥455 ng/mL independently predicts a worse prognosis in HCC patients with transplant surgery [5], while the EASL–EORTC guidelines recommend that an AFP cutoff of >200 and/or >400 ng/mL may be used to predict a worse prognosis [67]. In addition, according to the EASL-EORTC guidelines, the levels of AFP, vascular growth factor (VEGF), and angiopoietin-2 (Ang2) could all independently predict the survival of patients with untreated advanced HCC [67, 78].

Some gene signatures or biomarkers are being validated for HCC prognostication including EpCAM signature, G3-proliferation subclass, miR-26a, and poor-survival signature [79–82]. Before being validated by prospective, randomized trials, these gene signatures and biomarkers should be used carefully in clinical practice.

6.3.4 Liver Cancer Biomarker for Post-resection Surveillance

The updated or recently published guidelines agree that serum markers, commonly AFP, may be used to monitor the patients with resected HCC. The NCCN guidelines recommend to measure AFP levels, in the patients with initially elevated AFP, every 3 months for 2 years than every 6–12 months with or without surveillance by imaging studies (three-phase high-quality cross-sectional imaging for the same interval schedules), although it acknowledges that only limited data on the subject are available [5]. For the same patient population, the Korean guidelines instead recommend both AFP and imaging studies, without specifying optimal monitoring intervals [77]. The ESMO-ESDO and SEOM guidelines, on the other hand, recommends not to use serum markers alone for HCC post-resection surveillance and to use dynamic CT or MRI studies every 3 months for 2 years and every 6 months afterward [55, 68, 83].

6.4 Emerging Biomarkers for the Diagnosis, Prognosis, and Treatment of HCC

Genomic-wide molecular profiling of HCC and dysplasia was carried out as early as 2007 [84]. With the advancement in genomic medicine and our understanding of genomic data, it was hoped that genomic and genetic data could be incorporated into the HCC management as a biomarker [85–87]. Epigenetic markers are another group of emerging biomarkers for HCC prognostication and treatment-response prediction [88, 89]. Related epigenetic markers and proteomic-based approaches also reveal several interesting protein biomarkers for HCC [7, 54, 90]. Finally, microRNA is an increasingly expanding group of biomarkers [54, 91–93]. Several recent articles summarize the emerging biomarkers for the diagnosis, prognosis, and treatment of HCC [6, 7, 59, 85]. However, despite the enthusiasm in and potential promises of these emerging biomarkers, none of these biomarkers are supported by high-level clinical evidence for regular clinical use, endorsed by any clinical guidelines or reimbursed by insurers.

6.4.1 Serum Proteins

As the classic biomarkers for HCC, serum-based proteins are still one of major interests in the biomarker research field. Most of these biomarkers could be assessed using clinical chemistry methodology and appear clinically applicable.

Gypican 3
Gypican 3 (GPC-3) is a cell surface (plasma membrane)-bound heparan sulfate proteoglycan and was found expressed in 72% of HCC tissue by immunohistochemistry and elevated in 53% of HCC patients (no elevation seen in any healthy subjects of the same study) [94]. The sensitivity and specificity of GPC-3 were 61.33% and 41.82%, reportedly lower than that of AFP (68.57% and 94.55%) as shown in a study [95], while

another meta-analysis showed comparable sensitivity and specificity of GPC-3 and AFP [96]. Recently, GPC-HCC, a novel score based on combination of GPC-3 and routine laboratory tests, was developed for HCC diagnosis and could reach an even higher sensitivity of 93% and specificity of 93% [97]. The finding seems very promising.

Osteopontin

Osteopontin (OPN), a transformation-related protein phosphatase, is an integrin-binding glycophosphoprotein produced by several types of malignancies, including lung, breast, and colon cancers [6]. Its sensitivity and specificity for detecting early HCC ranged 72–83% and 62–63%, respectively [6, 7]. A prior report suggests OPN produces lower accuracy than GPC-3 and AFP [98]. However, a recent prospective, population study found that combination of OPN and liver function tests would increase its performance in detecting HCC, and more strikingly combination of AFP and OPN was best able to predict HCC risk in this low-risk population [99]. Despite the finding's potential significance, validation studies are needed.

Golgi Protein 73

Golgi protein 73 (GP73) is a type II Golgi-specific transmembrane protein and normally not present in hepatocytes [6, 7]. Its expression is increased in chronic liver diseases and substantially elevated in HCC patients [6, 7]. In 2005, GP73 was reportedly increased in the sera of 57% of HCC patients with low AFP serum levels, with a sensitivity better than AFP [100]. A larger study later also showed, using 8.5 relative units as a cutoff value, GP73 had the sensitivity of 74.6% and specificity of 97.4% [101]. However, as other emerging biomarkers, the highest sensitivity and specificity of GP73 would be achieved when combined with AFP [102, 103]. Some scholars also noticed the lower sensitivity of detecting GP73 using immunoblotting than using enzyme-linked immunosorbent assay [7, 100, 103, 104]. Therefore, detection methods may have some impact on the performance of GP73.

6.4.2 Liquid Biopsy for Liver Cancers

Current methods of liquid biopsy for cancers assess one of the three subjects, circulating DNA/RNA, tumor cells, and exosomes from the tumors in the blood [105]. Liquid biopsy offers patients the benefits of convenience, low costs, and avoidance of potential side effects caused by invasive biopsies. However, none of them is approved for primary diagnosis but monitoring disease progression or recurrence [105]. Many homebrewed and commercial products are available in the market, while much is not known about the HCC-related circulating DNA/RNA, circulating tumor cells, and exosomes in blood.

Circulating DNA/RNA

Circulating cell-free DNA (cfDNA) has been used as a cancer biomarker since the late 2000s, while many studies were underpowered, and the cfDNA sensitivity and specificity seemed limited at the time [106]. Using branched DNA as the marker of cfDNA, one group reported a sensitivity of 53% for cfDNA alone, comparable to the sensitivity of 53.8% and 66.7% for AFP and AFP-L3, respectively [107]. Combination of cfDNA and one of the two known HCC biomarkers (AFP or AFP-L3) reached a sensitivity higher than either alone, suggestive of a potential diagnostic value of cfDNA [107]. A recent circulating microRNA study in China showed promising diagnostic values of serum miR-10b, miR-106b, and miR-181a for early HCC detection, with area under the curve of >85% [91]. Recent works also show that circulating DNA and protein biomarkers jointly could predict clinical responsiveness of regorafenib and prognosis of patients with metastatic colorectal cancer [108]. It is hoped that circulating DNA may be used to serve a similar role in HCC. The major limitation of circulating DNA/RNA is low specificity [109]. Given its considerably high sensitivity, it is recommended to use circulating DNA/RNA as a screening tool for HCC detection, with or without additional cancer biomarker of AFP or AFP-L3 [91, 109].

Circulating Tumor Cells (CTC)

Ber-EP4 antibody was one of the first tools used to detect circulating HCC cells [110]. Many attempts were since then made to identify biomarkers for circulating HCC cells [111–114]. One study also identified CD90 + CXCR4+ cells as circulating tumor stem cells of HCC [114]. Nanotechnology was also employed to better isolate CTC of HCC [115]. Besides diagnosis and monitoring disease progression, CTC of HCC may help prognostication of HCC [116–118]. However, the known HCC biomarkers and other common epithelial markers were found not specific for HCC, including AFP, asialoglycoprotein receptor or epithelial cell adhesion molecule, and CD133 or CD90 [119]. Additional validation studies are needed to confirm these markers and clinical utilities of HCC CTC.

CTC may also help predict treatment outcomes [105]. The burden of epithelial cell adhesion molecule-positive (EpCAM+) CTC of HCC could predict prognosis of patients with resected HCC [120]. Moreover, IGFBP1 mRNA expression levels in the (EpCAM+) CTC of HCC could help choose patients who are more likely responsive to radiotherapy [121]. Furthermore, pERK/pAkt phenotyping in CTC may predict sorafenib efficacy for advanced HCC [122]. Recently, circulating breast cancer cells may be cultured in vitro and then used to assess the drug sensitivity for guiding clinical choice of chemotherapy agents [123]. For the similar application in HCC, microfluidic chips were developed to culture CTC and examine their drug sensitivity for clinical use [124].

Exosomes

Exosomes are a type of extracellular vesicles, ranging 40–150 nm in size. They contain DNAs, RNAs, and proteins [125]. Early interest in exosomes was focused on its role in therapeutic target discovery and immunotherapy [126, 127]. In 2012, a report showed that anticancer drug could induce secretion of exosomes from HCC [128]. Recent reports consider that circulating exosomes and their contents may serve as biomarkers for cancer diagnosis and progression surveillance [105, 125]. Several exosome-based biomarkers for HCC have been identified [129, 130]. For example, miR-718 in serum exosomes may predict HCC recurrence after liver transplant [131]. However, one caveat is that exosomes may be released at the stimulation of hepatitis B or C infection [130]. Additional specific markers in the exosomes appear needed for better diagnostic specificity.

6.5   Perspectives

6.5.1   Future Research Directions

The aforementioned emerging biomarkers definitely show great promises. More resources and efforts probably should be focused on them.

An often-understudied subject concerning cancer biomarkers is the barrier in technology diffusion. Such a barrier might be present in the adoption of new endoscopic technology and diagnostic tests of prostate cancer [132, 133]. In addition, technology diffusion of newer treatment modality may not necessarily lead to better care quality and clinical outcomes [134–136]. The driving cause(s) of the counterintuitive findings in prostate cancer is not clear but may be linked to the issues associated with the bona fide clinical efficacy of new technology and the adherence to the FDA-approved indications. It is also not clear how the removal of AFP as a recommended screening method will impact the long-term outcomes of the HCC high-risk population at large, despite its sound scientific/clinical merits. Moreover, much is not known about the economic and clinical effects of technology diffusion on liver cancer biomarker discovery, validation, and clinical utility.

Big data become increasingly important for epidemiological studies [137–141]. Due to the higher incidence of liver cancers in the low-income countries, they may offer significant advantages for these countries, while the improvements in the quality, quantity, storage, and analysis of health data seem to be the major challenges [137]. Moreover, cautions should be taken on how to methodologically minimize biases in the observational studies and trials using big data [138, 140]. Finally, harmonization of test platform and exchangeability of the results may also be considered for future development of liver cancer biomarkers using big data [141].

Meta-analyses and systematic reviews are underutilized in diagnostic pathologic studies [142]. Their values in aiding diagnostic pathology, including biomarker identification and utilization, have become gradually recognized in the recent years [142]. In fact, more than 50% of the meta-analyses and systematic reviews in diagnostic pathology are related to biomarker (unpublished data, Kinzler M and Zhang L). Marchevsky and Wick provided an elegant review on the evidence-based pathology with a focus on systematic review and meta-analysis [143], while our group attempted to share some practical tips regarding the use of meta-analysis for diagnostic pathology [144]. It is very likely that meta-analysis and systematic review will help improve liver cancer biomarker discovery and validation.

The adherences to the AASLD guidelines appear poor and will likely impact the clinical outcomes of the population with a diagnosis or a risk of liver cancers

[145–148]. More research efforts may have been focused on the problem of knowledge diffusion/guideline adherence, i.e., increasing the patient and physician's adherence to the guidelines.

6.5.2 Summary

Cancer biomarkers are critical for detecting HCC and guiding treatment of HCC. AFP is one of the classic and most widely used biomarkers for HCC detection and post-surgery surveillance; however, it is no longer recommended for screening high-risk patients by most of the current guidelines. The reason may be less desirable sensitivity and specificity and perhaps also increased diagnostic accuracy of noninvasive imaging study methods. Advancement in precision medicine, genomic medicine, microRNA, next-generation sequencing, computational biology, and other emerging technologies are shifting the paradigm of cancer biomarker discovery. On the other hand, the stringent validation methodology (largely epidemiology based) seems to remain the same and still adhere to its goal of providing the highest possible level of clinical evidence and statistical powers. Finally, cancer biomarkers largely rely on the development of new (precision medicine based) therapeutics; by the same token, cancer biomarkers are also increasingly used for selecting patients for a given new medicine or treatment modality. Anti-PD-1/PD-L1 therapy is one of the examples and will likely be applied in HCC patients in the near future.

References

1. Siegel RL, Miller KD, Jemal A. Cancer statistics, 2016. CA Cancer J Clin. 2016;66:7–30.
2. Chen W, Zheng R, Baade PD, Zhang S, Zeng H, Bray F, et al. Cancer statistics in China, 2015. CA Cancer J Clin. 2016;66:115–32.
3. Yu SJ. A concise review of updated guidelines regarding the management of hepatocellular carcinoma around the world: 2010-2016. Clin Mol Hepatol. 2016;22:7–17.
4. Sangiovanni A, Colombo M. Treatment of hepatocellular carcinoma: beyond international guidelines. Liver Int. 2016;36(Suppl 1):124–9.
5. NCCN. NCCN guidelines: hepatobiliary cancers. NNCN; 2016.
6. Tsuchiya N, Sawada Y, Endo I, Saito K, Uemura Y, Nakatsura T. Biomarkers for the early diagnosis of hepatocellular carcinoma. World J Gastroenterol. 2015;21:10573–83.
7. Chaiteerakij R, Addissie BD, Roberts LR. Update on biomarkers of hepatocellular carcinoma. Clin Gastroenterol Hepatol. 2015;13:237–45.
8. Simon R. Sensitivity, specificity, PPV, and NPV for predictive biomarkers. J Natl Cancer Inst. 2015;107:djv153.
9. Janes H, Pepe MS, McShane LM, Sargent DJ, Heagerty PJ. The fundamental difficulty with evaluating the accuracy of biomarkers for guiding treatment. J Natl Cancer Inst. 2015;107:djv157.
10. Sawyers CL. The cancer biomarker problem. Nature. 2008;452:548–52.
11. Birkeland ML, McClure JS. Optimizing the clinical utility of biomarkers in oncology: the NCCN biomarkers compendium. Arch Pathol Lab Med. 2015;139:608–11.
12. Fitzgibbons PL, Lazar AJ, Spencer S. Introducing new College of American Pathologists reporting templates for cancer biomarkers. Arch Pathol Lab Med. 2014;138:157–8.

13. Cagle PT, Sholl LM, Lindeman NI, Alsabeh R, Divaris DX, Foulis P, et al. Template for reporting results of biomarker testing of specimens from patients with non-small cell carcinoma of the lung. Arch Pathol Lab Med. 2014;138:171–4.
14. Chiosea S, Asa SL, Berman MA, Carty SE, Currence L, Hodak S, et al. Template for reporting results of biomarker testing of specimens from patients with thyroid carcinoma. Arch Pathol Lab Med. 2017;141(4):559–63.
15. Azuaje F, Devaux Y, Wagner D. Challenges and standards in reporting diagnostic and prognostic biomarker studies. Clin Transl Sci. 2009;2:156–61.
16. Ransohoff DF. How to improve reliability and efficiency of research about molecular markers: roles of phases, guidelines, and study design. J Clin Epidemiol. 2007;60:1205–19.
17. Collins GS, Reitsma JB, Altman DG, Moons KG. Transparent Reporting of a multivariable prediction model for Individual Prognosis or Diagnosis (TRIPOD): the TRIPOD statement. Ann Intern Med. 2015;162:55–63.
18. Bossuyt PM, Reitsma JB, Bruns DE, Gatsonis CA, Glasziou PP, Irwig L, et al. STARD 2015: an updated list of essential items for reporting diagnostic accuracy studies. BMJ. 2015;351:h5527.
19. McShane LM, Altman DG, Sauerbrei W, Taube SE, Gion M, Clark GM. Reporting recommendations for tumor marker prognostic studies (REMARK). J Natl Cancer Inst. 2005;97:1180–4.
20. Duffy MJ, Sturgeon CM, Soletormos G, Barak V, Molina R, Hayes DF, et al. Validation of new cancer biomarkers: a position statement from the European group on tumor markers. Clin Chem. 2015;61:809–20.
21. Soletormos G, Duffy MJ, Hayes DF, Sturgeon CM, Barak V, Bossuyt PM, et al. Design of tumor biomarker-monitoring trials: a proposal by the European Group on Tumor Markers. Clin Chem. 2013;59:52–9.
22. Andre F, McShane LM, Michiels S, Ransohoff DF, Altman DG, Reis-Filho JS, et al. Biomarker studies: a call for a comprehensive biomarker study registry. Nat Rev Clin Oncol. 2011;8:171–6.
23. Fine JP, Pencina M. On the quantitative assessment of predictive biomarkers. J Natl Cancer Inst. 2015;107:djv187.
24. Simon R. Stratification and partial ascertainment of biomarker value in biomarker-driven clinical trials. J Biopharm Stat. 2014;24:1011–21.
25. Rundle A, Ahsan H, Vineis P. Better cancer biomarker discovery through better study design. Eur J Clin Invest. 2012;42:1350–9.
26. McShane LM, Hayes DF. Publication of tumor marker research results: the necessity for complete and transparent reporting. J Clin Oncol. 2012;30:4223–32.
27. Kern SE. Why your new cancer biomarker may never work: recurrent patterns and remarkable diversity in biomarker failures. Cancer Res. 2012;72:6097–101.
28. Baker SG, Kramer BS, Sargent DJ, Bonetti M. Biomarkers, subgroup evaluation, and clinical trial design. Discov Med. 2012;13:187–92.
29. Ahern TP, Hankinson SE. Re: use of archived specimens in evaluation of prognostic and predictive biomarkers. J Natl Cancer Inst. 2011;103:1558–9; author reply 9–60.
30. Vaught JB, Hsing AW. Methodologic data: important foundation for molecular and biomarker studies. Cancer Epidemiol Biomarkers Prev. 2010;19:901–2.
31. Diamandis EP. Cancer biomarkers: can we turn recent failures into success? J Natl Cancer Inst. 2010;102:1462–7.
32. Pepe MS, Feng Z, Janes H, Bossuyt PM, Potter JD. Pivotal evaluation of the accuracy of a biomarker used for classification or prediction: standards for study design. J Natl Cancer Inst. 2008;100:1432–8.
33. Diamandis EP, Hoffman BR, Sturgeon CM. National Academy of Clinical Biochemistry laboratory medicine practice guidelines for the use of tumor markers. Clin Chem. 2008;54:1935–9.
34. Administration USFaD. In vitro companion diagnostic devices: guidance for industry and food and drug administration staff. In: Services DoHaH, editor. U.S. Food and Drug Administration; 2014.

35. Administration USFaD. Administration, hematology/oncology (cancer) approvals & safety notifications. 2016.
36. Sholl LM, Aisner DL, Allen TC, Beasley MB, Borczuk AC, Cagle PT, et al. Programmed death Ligand-1 immunohistochemistry—a new challenge for pathologists: a perspective from Members of the Pulmonary Pathology Society. Arch Pathol Lab Med. 2016;140:341–4.
37. Reck M, Rodriguez-Abreu D, Robinson AG, Hui R, Csoszi T, Fulop A, et al. Pembrolizumab versus chemotherapy for PD-L1-positive non-small-cell lung cancer. N Engl J Med. 2016;375:1823–33.
38. Ferris RL, Blumenschein G Jr, Fayette J, Guigay J, Colevas AD, Licitra L, et al. Nivolumab for recurrent squamous-cell carcinoma of the head and neck. N Engl J Med. 2016;375:1856–67.
39. Garon EB, Rizvi NA, Hui R, Leighl N, Balmanoukian AS, Eder JP, et al. Pembrolizumab for the treatment of non-small-cell lung cancer. N Engl J Med. 2015;372:2018–28.
40. Brahmer J, Reckamp KL, Baas P, Crino L, Eberhardt WE, Poddubskaya E, et al. Nivolumab versus docetaxel in advanced squamous-cell non-small-cell lung cancer. N Engl J Med. 2015;373:123–35.
41. Borghaei H, Paz-Ares L, Horn L, Spigel DR, Steins M, Ready NE, et al. Nivolumab versus docetaxel in advanced nonsquamous non-small-cell lung cancer. N Engl J Med. 2015;373:1627–39.
42. Kazandjian D, Suzman DL, Blumenthal G, Mushti S, He K, Libeg M, et al. FDA approval summary: nivolumab for the treatment of metastatic non-small cell lung cancer with progression on or after platinum-based chemotherapy. Oncologist. 2016;21:634–42.
43. Novotny JF Jr, Cogswell J, Inzunza H, Harbison C, Horak C, Averbuch S. Establishing a complementary diagnostic for anti-PD-1 immune checkpoint inhibitor therapy. Ann Oncol. 2016;27:1966–9.
44. Meng X, Huang Z, Teng F, Xing L, Yu J. Predictive biomarkers in PD-1/PD-L1 checkpoint blockade immunotherapy. Cancer Treat Rev. 2015;41:868–76.
45. Administration USFaD. FDA expands approved use of Opdivo in advanced lung cancer. 2015.
46. Milne CP, Bryan C, Garafalo S, McKiernan M. Complementary versus companion diagnostics: apples and oranges? Biomark Med. 2015;9:25–34.
47. Administration USFaD. VENTANA PD-L1 (SP142) Assay: insert. 1015005EN Rev A ed2016.
48. Administration USFaD. DAKO PD-L1 IHC 22C3 pharmDx: Insert. P03951_02/SK00621-5/2015.09 ed2015.
49. Scheel AH, Dietel M, Heukamp LC, Johrens K, Kirchner T, Reu S, et al. Harmonized PD-L1 immunohistochemistry for pulmonary squamous-cell and adenocarcinomas. Mod Pathol. 2016;29:1165–72.
50. Gaule P, Smithy JW, Toki M, Rehman J, Patell-Socha F, Cougot D, et al. A quantitative comparison of antibodies to programmed cell death 1 ligand 1. JAMA Oncol. 2016 Aug 18. doi: 10.1001/jamaoncol.2016.3015. [Epub ahead of print]
51. Chow PK, Choo SP, Ng DC, Lo RH, Wang ML, Toh HC, et al. National Cancer Centre Singapore consensus guidelines for hepatocellular carcinoma. Liver Cancer. 2016;5:97–106.
52. Kokudo N, Hasegawa K, Akahane M, Igaki H, Izumi N, Ichida T, et al. Evidence-based clinical practice guidelines for hepatocellular carcinoma: the Japan Society of Hepatology 2013 update (3rd JSH-HCC Guidelines). Hepatol Res. 2015;45:123–7.
53. Burak KW, Sherman M. Hepatocellular carcinoma: consensus, controversies and future directions. A report from the Canadian Association for the Study of the Liver Hepatocellular Carcinoma Meeting. Can J Gastroenterol Hepatol. 2015;29:178–84.
54. Lee SC, Tan HT, Chung MC. Prognostic biomarkers for prediction of recurrence of hepatocellular carcinoma: current status and future prospects. World J Gastroenterol. 2014;20:3112–24.
55. Verslype C, Rosmorduc O, Rougier P. Hepatocellular carcinoma: ESMO-ESDO Clinical Practice Guidelines for diagnosis, treatment and follow-up. Ann Oncology. 2012;23(Suppl 7):vii41–8.
56. Sherman M, Bruix J, Porayko M, Tran T. Screening for hepatocellular carcinoma: the rationale for the American Association for the Study of Liver Diseases recommendations. Hepatology (Baltimore, MD). 2012;56:793–6.

57. Qin S. Guidelines on the diagnosis and treatment of primary liver cancer (2011 edition). Chin Clin Oncol. 2012;1:10.
58. 2011 European Association of the Study of the Liver hepatitis C virus clinical practice guidelines. Liver Int. 2012;32 Suppl 1:2–8.
59. Sturgeon CM, Duffy MJ, Hofmann BR, Lamerz R, Fritsche HA, Gaarenstroom K, et al. National Academy of Clinical Biochemistry Laboratory Medicine Practice Guidelines for use of tumor markers in liver, bladder, cervical, and gastric cancers. Clin Chem. 2010;56:e1–48.
60. Benson AB 3rd, Abrams TA, Ben-Josef E, Bloomston PM, Botha JF, Clary BM, et al. NCCN clinical practice guidelines in oncology: hepatobiliary cancers. J Natl Compr Canc Netw. 2009;7:350–91.
61. Zhao C, Nguyen MH. Hepatocellular carcinoma screening and surveillance: practice guidelines and real-life practice. J Clin Gastroenterol. 2016;50(2):120–33.
62. Clinical Practice Guidelines for Hepatocellular Carcinoma Differ between Japan, United States, and Europe. Liver Cancer. 2015;4:85–95.
63. Song DS, Bae SH. Changes of guidelines diagnosing hepatocellular carcinoma during the last ten-year period. Clin Mol Hepatol. 2012;18:258–67.
64. Bota S, Piscaglia F, Marinelli S, Pecorelli A, Terzi E, Bolondi L. Comparison of international guidelines for noninvasive diagnosis of hepatocellular carcinoma. Liver Cancer. 2012;1:190–200.
65. McPherson RA, Pincus MR, Henry JB. Henry's clinical diagnosis and management by laboratory methods. 22nd ed. Philadelphia: Elsevier Saunders; 2011.
66. Bruix J, Sherman M. Management of hepatocellular carcinoma: an update. Hepatology (Baltimore, MD). 2011;53:1020–2.
67. European Association For The Study Of The Liver, European Organisation For Research And Treatment Of Cancer. EASL-EORTC clinical practice guidelines: management of hepatocellular carcinoma. J Hepatol. 2012;56:908–43.
68. Sastre J, Diaz-Beveridge R, Garcia-Foncillas J, Guardeno R, Lopez C, Pazo R, et al. Clinical guideline SEOM: hepatocellular carcinoma. Clin Transl Oncol. 2015;17:988–95.
69. Omata M, Lesmana LA, Tateishi R, Chen PJ, Lin SM, Yoshida H, et al. Asian Pacific Association for the Study of the Liver consensus recommendations on hepatocellular carcinoma. Hepatol Int. 2010;4:439–74.
70. 2014 Korean Liver Cancer Study Group-National Cancer Center Korea practice guideline for the management of hepatocellular carcinoma. Korean J Radiol. 2015;16:465–522.
71. Kudo M, Matsui O, Izumi N, Iijima H, Kadoya M, Imai Y, et al. JSH consensus-based clinical practice guidelines for the Management of Hepatocellular Carcinoma: 2014 Update by the Liver Cancer Study Group of Japan. Liver Cancer. 2014;3:458–68.
72. Mendez-Sanchez N, Ridruejo E, Alves de Mattos A, Chavez-Tapia NC, Zapata R, Parana R, et al. Latin American Association for the Study of the Liver (LAASL) clinical practice guidelines: management of hepatocellular carcinoma. Ann Hepatol. 2014;13(Suppl 1):S4–40.
73. Marrero JA, El-Serag HB. Alpha-fetoprotein should be included in the hepatocellular carcinoma surveillance guidelines of the American Association for the Study of Liver Diseases. Hepatology (Baltimore, MD). 2011;53:1060–1; author reply 1–2.
74. Marrero JA, Feng Z, Wang Y, Nguyen MH, Befeler AS, Roberts LR, et al. Alpha-fetoprotein, des-gamma carboxyprothrombin, and lectin-bound alpha-fetoprotein in early hepatocellular carcinoma. Gastroenterology. 2009;137:110–8.
75. Leerapun A, Suravarapu SV, Bida JP, Clark RJ, Sanders EL, Mettler TA, et al. The utility of Lens culinaris agglutinin-reactive alpha-fetoprotein in the diagnosis of hepatocellular carcinoma: evaluation in a United States referral population. Clin Gastroenterol Hepatol. 2007;5:394–402; quiz 267.
76. Ono M, Ohta H, Ohhira M, Sekiya C, Namiki M. Measurement of immunoreactive prothrombin precursor and vitamin-K-dependent gamma-carboxylation in human hepatocellular carcinoma tissues: decreased carboxylation of prothrombin precursor as a cause of des-gamma-carboxyprothrombin synthesis. Tumour Biol. 1990;11:319–26.

77. Korean Liver Cancer Study Group, National Cancer Center, Korea. 2014 KLCSG-NCC Korea Practice Guideline for the Management of Hepatocellular Carcinoma. Gut Liver. 2015;9:267–317.
78. Miyahara K, Nouso K, Tomoda T, Kobayashi S, Hagihara H, Kuwaki K, et al. Predicting the treatment effect of sorafenib using serum angiogenesis markers in patients with hepatocellular carcinoma. J Gastroenterol Hepatol. 2011;26:1604–11.
79. Yamashita T, Forgues M, Wang W, Kim JW, Ye Q, Jia H, et al. EpCAM and alpha-fetoprotein expression defines novel prognostic subtypes of hepatocellular carcinoma. Cancer Res. 2008;68:1451–61.
80. Ji J, Shi J, Budhu A, Yu Z, Forgues M, Roessler S, et al. MicroRNA expression, survival, and response to interferon in liver cancer. N Engl J Med. 2009;361:1437–47.
81. Villanueva A, Hoshida Y, Battiston C, Tovar V, Sia D, Alsinet C, et al. Combining clinical, pathology, and gene expression data to predict recurrence of hepatocellular carcinoma. Gastroenterology. 2011;140:1501–12.e2.
82. Hoshida Y, Villanueva A, Kobayashi M, Peix J, Chiang DY, Camargo A, et al. Gene expression in fixed tissues and outcome in hepatocellular carcinoma. N Engl J Med. 2008;359:1995–2004.
83. Hatzaras I, Bischof DA, Fahy B, Cosgrove D, Pawlik TM. Treatment options and surveillance strategies after therapy for hepatocellular carcinoma. Ann Surg Oncol. 2014;21:758–66.
84. Wurmbach E, Chen YB, Khitrov G, Zhang W, Roayaie S, Schwartz M, et al. Genome-wide molecular profiles of HCV-induced dysplasia and hepatocellular carcinoma. Hepatology (Baltimore, MD). 2007;45:938–47.
85. Zucman-Rossi J, Villanueva A, Nault JC, Llovet JM. Genetic landscape and biomarkers of hepatocellular carcinoma. Gastroenterology. 2015;149:1226–39.e4.
86. Llovet JM, Villanueva A, Lachenmayer A, Finn RS. Advances in targeted therapies for hepatocellular carcinoma in the genomic era. Nat Rev Clin Oncol. 2015;12:436.
87. Quetglas IM, Moeini A, Pinyol R, Llovet JM. Integration of genomic information in the clinical management of HCC. Best Pract Res Clin Gastroenterol. 2014;28:831–42.
88. Villanueva A, Portela A, Sayols S, Battiston C, Hoshida Y, Mendez-Gonzalez J, et al. DNA methylation-based prognosis and epidrivers in hepatocellular carcinoma. Hepatology (Baltimore, MD). 2015;61:1945–56.
89. Banaudha KK, Verma M. Epigenetic biomarkers in liver cancer. Methods Mol Biol (Clifton, NJ). 2015;1238:65–76.
90. Committee on the Review of Omics-Based Tests for Predicting Patient Outcomes in Clinical Trials, Board on Health Care Services, Board on Health Sciences Policy, Institute of Medicine. Evolution of translational omics: lessons learned and the path forward. Washington (DC): National Academies Press (US); 2012. Copyright 2012 by the National Academy of Sciences. All rights reserved; 2012.
91. Jiang L, Cheng Q, Zhang BH, Zhang MZ. Circulating microRNAs as biomarkers in hepatocellular carcinoma screening: a validation set from China. Medicine (Baltimore). 2015;94:e603.
92. Anwar SL, Lehmann U. MicroRNAs: emerging novel clinical biomarkers for hepatocellular carcinomas. J Clin Med. 2015;4:1631–50.
93. Li X, Yang W, Lou L, Chen Y, Wu S, Ding G. microRNA: a promising diagnostic biomarker and therapeutic target for hepatocellular carcinoma. Dig Dis Sci. 2014;59:1099–107.
94. Capurro M, Wanless IR, Sherman M, Deboer G, Shi W, Miyoshi E, et al. Glypican-3: a novel serum and histochemical marker for hepatocellular carcinoma. Gastroenterology. 2003;125:89–97.
95. Ozkan H, Erdal H, Kocak E, Tutkak H, Karaeren Z, Yakut M, et al. Diagnostic and prognostic role of serum glypican 3 in patients with hepatocellular carcinoma. J Clin Lab Anal. 2011;25:350–3.
96. Xu C, Yan Z, Zhou L, Wang Y. A comparison of glypican-3 with alpha-fetoprotein as a serum marker for hepatocellular carcinoma: a meta-analysis. J Cancer Res Clin Oncol. 2013;139:1417–24.
97. Attallah AM, El-Far M, Omran MM, Abdelrazek MA, Attallah AA, Saeed AM, et al. GPC-HCC model: a combination of glybican-3 with other routine parameters improves the diagnostic efficacy in hepatocellular carcinoma. Tumour Biol. 2016;37:12571–7.

98. Lee HJ, Yeon JE, Suh SJ, Lee SJ, Yoon EL, Kang K, et al. Clinical utility of plasma glypican-3 and osteopontin as biomarkers of hepatocellular carcinoma. Gut Liver. 2014;8:177–85.

99. Duarte-Salles T, Misra S, Stepien M, Plymoth A, Muller D, Overvad K, et al. Circulating osteopontin and prediction of hepatocellular carcinoma development in a large European population. Cancer Prev Res (Phila). 2016;9:758–65.

100. Marrero JA, Romano PR, Nikolaeva O, Steel L, Mehta A, Fimmel CJ, et al. GP73, a resident Golgi glycoprotein, is a novel serum marker for hepatocellular carcinoma. J Hepatol. 2005;43:1007–12.

101. Mao Y, Yang H, Xu H, Lu X, Sang X, Du S, et al. Golgi protein 73 (GOLPH2) is a valuable serum marker for hepatocellular carcinoma. Gut. 2010;59:1687–93.

102. Dai M, Chen X, Liu X, Peng Z, Meng J, Dai S. Diagnostic value of the combination of Golgi protein 73 and alpha-fetoprotein in hepatocellular carcinoma: a meta-analysis. PLoS One. 2015;10:e0140067.

103. Tian L, Wang Y, Xu D, Gui J, Jia X, Tong H, et al. Serological AFP/Golgi protein 73 could be a new diagnostic parameter of hepatic diseases. Int J Cancer. 2011;129:1923–31.

104. Wang M, Long RE, Comunale MA, Junaidi O, Marrero J, Di Bisceglie AM, et al. Novel fucosylated biomarkers for the early detection of hepatocellular carcinoma. Cancer Epidemiol Biomarkers Prev. 2009;18:1914–21.

105. Chi KR. The tumour trail left in blood. Nature. 2016;532:269–71.

106. Jung K, Fleischhacker M, Rabien A. Cell-free DNA in the blood as a solid tumor biomarker—a critical appraisal of the literature. Clin Chim Acta. 2010;411:1611–24.

107. Chen K, Zhang H, Zhang LN, Ju SQ, Qi J, Huang DF, et al. Value of circulating cell-free DNA in diagnosis of hepatocellular carcinoma. World J Gastroenterol. 2013;19:3143–9.

108. Tabernero J, Lenz HJ, Siena S, Sobrero A, Falcone A, Ychou M, et al. Analysis of circulating DNA and protein biomarkers to predict the clinical activity of regorafenib and assess prognosis in patients with metastatic colorectal cancer: a retrospective, exploratory analysis of the CORRECT trial. Lancet Oncol. 2015;16:937–48.

109. Su YH, Lin SY, Song W, Jain S. DNA markers in molecular diagnostics for hepatocellular carcinoma. Expert Rev Mol Diagn. 2014;14:803–17.

110. Sabile A, Louha M, Bonte E, Poussin K, Vona G, Mejean A, et al. Efficiency of Ber-EP4 antibody for isolating circulating epithelial tumor cells before RT-PCR detection. Am J Clin Pathol. 1999;112:171–8.

111. Zhang Y, Li J, Cao L, Xu W, Yin Z. Circulating tumor cells in hepatocellular carcinoma: detection techniques, clinical implications, and future perspectives. Semin Oncol. 2012;39:449–60.

112. Chiappini F. Circulating tumor cells measurements in hepatocellular carcinoma. Int J Hepatol. 2012;2012:684802.

113. Liu YK, Hu BS, Li ZL, He X, Li Y, Lu LG. An improved strategy to detect the epithelial-mesenchymal transition process in circulating tumor cells in hepatocellular carcinoma patients. Hepatol Int. 2016;10:640–6.

114. Zhu L, Zhang W, Wang J, Liu R. Evidence of CD90+CXCR4+ cells as circulating tumor stem cells in hepatocellular carcinoma. Tumour Biol. 2015;36:5353–60.

115. Wang S, Zhang C, Wang G, Cheng B, Wang Y, Chen F, et al. Aptamer-mediated transparent-biocompatible nanostructured surfaces for hepotocellular circulating tumor cells enrichment. Theranostics. 2016;6:1877–86.

116. Fan JL, Yang YF, Yuan CH, Chen H, Wang FB. Circulating tumor cells for predicting the prognostic of patients with hepatocellular carcinoma: a meta analysis. Cell Physiol Biochem. 2015;37:629–40.

117. Huang JW, Liu B, Hu BS, Li Y, He X, Zhao W, et al. Clinical value of circulating tumor cells for the prognosis of postoperative transarterial chemoembolization therapy. Med Oncol. 2014;31:175.

118. Zhou Y, Wang B, Wu J, Zhang C, Zhou Y, Yang X, et al. Association of preoperative EpCAM Circulating Tumor Cells and peripheral Treg cell levels with early recurrence of hepatocellular carcinoma following radical hepatic resection. BMC Cancer. 2016;16:506.

119. Wu LJ, Pan YD, Pei XY, Chen H, Nguyen S, Kashyap A, et al. Capturing circulating tumor cells of hepatocellular carcinoma. Cancer Lett. 2012;326:17–22.
120. Sun YF, Xu Y, Yang XR, Guo W, Zhang X, Qiu SJ, et al. Circulating stem cell-like epithelial cell adhesion molecule-positive tumor cells indicate poor prognosis of hepatocellular carcinoma after curative resection. Hepatology (Baltimore, MD). 2013;57:1458–68.
121. Nel I, Baba HA, Weber F, Sitek B, Eisenacher M, Meyer HE, et al. IGFBP1 in epithelial circulating tumor cells as a potential response marker to selective internal radiation therapy in hepatocellular carcinoma. Biomark Med. 2014;8:687–98.
122. Li J, Shi L, Zhang X, Sun B, Yang Y, Ge N, et al. pERK/pAkt phenotyping in circulating tumor cells as a biomarker for sorafenib efficacy in patients with advanced hepatocellular carcinoma. Oncotarget. 2016;7:2646–59.
123. Yu M, Bardia A, Aceto N, Bersani F, Madden MW, Donaldson MC, et al. Cancer therapy. Ex vivo culture of circulating breast tumor cells for individualized testing of drug susceptibility. Science. 2014;345:216–20.
124. Zhang Y, Zhang X, Zhang J, Sun B, Zheng L, Li J, et al. Microfluidic chip for isolation of viable circulating tumor cells of hepatocellular carcinoma for their culture and drug sensitivity assay. Cancer Biol Ther. 2016;17:1177–87.
125. Kalluri R. The biology and function of exosomes in cancer. J Clin Invest. 2016;126:1208–15.
126. Iero M, Valenti R, Huber V, Filipazzi P, Parmiani G, Fais S, et al. Tumour-released exosomes and their implications in cancer immunity. Cell Death Differ. 2008;15:80–8.
127. Mignot G, Roux S, Thery C, Segura E, Zitvogel L. Prospects for exosomes in immunotherapy of cancer. J Cell Mol Med. 2006;10:376–88.
128. Lv LH, Wan YL, Lin Y, Zhang W, Yang M, Li GL, et al. Anticancer drugs cause release of exosomes with heat shock proteins from human hepatocellular carcinoma cells that elicit effective natural killer cell antitumor responses in vitro. J Biol Chem. 2012;287:15874–85.
129. Wu Z, Zeng Q, Cao K, Sun Y. Exosomes: small vesicles with big roles in hepatocellular carcinoma. Oncotarget. 2016;7:60687–97.
130. Cai S, Cheng X, Pan X, Li J. Emerging role of exosomes in liver physiology and pathology. Hepatol Res. 2016 Aug 18. doi: 10.1111/hepr.12794. [Epub ahead of print]
131. Sugimachi K, Matsumura T, Hirata H, Uchi R, Ueda M, Ueo H, et al. Identification of a bona fide microRNA biomarker in serum exosomes that predicts hepatocellular carcinoma recurrence after liver transplantation. Br J Cancer. 2015;112:532–8.
132. Schroeck FR, Kaufman SR, Jacobs BL, Skolarus TA, Miller DC, Weizer AZ, et al. Technology diffusion and diagnostic testing for prostate cancer. J Urol. 2013;190:1715–20.
133. Kasumi WT, Kasumi A, Ishikawa B. The spread of upper gastrointestinal endoscopy in Japan and the United States. An international comparative analysis of technology diffusion. Int J Technol Assess Health Care. 1993;9:416–25.
134. Shen C, Tina Shih YC. Therapeutic substitutions in the midst of new technology diffusion: the case of treatment for localized prostate cancer. Soc Sci Med (1982). 2016;151:110–20.
135. Schroeck FR, Kaufman SR, Jacobs BL, Skolarus TA, Zhang Y, Hollenbeck BK. Technology diffusion and prostate cancer quality of care. Urology. 2014;84:1066–72.
136. Schroeck FR, Kaufman SR, Jacobs BL, Zhang Y, Weizer AZ, Montgomery JS, et al. The impact of technology diffusion on treatment for prostate cancer. Med Care. 2013;51:1076–84.
137. Wyber R, Vaillancourt S, Perry W, Mannava P, Folaranmi T, Celi LA. Big data in global health: improving health in low- and middle-income countries. Bull World Health Organ. 2015;93:203–8.
138. Tanaka S, Tanaka S, Kawakami K. Methodological issues in observational studies and non-randomized controlled trials in oncology in the era of big data. Jpn J Clin Oncol. 2015;45:323–7.
139. Mooney SJ, Westreich DJ, El-Sayed AM. Commentary: epidemiology in the era of big data. Epidemiology (Cambridge, MA). 2015;26:390–4.
140. Kaplan RM, Chambers DA, Glasgow RE. Big data and large sample size: a cautionary note on the potential for bias. Clin Transl Sci. 2014;7:342–6.

141. Dutruel C, Thole J, Geels M, Mollenkopf HJ, Ottenhoff T, Guzman CA, et al. TRANSVAC workshop on standardisation and harmonisation of analytical platforms for HIV, TB and malaria vaccines: 'how can big data help?'. Vaccine. 2014;32:4365–8.
142. Kinzler M, Zhang L. Underutilization of meta-analysis in diagnostic pathology. Arch Pathol Lab Med. 2015;139:1302–7.
143. Marchevsky AM, Wick MR. Evidence-based pathology: systematic literature reviews as the basis for guidelines and best practices. Arch Pathol Lab Med. 2015;139:394–9.
144. Mayo E, Kinzler M, Zhang L. Considerations for conducting meta-analysis in diagnostic pathology. Arch Pathol Lab Med. 2015;139:1331.
145. Wu Y, Johnson KB, Roccaro G, Lopez J, Zheng H, Muiru A, et al. Poor adherence to AASLD guidelines for chronic hepatitis B Management and treatment in a large academic medical center. Am J Gastroenterol. 2014;109:867–75.
146. Leoni S, Piscaglia F, Serio I, Terzi E, Pettinari I, Croci L, et al. Adherence to AASLD guidelines for the treatment of hepatocellular carcinoma in clinical practice: experience of the Bologna Liver Oncology Group. Dig Liver Dis. 2014;46:549–55.
147. Borzio M, Fornari F, De Sio I, Andriulli A, Terracciano F, Parisi G, et al. Adherence to American Association for the Study of Liver Diseases guidelines for the management of hepatocellular carcinoma: results of an Italian field practice multicenter study. Future Oncol (London, England). 2013;9:283–94.
148. Sharma P, Saini SD, Kuhn LB, Rubenstein JH, Pardi DS, Marrero JA, et al. Knowledge of hepatocellular carcinoma screening guidelines and clinical practices among gastroenterologists. Dig Dis Sci. 2011;56:569–77.

Imaging of Hepatocellular Carcinoma

7

Naziya Samreen and Joseph R. Grajo

7.1 Introduction

Hepatocellular carcinoma (HCC), the sixth most common cancer worldwide, is a frequent cause of diagnostic liver imaging [1]. It causes approximately 250,000 deaths per year worldwide [2]. Given the high prevalence of the disease, accurate screening and diagnosis of this tumor are critical for possible early intervention.

Liver cirrhosis increases the risk of HCC. The annual risk of HCC in patients with cirrhosis is approximately 1–6% [3]. Although there are a myriad of causative factors for cirrhosis including alcohol, autoimmune hepatitis, nonalcoholic fatty liver disease, and specific metabolic disorders, hepatitis B and C are responsible for a majority of causes of cirrhosis and subsequent HCC [4]. There is evidence to suggest that viral hepatitis is responsible for 75% of HCC worldwide. Given that up to 90% of HCC occurs in patients with a background of cirrhotic liver disease, screening for HCC in this patient population is critical [4].

7.2 Screening of HCC

The purpose of screening is to allow early detection of HCC in at-risk, asymptomatic individuals in order to decrease HCC-related mortality. Since the HCC tumor doubling time is 6–12 months, the American Association for the Study of Liver Diseases (AASLD) recommends HCC screening every 6 months. Ultrasound has a

N. Samreen, M.D. (✉) • J.R. Grajo, M.D.
Department of Radiology, University of Florida, Gainesville, FL, USA
e-mail: SAMREN@radiology.ufl.edu

© Springer International Publishing AG 2018
C. Liu (ed.), *Precision Molecular Pathology of Liver Cancer*,
Molecular Pathology Library, https://doi.org/10.1007/978-3-319-68082-8_7

sensitivity of 65–80% and a specificity of greater than 90% for screening of HCC [5]. It has replaced serum alpha-fetoprotein (AFP) marker as the predominant screening test for HCC.

Screening recommendations apply to patients with chronic hepatitis C who have developed cirrhosis. Some experts also recommend screening HCV-infected patients who have liver fibrosis but not cirrhosis. HCC surveillance is not recommended in HCV-infected patients without fibrosis or cirrhosis [6].

Hepatitis B is considered more oncogenic compared to hepatitis C, and, therefore, screening recommendations in patients with hepatitis B are more aggressive. In patients with hepatitis B infection, screening for HCC is recommended in patients with cirrhosis, patients with family history of HCC, Asian males >40 years, Asian females >50 years, and Africans >20 years [6].

HCC screening is also recommended in other patients with cirrhosis, including those with stage 4 primary biliary cirrhosis (PBC), genetic hemochromatosis, alpha 1 antitrypsin deficiency, or other causes of cirrhosis [6]. Surveillance is also performed in patients listed for liver transplantation because the development of HCC increases the priority of these patients on the transplant list [5].

Once a small nodule is identified on screening ultrasound, further imaging recommendations are based on the size of the nodule. If the nodule is less than 1 cm, repeat ultrasound in 3 months is recommended to assess for stability. If the nodule increases in size during the 3-month period, further investigation is recommended. If the initial nodule is greater than 1 cm, evaluation with multiphase multidetector CT or dynamic contrast-enhanced MRI is recommended [5].

7.3 Altered Hemodynamics

The physiologic and pathologic alterations that occur in a cirrhotic liver are critical to understanding the imaging findings of HCC. With cirrhosis, the liver becomes more fibrotic. There is hypertrophy of the caudate lobe (segment I) as well as the lateral segments of the left hepatic lobe (segments II and III). The portal blood flow is altered as the portal veins become more tortuous and subsequently diminutive, which may ultimately lead to reversal of portal flow. There are multiple regenerative nodules that emerge as the liver tries to regenerate its parenchyma. The umbilical vein is recanalized, and multiple varices form in an effort to divert portal flow away from the liver tissue, which now has increased parenchymal resistance. With time, dysplastic nodules can emerge, which are precancerous and can serve as precursors to HCC [7]. Stromal invasion and alteration of arterial supply to the nodule then occur, allowing the dysplastic nodule to develop into HCC. While most of the liver is supplied by the portal system (75%) in normal hepatic physiology, the predominant supply to a HCC is from the hepatic arterial system. This altered hemodynamic system is the basis of radiologic imaging as it helps differentiate background liver parenchyma from HCC.

7.4   Ultrasound

As stated previously, ultrasound is the predominant screening tool for HCC. Unenhanced brightness mode (B-mode) ultrasound is most commonly used for HCC screening. Additional sonographic tools that can be used in the detection of HCC are Doppler imaging and contrast-enhanced ultrasound.

HCC does not have a specific appearance on ultrasound (Fig. 7.1). Well-differentiated HCC less than 3 cm usually appears as a well-circumscribed hypoechoic mass [8]. There are studies to suggest that small HCCs that are less than 5 cm are hypoechoic on ultrasound approximately 75% of the time [9]. However, HCC can be hyperechoic or of mixed echogenicity on ultrasound [10]. As the tumor grows, a hypoechoic rim can develop [11]. The HCC can also become more heterogeneous with growth. If there is a fatty component to the tumor, or if there is hemorrhage within the tumor, these can lead to a hyperechoic signal as well.

Doppler ultrasound is an adjunct to B-mode ultrasound for detection of HCC. Approximately 75% of HCC tumors demonstrate internal vascularity on Doppler ultrasound. This is in contrast to liver metastatic lesions, which

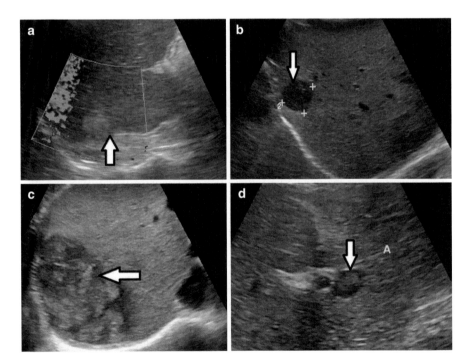

Fig. 7.1 HCC can have variable appearances on ultrasound. (**a**) *Arrow* points to a HCC lesion, which is hyperechoic relative to liver parenchyma. (**b**) *Arrow* points to a HCC lesion that is hypoechoic on ultrasound. (**c**) *Arrow* points to a HCC, which is heterogeneous and large on ultrasound. (**d**) *Arrow* points to a HCC lesion, which has a target appearance. A target appearance is used to describe a lesion that has a hyperechoic center and a hypoechoic rim

demonstrate internal vascularity only approximately 25% of the time [8]. Invasion of the hepatic or portal veins is also strongly suggestive of HCC.

Contrast-enhanced ultrasound (CEUS) is an emerging technique that can potentially detect HCC. The technique involves administration of intravenous contrast and obtaining images in the arterial, venous, and delayed phases. After administration of contrast, the arterial phase images are obtained at 15–30 s, the venous phase images are obtained at 50–80 s, and the delayed phase images are obtained at 180–240 s [12]. Since HCC obtains most of its blood flow from the hepatic arterial system, contrast flows into the tumor in the arterial phase, and the tumor appears hyperechoic on ultrasound compared to the rest of the liver parenchyma. Subsequently, when the rest of the liver parenchyma enhances with contrast in the venous and delayed phases, the contrast within the HCC lesion washes out. This is because the predominant blood supply to the liver is from the portal veins, while the tumor predominantly gets its blood supply from the hepatic arteries. The lesion therefore becomes isoechoic and subsequently hypoechoic compared to the rest of the liver parenchyma with time.

While this can potentially play an important role in identifying HCC and has an advantage of avoiding the radiation risk that patients obtain with CT, the AASLD excludes CEUS as a diagnostic tool in patients with cirrhosis due to its high false positive rate. There are, however, societies such as the Italian Association for the Study of the Liver (AISF) who maintain a role for CEUS in identifying HCC nodules that are specifically greater than 1 cm [12].

7.5   Ultrasound Surveillance Algorithm

Although any nodule detected on ultrasound in a patient undergoing surveillance could potentially represent HCC, there are guidelines by the AASLD for subsequent management based on size. If a nodule <1 cm is detected on screening ultrasound, it is suggested that the nodule be followed every 3 months with ultrasound. If it increases in size within this time period, further imaging using multiphase contrast-enhanced CT or MRI is recommended. If the nodule initially detected on screening ultrasound is greater than 1 cm in size, multiphase contrast-enhanced CT or MRI are directly recommended as the next step in management [5].

7.6   Computed Tomography (CT)

Multiphase CT is an option used to further characterize liver lesions noted on ultrasound or single-phase CT (Fig. 7.2). After the administration of intravenous contrast, CT scans are usually performed in the late arterial phase, portal venous phase, and delayed phase. The arterial phase is usually performed at 15–30 s [13] and represents the enhancement of the hepatic arteries with some early enhancement of the portal veins. The portal venous phase is performed at approximately 60–80 s and represents enhancement of the entire portal venous system as well

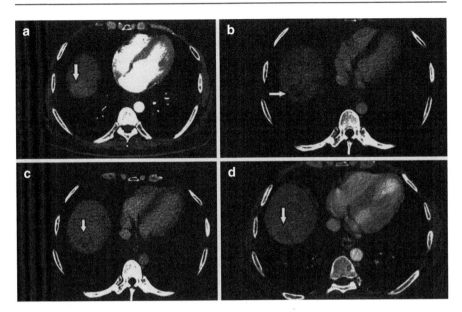

Fig. 7.2 (**a**) CT of the liver during the arterial phase demonstrates a lesion in the liver dome that is hyperenhancing relative to the rest of the liver parenchyma. (**b**) Venous phase demonstrates that the lesion is hypoenhancing compared to surrounding liver parenchyma. This is referred to as "washout." There is a faint area of enhancement around the lesion, which is the pseudocapsule. (**c**) Delayed phase imaging demonstrates persistent washout of the lesion relative to surrounding liver parenchyma. (**d**) Initial single-phase scan obtained during the early venous phase, which better demonstrates the peripherally enhancing pseudocapsule. Collectively, this multiphase exam demonstrates characteristics highly suspicious for HCC, which are arterial enhancement, venous phase washout, and pseudocapsule formation

as the hepatic veins [14]. A delayed scan is obtained at approximately 3–5 min and represents the equilibrium phase when contrast has mostly washed out of the liver parenchyma.

Hepatocellular carcinoma is an epithelial tumor composed of cells similar to normal hepatocytes. In the process of hepatocarcinogenesis, there is development of increased arterial supply to the tumor [7]. The purpose of the late arterial phase therefore is to identify intrahepatic lesions that demonstrate hypervascularity compared to the rest of the liver parenchyma. Studies have shown that approximately 78% of HCCs demonstrate arterial enhancement [15]. Findings, however, do vary depending on tumor differentiation and size. Although the majority of HCC lesions demonstrate hypervascularity regardless of differentiation, moderately differentiated HCCs are noted to have the highest proportion of arterial enhancement. The number of well-differentiated HCCs demonstrating hyperenhancement is slightly less, and poorly differentiated HCCs are proportionally the least in terms of arterial enhancement [15, 16]. The variation of arterial enhancement is again secondary to the degree of tumoral neoangiogenesis in the various levels of differentiation [15]. Tumoral size also plays a role in the visualization of arterial enhancement. Studies have shown that arterial enhancement is more commonly found in HCCs that are

1–2.9 cm (70–75%) compared to HCCs that are less than 1 cm (52%) [16]. However, when tumors significantly increase in size to greater than 5 cm, arterial flow may diminish, likely secondary to increased cell proliferation causing increased interstitial pressure and regression of neoarteries [7].

There are a few lesions in addition to HCC that also may demonstrate hyperenhancement in the arterial phase. These include benign perfusion alterations, small hemangiomas, small focal nodular hyperplasia-type lesions, atypical cirrhotic or dysplastic nodules, atypical focal/confluent fibrosis, and other malignancies such as small intrahepatic cholangiocarcinomas or hypervascular metastases such as neuroendocrine tumors [14]. Additionally, since HCC commonly occurs on a background of cirrhosis or chronic hepatitis where arterioportal shunting is common, a large majority of focal enhancing areas less than 2 cm that are only identified on the arterial phase and are predominantly wedge shaped and subcapsular are actually nonneoplastic [14]. The other phases of multiphase CT therefore are important to further characterize lesions that are hyperenhancing in the arterial phase and well as to identify HCC lesions that may not arterially enhance.

The portal venous phase and delayed phases also play a critical role in the evaluation of HCC. HCC predominantly (approximately 72% of the time) demonstrates a washout pattern on these two phases, which means it is hypoenhancing compared to the rest of the background liver parenchyma [15]. This occurs because, with hepatocarcinogenesis, there is a decrease in the number of portal tracts that contain the portal veins. This leads to a gradual decrease in blood flow to the tumor during the portal venous phase. The reduction in portal flow parallels the progression of HCC such that the more advanced the HCC, the more likely it is to have reduced or absent portal blood flow [15].

As with arterial phase imaging, tumoral differentiation plays a role in the imaging pattern of HCC during the portal venous and delayed phases. Moderately differentiated and poorly differentiated HCCs are more likely to demonstrate washout on these phases (75–76%, respectively). This is in contrast to well-differentiated tumors which were shown to demonstrate washout only 50% of the time according to some studies [15]. There is also evidence to suggest that with progression from well to moderate to poor differentiation of HCC, there is a shift in the timing of washout pattern during the portal venous phase. Well-differentiated HCC tends to washout relatively late compared to poorly differentiated tumors [15]. Additionally, a minority of HCC tumors are iso- or hyperattenuating during the portal venous phase. It is important to note that there are other liver lesions that can be hypoattenuating relative to the rest of the liver parenchyma on the portal venous or delayed phases, making it important to look at the enhancement pattern of the lesion on all three phases of imaging.

The delayed phase is especially important in HCC tumors that demonstrate slow washout, as this may not be apparent on the initial portal venous phase. This is in part because with cirrhosis, the increased hepatic tissue resistance causes delayed background parenchymal enhancement. The delayed phase imaging is also important in differentiating HCC from other tumors like cholangiocarcinoma, which demonstrate progressively increased enhancement on the portal venous and delayed phases.

There are additional characteristics of HCC that can be present on CT, including capsule formation and portal vein invasion. Capsule formation is a feature of HCC that occurs with disease progression and is suggestive of tumor with increased malignant potential compared to early HCC. Progressed HCC tumors are noted to have capsule formation and internal fibrous septa approximately 70% of the time [14]. Capsule enhancement appears as a complete or partial peripheral hyperenhancing rim around the tumor. It is classically seen a few seconds after tumoral enhancement and is best visualized in the late arterial or early portal venous phase. Visualization of a capsule suggests that tumor venous drainage has progressed from the hepatic veins to the portal veins [14].

Invasion into the venous system, predominantly into the portal veins, is another characteristic of HCC that helps differentiate it from other tumors. It is more frequently found in tumors of increased size and histologic grade. Vascular invasion carries a poorer prognosis as it represents a means by which HCC metastasizes to other areas of the liver as well as to different parts of the body [7]. Tumor thrombus within a lumen of a vein can also demonstrate enhancement on the arterial phase and appear hypodense on the portal venous phase. If present, these characteristics help differentiate it from bland venous thrombosis, which can also occur in this patient population.

Intratumoral fat, or hepatosteatosis, is another characteristic feature of HCC. It represents a process by which abnormal hepatocytes accumulate more intracellular fat and is seen in approximately 40% of early HCCs [7]. However, this finding is most commonly seen in HCCs that are approximately 1.5 cm in diameter. It is uncommon with further increase in tumor size and grade and not frequently seen in HCCs larger than 3 cm [7]. Intratumoral fat however is better recognized on MRI as it is difficult to characterize well on CT.

7.7   Magnetic Resonance Imaging (MRI)

Given technical advancements, HCC has now become an imaging diagnosis. The criteria include any nodule greater than 1 cm that demonstrates arterial enhancement and subsequent washout on CT or MRI. Although many meta-analyses found CT and MRI to have comparable specificities for the diagnosis of HCC in a cirrhotic liver, MRI is noted to have a higher sensitivity than CT, with MRI sensitivities ranging from 70 to 85% and CT sensitivities ranging from 50 to 68% [17]. The sensitivity for MRI detection of HCC, however, does vary depending on the size of tumor. A HCC larger than 2 cm was noted to have 100% sensitivity on MRI, while a HCC less than 1 cm had only a 4% sensitivity on one study [17].

The typical MRI protocol for HCC includes multiple T1-weighted imaging sequences and T2-weighted imaging sequences, including diffusion-weighted imaging. The T1 sequences are preferably obtained both pre- and postcontrast if the patient is able to receive intravenous contrast. There are several contrast agents that can be used for liver imaging, the most common being extracellular agents, hepatobiliary agents, or reticuloendothelial agents.

Gadolinium chelates are common extracellular contrast agents used in the MRI detection of HCC. Gadolinium demonstrates pharmacokinetics similar to the iodinated contrast media used in CT. As an extracellular agent, it leaves the vasculature and enters the interstitial space after it is administered intravenously. It causes relaxation of adjacent water protons since it is highly paramagnetic and has seven unpaired electrons. This in turn shortens the T1 and T2 times, leading to enhanced T1 signal and hypointense T2 signal on MRI. A single gadolinium atom has the potential to relax multiple adjacent protons, allowing better visualization of subtle small areas of contrast enhancement, which makes MRI more sensitive than CT [18]. The T1 postcontrast images, therefore, are a primary tool for evaluating HCC. A similar enhancement pattern as CT is used to characterize HCC on MRI, which includes arterial enhancement and subsequent washout on the venous and/or delayed imaging.

Gadoxetate disodium (Eovist) is a hepatobiliary (or hepatocyte-specific) agent that is used for MRI evaluation of liver lesions, including HCC (Fig. 7.3). After intravenous administration, it enters the extracellular space similar to extracellular

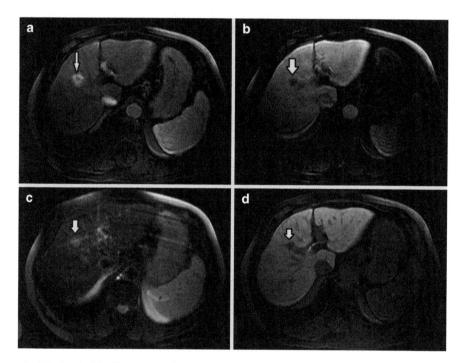

Fig. 7.3 MRI of the liver was performed using Eovist. (**a**) T1-weighted image of a HCC during the arterial phase demonstrates hyperenhancement of the lesion relative to liver parenchyma as demonstrated by the *arrow*. (**b**) T1-weighted image of the HCC during the delayed phase demonstrates washout relative to liver parenchyma. There is also a visible pseudocapsule around the lesion. (**c**) T2-weighted image of the HCC lesion demonstrates mild hyperintensity relative to the rest of the liver parenchyma. (**d**) 20 min hepatocyte phase demonstrates no uptake of contrast by the tumor, while the rest of the liver parenchyma is able to uptake the Eovist and demonstrate increased signal

agents. However, it is unique in that it is subsequently transported into the hepatocyte by an ATP-dependent receptor called organic anion transporting polypeptide (OATP1). Once inside the hepatocyte, it is excreted into the biliary canaliculi by another transporter known as canalicular multispecific organic anion transporter (cMOAT). Excretion of Eovist into the biliary system therefore is dependent on the overall liver function. In patients with normal liver function, approximately 50% of Eovist is excreted via the hepatobiliary system, and the rest is excreted by the kidneys [7]. Since it has a half-life of 56 min, hepatic phase imaging for Eovist is usually done 20 min after intravenous administration of the contrast agent. By 20 min, the contrast is taken up by the hepatocytes where it reversibly interacts with intracellular proteins and leads to increased T1 relaxivity compared to other contrast agents. The 20 min hepatocyte sequence is unique to Eovist and is simply an addition to the usual hepatic imaging sequences. Since HCC has altered hepatocyte function, the tumor cells are not able to take up Eovist. The HCC therefore appears hypointense on the 20 min phase compared to the surrounding liver parenchyma where the hepatocytes are able to uptake Eovist and demonstrate increased signal.

A third agent used for imaging HCC is superparamagnetic iron oxide (SPIO) particles. These are iron-based particles designed to target the reticuloendothelial system, specifically the liver and the spleen. Only one of these agents, ferumoxide, is approved for use in the United States. In the liver, SPIO particles are phagocytosed by a type of macrophages known as Kupffer cells which line the sinusoids [18]. Subsequently, the particles cause inhomogeneities in the magnetic field leading to T2 and T2* shortening which is reflected on MRI as hypointense signal. Tissues containing these particles also demonstrate mildly decreased T1 signal. SPIO particles are helpful in the imaging of HCC because while background liver parenchyma contains Kupffer cells and is able to take up these particles, most HCC tumors are deficient in Kupffer cells. HCC tumors, therefore, appear hyperintense relative to the surrounding hypointense liver parenchyma. The degree to which SPIO particles are used is variable. In terms of accuracy, it was reported in one series that gadolinium was better than SPIO particles for the detection of small HCC tumors [18]. SPIO particles are also more expensive and take a longer time to image than gadolinium. However, in patients with significant cirrhosis and alteration in liver perfusion, gadolinium enhancement of HCC may be poor. SPIO particles therefore can be used as an adjunct in such situations to help in the detection of HCC. It has been proposed that SPIO particles are most useful when administered along with gadolinium to increase contrast between HCC and background liver parenchyma and thereby improve the detection of HCC [18].

In addition to the three-phase enhancement pattern that characterizes HCC on CT, MRI offers additional tools to aid in the diagnosis of HCC. T2-weighted imaging sequences are an important part of HCC diagnosis on MRI. These are fluid sensitive sequences. So, lesions with high intracellular or extracellular water content demonstrate increased signal, while lesions with low water content appear hypointense. Although many liver lesions can demonstrate increased signal on T2-weighted images, mild-to-moderate T2 hyperintensity is typical of HCC [14]. Most HCCs that demonstrate these findings are of advanced grade. It has been shown that 77% of HCC lesions greater than 3 cm demonstrate this characteristic signal intensity [14].

A specific combination of imaging sequences known as T1 gradient echo in-phase and out-of-phase imaging is a useful adjunct for the diagnosis of HCC on MRI. These sequences are based on the premise that HCC tumors, especially during early development, often contain intralesional fat (Fig. 7.4). Since intralesional fat is a more characteristic of early HCC than progressed HCC, if detected, it can serve as a good prognostic feature. The imaging sequences are based on the principle that in the presence of intralesional fat, lipid and water protons occupy the same voxel. Lipid and water protons, however, inherently precess at different frequencies. In-phase imaging is obtained when lipid and water protons are precessing at a similar frequency. At this time, which occurs approximately every 4.2 ms on a 1.5 T magnet, their signal is additive. When lipid and water proton signals are out of phase with each other, there is cancellation of signal resulting in signal loss. Therefore, loss of intralesional signal on out-of-phase images compared to in-phase images is helpful for diagnosis of intralesional fat when there is a lesion suspicious for HCC, especially during the early stage [19].

Diffusion-weighted imaging (DWI) is another tool that is being increasingly used in liver imaging to diagnose HCC (Fig. 7.5). It is based on the phenomenon of

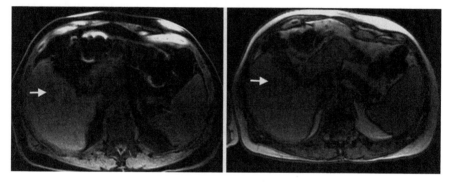

Fig. 7.4 In-phase (*left*) and out-of-phase (*right*) imaging. A lesion appears more hypointense on out-of-phase imaging compared to the in-phase imaging. This is suggestive of intralesional fat, which demonstrates signal dropout, another characteristic that can be seen with HCC tumors

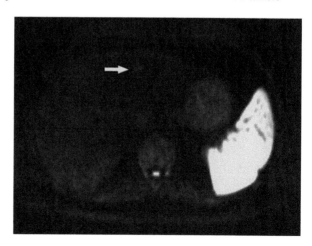

Fig. 7.5 Diffusion-weighted image of a HCC lesion shows mild hyperintensity in the region of the tumor suggestive of diffusion restriction

random movement of water molecules driven by their internal thermal energy, a concept known as Brownian motion. DWI is governed by inherent tissue properties, which can allow relatively free movement of water in certain areas and impede diffusion of water molecules in other areas. DWI is a T2-based imaging sequence. Tissues with high cellularity restrict the motion of water molecules within them, while tissues with lower cellularity cause less impedance to the movement of water molecules. Imaging is obtained using two strong gradients, one of which dephases the protons and the other rephases the protons. In tissues with restricted motion, water protons experience both the dephasing and rephasing gradients, thereby producing a hyperintense T2 signal. If there is movement of water molecules between the dephasing and rephasing gradients, there is a reduction in overall T2 signal intensity on imaging. Apparent diffusion coefficient (ADC) is a quantitative expression of diffusion, which is automatically calculated by the software. Low ADC values represent diffusion restriction, whereas high ADC values reflect relatively free diffusion of water molecules [20].

HCC can have a variable appearance on diffusion-weighted imaging depending on histologic makeup. Moderate to poorly differentiated HCC tumors are often hyperintense on DWI, whereas well-differentiated tumors often appear isointense on diffusion-weighted imaging [21]. Diffusion-weighted imaging has been shown to be especially helpful in HCCs measuring less than 2 cm. In a study by Zech et al., conventional MRI demonstrated a sensitivity of 67.6% and a positive predictive value of 59%, while diffusion-weighted imaging had a sensitivity of 91.2% and a positive predictive value of 81.6% in HCC tumors less than 2 cm. In HCC lesions greater than 2 cm, DWI did not appear to be significantly better than conventional MRI [20]. A limitation of DWI is that in cirrhotic livers, the value of ADC might be limited as both cirrhotic liver and HCCs can have low ADC values.

7.8   Emerging Imaging Techniques

7.8.1   Elastography

MR elastography is becoming increasingly utilized for the assessment of liver fibrosis. The concept involves applying a stress to tissue and measuring the resultant response. The first step is causing tissue vibration, which is most commonly done using an audio source located outside the scanner room. These tissue vibrations produce low-frequency shear waves. Typically, a frequency of 60 Hz is used. A motion-sensitive dynamic MRI sequence is then used to image the liver. Spatial information is reflected in quantitative shear stiffness maps using an inversion algorithm. Mechanical shear waves travel more slowly in softer tissues and have a shorter wavelength. Conversely, in stiffer tissues, shear waves travel faster and have a longer wavelength. Since the measured stiffness depends on frequency, the imaging can be done on a 1.5 or 3 T magnet strength given that the frequency is similar [22].

Tissue stiffness in vivo depends on tissue components, structural organization, and blood perfusion. Pathology in the liver therefore alters tissue structure causing the abnormal tissue to respond differently under stress than normal tissue. At 60 Hz, normal liver tissue has a mean stiffness of 1.54–2.87 kPa [22]. In chronic liver disease, collagen is deposited in the extracellular matrix causing liver fibrosis. Given that liver fibrosis demonstrates a linear increase in liver stiffness, MR elastography is a great tool for staging liver fibrosis. It has been shown to have a high accuracy in differentiating liver fibrosis from normal liver and/or liver with inflammation but no fibrosis. Preliminary studies have also shown that malignant liver tumors such as HCC have a higher liver stiffness compared to benign tumors and normal liver [23]. Using a cutoff value of 5 kPa, one study demonstrated a 100% accuracy of MR elastography in differentiating malignant tumors from benign tumors [22].

Ultrasound elastography is another method used to evaluate liver fibrosis. It can be performed using different techniques such as transient elastography (TE), real-time/static elastography (RTE), acoustic radiation force impulse (ARFI), or real-time shear wave elastography (SWE). TE is performed by using a mechanical actuator to cause skin vibrations which induces low-frequency mechanical waves to propagate through the liver. The velocity of these waves is measured with ultrasound and used to calculate liver stiffness, which is expressed in kilopascals (kPa). ARFI and SWE are shear wave techniques that use acoustic radiation force to cause microscopic tissue movements and thereby produce shear waves. The waves are studied to estimate tissue stiffness and shear wave velocity.

Both TE and SWE appear promising for the diagnosis of cirrhosis. In a large multicenter study, ARFI-based SWE showed a sensitivity of 69.1% and a specificity of 79.8% to diagnose fibrosis greater than METAVIR F2 stage (defined as moderate liver damage) [24]. TE was also shown to be better than ARFI for predicting the presence of cirrhosis and fibrosis at the F1 stage or greater. Another study demonstrated TE as an ideal method to diagnose cirrhosis in patients with hepatitis C virus as it could potentially decrease the number of liver biopsies [25]. In patients with hepatitis B virus, ARFI and TE had similar diagnostic accuracies of diagnosing stage two fibrosis or greater, with areas under the curve of 0.75 and 0.83, respectively [25]. Several studies have been performed to evaluate the ability of ultrasound elastography to differentiate between benign and malignant lesions. A meta-analysis of RTE and ARFI in 2013 showed a sensitivity of 85% and specificity of 84% of these modalities to distinguish benign from malignant lesions [25]. Other studies, however, have shown no statistically significant difference in differentiating benign and malignant liver lesions using ultrasound elastography [25].

7.8.2 Dual-Energy CT

Dual-energy CT (DECT) is an emerging technique that can be used to characterize liver lesions. While conventional CT uses a single polychromatic x-ray beam ranging from 70 to 140 kVp (standard of 120 kVp), dual-energy CT uses two energy levels, typically 80 and 140 kVp [26]. Dual-energy CT allows for improved conspicuity/enhancement of iodine in parenchymal tissue. Given its high atomic number of 53, iodine attenuates differently when exposed to a lower-energy beam compared to normal soft tissues such as the liver, which are made up of substances with low atomic numbers [27]. The low-energy acquisition from the 80 kVp energy datasets is noted to be more sensitive in detection of hypervascular liver lesions such as HCC due to improved contrast-to-noise ratio [28].

7.9   Imaging Implications on Patient Care Including Transplant Eligibility

In order to have a systematic way of reporting imaging findings on CT and MRI in patients at risk for HCC, the Liver Imaging Reporting and Data System (LI-RADS) was formulated in 2011. It was developed by a committee of international experts in medicine, surgery, and radiology with the ultimate goal of providing an estimated probability of a liver nodule representing a HCC. In patients at high risk for developing HCC, it categorizes liver lesions noted on CT or MRI into LI-RADS category 1–5. These categories represent benign, probably benign, intermediate probability of being HCC, probably HCC, and definitively HCC respectively. The four major imaging features used to assign a LI-RADS category include arterial phase hyperenhancement, washout appearance following hyperenhancement, capsule enhancement, and threshold growth compared to previous imaging [29]. A category of LR-M is reserved for a mass thought to be a malignancy other than HCC. LR-5V is reserved for tumor in a vein.

The highlights of the LI-RADS classification system as outlined by the ACR are discussed below [29, 30]. A LI-RADS 1 is assigned to a lesion that either has diagnostic benign imaging features or resolves without treatment. LI-RADS 1 is benign and LI-RADS 5 has a 100% certainty of a lesion being HCC. A LI-RADS 2 is assigned to a lesion that has imaging features suggestive of a benign entity; the imaging features remain stable for ≥2 years or if the lesion likely disappeared without treatment. LI-RADS 3, LI-RADS 4, and LI-RADS 5 are further subdivided based on size and presence of additional major features which include hypoenhancement during portal venous or delayed phase or increase in diameter of at least 1 cm in 1 year. In a mass-like lesion less than 2 cm, mass-like configuration, and arterial *hyper*enhancement, a LI-RADS 3 is assigned if there are no additional major features, a LI-RADS 4 is assigned if there is one additional major feature, and LI-RADS 5 if there are two additional major features. In a mass-like lesion less than 2 cm, mass-like configuration, and arterial *hypo*enhancement, a LI-RADS 3 is assigned if there are zero or one additional major features and a LI-RADS 4 is assigned if there are two additional major features. A LI-RADS 5 does not include arterially iso- or hypoenhancing lesions. In a mass-like lesion ≥2 cm, a LI-RADS 3 is assigned if it is hypoenhancing and a LI-RADS 4 if it is arterially enhancing with no additional major features or if it is arterially hypo- or isoenhancing with one or two major features. In such a lesion, a LI-RADS 5 is assigned if it demonstrates arterial hyperenhancement with one or two major features. If there is probable tumor within a vein, the lesion is assigned a LI-RADS 4, and if there is definite tumor within a vein, the lesion is assigned a LI-RADS 5 [29]. The LI-RADS categories 2, 3, and 4 are not definitely benign and not definitely HCC, and further evaluation may be needed to characterize these lesions [30].

In 2011, the United Network for Organ Sharing and Organ Procurement and Transplant Network (UNOS-OPTN) established imaging criteria to diagnose HCC using dynamic CT and MRI. These criteria were used to determine liver transplantation eligibility of patients with HCC who did not have extrahepatic spread and/or macrovascular involvement of tumor on imaging. The UNOS-OPTN classification system is as follows: 5A, 5A-g, 5B, 5X, and 5T. A 5A lesion measures 10–20 mm, demonstrates hypervascularity during the late arterial phase, and demonstrates both portal venous or delayed washout and capsule formation. A 5A-g lesion measures 10–20 mm, demonstrates hypervascularity during the late arterial phase, and has ≥50% diameter growth on serial MRI or CT ≤6 months apart. A 5B lesion measures 20–50 mm, is hypervascular during the late arterial phase, and has one of the following: portal venous or delayed washout, late capsule or pseudocapsule enhancement, ≥50% diameter growth on serial MRI or CT ≤6 months apart, or biopsy-proven HCC. A 5T lesion includes a biopsy-proven HCC, a class 5 lesion treated with locoregional therapy, or persistent/recurrent HCC at a prior treatment site. A class 5X lesion is one that meets radiologic criteria for HCC but is outside stage T2, including a lesion greater than 5 cm in diameter or more than two lesions, each of which are greater than 3 cm in diameter [31]. The UNOS-OPTN criteria do not include lesions less than 1 cm and those that do not demonstrate arterial hyperenhancement. The UNOS-OPTN criteria also defer to the LI-RADS for categorizing nodules that are not included within its imaging criteria for HCC [31].

Conclusion

In summary, various imaging techniques are currently being utilized for the noninvasive diagnosis of HCC including ultrasound, CT, and MRI. Many novel variations of these modalities are emerging for potential of increased utility in the future, including contrast-enhanced ultrasound, ultrasound elastography, dual-energy CT, and MRI elastography, which has already shown promising results. These imaging modalities, along with imaging criteria developed by expert panels using a multidisciplinary approach, share the ultimate goal of identifying patients with HCC at an earlier stage and thereby allowing for early intervention.

References

1. Lencioni R, Crocetti L. Local-regional treatment of hepatocellular carcinoma. Radiology. 2012;262(1):43–58.
2. Clark HP, Forrest Carson W, Kavanagh PV, Ho CPH, Shen P, Zagoria RJ. Staging and current treatment of hepatocellular carcinoma. RadioGraphics. 2005;25(Suppl 1):S3–S23.
3. Miller JC, et al. Screening for hepatocellular carcinoma in cirrhotic patients. J Am Coll Radiol. 2008;5(9):1012–4.
4. Hussain SM, Reinhold C, Mitchell DG. Cirrhosis and lesion characterization at MR imaging. RadioGraphics. 2009;29(6):1637–52.

5. Bruix J, Sherman M, American Association for the Study of Liver Diseases. Management of hepatocellular carcinoma: an update. Hepatology. 2011;53:1020–2.
6. El-Serag HB, Marrero JA, Rudolph L, Reddy KR. Diagnosis and treatment of hepatocellular carcinoma. Gastroenterology. 2008;134(6):1752–63. https://doi.org/10.1053/j.gastro.2008.02.090. Review.
7. Choi J-Y, Lee J-M, Sirlin CB. CT and MR imaging diagnosis and staging of hepatocellular carcinoma: part I. Development, growth, and spread: key pathologic and imaging aspects. Radiology. 2014;272(3):635–54.
8. Bhosale P, Szkaruk J, Silverman PM. Current staging of hepatocellular carcinoma: imaging implications. Cancer Imaging. 2006;6(1):83–94. https://doi.org/10.1102/1470-7330.2006.0014.
9. Takayasu K, Moriyama N, Muramatsu Y, et al. The diagnosis of small hepatocellular carcinomas: efficacy of various imaging procedures in 100 patients. AJR Am J Roentgenol. 1990;155:49–54.
10. McEvoy SH, McCarthy CJ, Lavelle LP, Moran DE, Cantwell CP, Skehan SJ, Gibney RG, Malone DE. Hepatocellular carcinoma: illustrated guide to systematic radiologic diagnosis and staging according to guidelines of the American Association for the Study of Liver Diseases. RadioGraphics. 2013;33(6):1653–68.
11. Tchelepi H, Ralls PW, Radin R, Grant E. Sonography of diffuse liver disease. J Ultrasound Med. 2002;21:1023–32.
12. Palmieri VO, Santovito D, Marano G, Minerva F, Ricci L, D'Alitto F, Angelelli G, Palasciano G. Contrast-enhanced ultrasound in the diagnosis of hepatocellular carcinoma. Radiol Med. 2015;120(7):627–33. https://doi.org/10.1007/s11547-014-0494-9. Epub 20 Jan 2015.
13. Hwang GJ, Kim MJ, Yoo HS, Lee JT. Nodular hepatocellular carcinomas: detection with arterial-, portal-, and delayed-phase images at spiral CT. Radiology. 1997;202:383–8. https://doi.org/10.1148/radiology.202.2.9015062.
14. Choi J-Y, Lee J-M, Sirlin CB. CT and MR imaging diagnosis and staging of hepatocellular carcinoma: part II. Extracellular agents, hepatobiliary agents, and ancillary imaging features. Radiology. 2014;273(1):30–50.
15. Lee JH, Lee JM, Kim SJ, et al. Enhancement patterns of hepatocellular carcinomas on multiphasic multidetector row CT: comparison with pathological differentiation. Br J Radiol. 2012;85(1017):e573–83. https://doi.org/10.1259/bjr/86767895.
16. Yoon SH, Lee JM, So YH, Hong SH, Kim SJ, Han JK, Choi BI. Multiphasic MDCT enhancement pattern of hepatocellular carcinoma smaller than 3 cm in diameter: tumor size and cellular differentiation. Am J Roentgenol. 2009;193(6):W482–9.
17. Parente DB, Perez RM, Eiras-Araujo A, Oliveira Neto JA, Marchiori E, Constantino CP, Amorim VB, Rodrigues RS. MR imaging of hypervascular lesions in the cirrhotic liver: a diagnostic dilemma. RadioGraphics. 2012;32(3):767–87.
18. Gandhi SN, Brown MA, Wong JG, Aguirre DA, Sirlin CB. MR contrast agents for liver imaging: what, when, how. RadioGraphics. 2006;26(6):1621–36.
19. Prasad SR, Wang H, Rosas H, Menias CO, Narra VR, Middleton WD, Heiken JP. Fat-containing lesions of the liver: radiologic-pathologic correlation. RadioGraphics. 2005;25(2):321–31.
20. Kele PG, van der Jagt EJ. Diffusion weighted imaging in the liver. World J Gastroenterol. 2010;16(13):1567–76.
21. Silva AC, Evans JM, McCullough AE, Jatoi MA, Vargas HE, Hara AK. MR imaging of hypervascular liver masses: a review of current techniques. RadioGraphics. 2009;29(2):385–402.
22. Venkatesh SK, Ehman RL. Magnetic resonance elastography of liver. Magn Reson Imaging Clin N Am. 2014;22:433–46.
23. Venkatesh SK, Yin M, Glockner JF, Takahashi N, Araoz PA, Talwalkar JA, Ehman RL. MR elastography of liver tumors: preliminary results. AJR Am J Roentgenol. 2008;190(6):1534–40. https://doi.org/10.2214/AJR.07.3123.
24. Sporea I, Bota S, Peck-Radosavljevic M, Sirli R, Tanaka H, Iijima H, Badea R, Lupsor M, Fierbinteanu-Braticevici C, Petrisor A, Saito H, Ebinuma H, Friedrich-Rust M, Sarrazin C, Takahashi H, Ono N, Piscaglia F, Borghi A, D'Onofrio M, Gallotti A, Ferlitsch A, Popescu A,

Danila M. Acoustic Radiation Force Impulse elastography for fibrosis evaluation in patients with chronic hepatitis C: an international multicenter study. Eur J Radiol. 2012;81(12):4112–8. https://doi.org/10.1016/j.ejrad.2012.08.018. Epub 20 Sept 2012.

25. Dhyani M, Anvari A, Samir AE. Ultrasound elastography: liver. Abdom Imaging. 2015;40:698–708.

26. Grajo JR, Patino M, Prochowski A, Sahani DV. Dual energy in practice: basic principles and applications. Radiographics. 2016;36(4):1087–105.

27. Agrawal MD, Pinho DF, Kulkarni NM, Hahn PF, Guimaraes AR, Sahani DV. Oncologic applications of dual-energy CT in the abdomen. RadioGraphics. 2014;34(3):589–612.

28. Altenbernd J, Heusner TA, Ringelstein A, Ladd SC, Forsting M, Antoch G. Dual-energy-CT of hypervascular liver lesions in patients with HCC: investigation of image quality and sensitivity. Eur Radiol. 2011;21(4):738–43. https://doi.org/10.1007/s00330-010-1964-7. Epub 10 Oct 2010.

29. Purysko AS, Remer EM, Coppa CP, Leão Filho HM, Thupili CR, Veniero JC. LI-RADS: a case-based review of the new categorization of liver findings in patients with end-stage liver disease. Radiographics. 2012;32(7):1977–95. https://doi.org/10.1148/rg.327125026.

30. Mitchell DG, Bruix J, Sherman M, Sirlin CB. LI-RADS (Liver Imaging Reporting and Data System): summary, discussion, and consensus of the LI-RADS Management Working Group and future directions. Hepatology. 2015;61(3):1056–65.

31. Cruite I, Tang A, Sirlin CB. Imaging-based diagnostic systems for hepatocellular carcinoma. Am J Roentgenol. 2013;201(1):41–55.

Epithelial-to-Mesenchymal Transition in Hepatocellular Carcinoma

8

Jeannette Huaman, Cuong Bach, Adeodat Ilboudo, and Olorunseun O. Ogunwobi

8.1 Introduction

8.1.1 Hepatocellular Carcinoma and the Urgent Need for Alternative Treatment Options

Hepatocellular carcinoma (HCC) is the most common type of liver cancer and one of the leading causes of cancer-related mortality worldwide [1]. It is commonly referred to as hepatoma and it is an important public health problem. It occurs more frequently in men than in women and much more frequently in people with a history of liver problems such as hepatitis B and C viral infections [2]. Symptoms are more pronounced and specific during advanced stages of the disease, at which time treatment options and the extent to which these treatment options will be effective are limited. In focal localized hepatocellular carcinoma, partial hepatectomy is

J. Huaman, Ph.D.
Department of Biological Sciences, Hunter College of The City University of New York, New York, NY, USA

Department of Biology, The Graduate Center of The City University of New York, New York, NY, USA

C. Bach, Ph.D. • A. Ilboudo, Ph.D.
Department of Biological Sciences, Hunter College of The City University of New York, New York, NY, USA

O.O. Ogunwobi, M.D., Ph.D. (✉)
Department of Biological Sciences, Hunter College of The City University of New York, New York, NY, USA

Department of Biology, The Graduate Center of The City University of New York, New York, NY, USA

Joan and Sanford I. Weill Department of Medicine, Weill Cornell Medicine, Cornell University, New York, NY, USA
e-mail: Ogunwobi@GENECTR.HUNTER.CUNY.EDU

© Springer International Publishing AG 2018
C. Liu (ed.), *Precision Molecular Pathology of Liver Cancer*,
Molecular Pathology Library, https://doi.org/10.1007/978-3-319-68082-8_8

possible. In patients with intrahepatic metastasis, complete hepatectomy and liver transplantation (which involves a long wait-list, is surgically invasive, and is not optimal for certain people) are options available [3, 4]. These patients with intrahepatic metastasis as well as those with extrahepatic metastasis may also need systemic therapy with agents such as sorafenib. Unfortunately, targeted therapy with sorafenib only extends life by about 6 months [5]. Currently, the 5-year relative survival rate for patients with liver cancer is only 17%, mainly because of its late diagnosis [6]. As such, better tools are needed for earlier diagnosis and for treatment of advanced HCC.

8.1.2 Epithelial-to-Mesenchymal Transition

Diagnostic and therapeutic approaches can exploit biological mechanisms or processes that may be important in normal healthy cells and tissues but may be aberrant in cancer cells and tissues. A biological process that is normal and physiological in certain cells and tissues but that is hijacked by cancer cells is epithelial-to-mesenchymal transition (EMT) [7]. EMT is a process during which epithelial cells gradually change to become "mesenchymal-like" in nature. During this process, they also become more motile and invasive [8]. To understand this, it is helpful to distinguish between two distinct types of cells: epithelial and mesenchymal. As shown in Fig. 8.1, epithelial cells are cells that typically line the walls of blood vessels, body cavities, and organs (such as the lungs, stomach, small intestine, pancreas, and kidneys). They are normally polarized, attached to a basement membrane, and closely interconnected with one another. Epithelial cells are held together tightly at junctions via cadherin, catenin, and integrin molecules [9]. In contrast, mesenchymal cells are loosely associated cells that lack polarity and are characterized by greater migratory properties [10]. The transition of cells from epithelial to

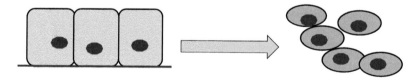

Epithelial cells

- Are attached to a basement membrane
- Are stationary
- Exhibit polarity
- Have high levels of E-Cadherin
- Have high levels of cytokeratin intermediate filaments
- Have high levels of claudins and occludins
- Have low levels of Fibronectin, Snail, Slug, Twist, Zeb1/2, MMPs

Mesenchymal cells

- Deattach from basement membrane & lose cell adhesion
- Are migratory and invasive
- Lose polarity
- Exhibit a switch from E-Cadherin to N-Cadherin
- Exhibit a switch from cytokeratin to vimentin filaments
- Exhibit repression of claudins and occludins
- Exhibit INCREASED levels of Fibronectin, Snail, Slug, Twist, Zeb1/2, MMPs
- Exhibit a gain of anti-apoptotic activities, self-renewal, and chemoresistance

Fig. 8.1 Epithelial versus mesenchymal characteristics

mesenchymal phenotype requires several biochemical changes and takes place normally during the development of the embryo. It is required for the formation of the mesoderm which occurs during the third week of the developing embryo [11] and neural crest formation which occurs after the formation of the three germ layers, a process otherwise known as gastrulation [12]. There are several things that must happen—specification of the area where EMT will occur, detachment of the epithelial cells from the basement membrane, and conversion to the mesenchymal cell structure/phenotype [13]. In adults, EMT also normally occurs during wound healing [14] and, in women, the formation of the mammary gland [15]. Although EMT is important in embryogenesis and some normal physiological processes in adult humans, EMT has been implicated and demonstrated to be involved in pathological conditions like fibrosis, inflammation, and cancer [16], raising the possibility of exploiting aspects of EMT for diagnostic or therapeutic applications, in HCC.

8.1.3   Classification of EMT

Depending on the settings in which EMT occurs and its functional consequences, EMT could be classified into three categories: type I, type II, and type III [8]. Type I EMT occurs in the context of implantation of the embryo to the uterine wall; formation of the placenta, in several instances during embryonic development (including mesoderm and neural crest formation); and organ development. EMT in these contexts results in a diverse population of cells sharing a common mesenchymal phenotype, which is neither induced by inflammation nor results in fibrosis or metastasis [17, 18]. It is important to note that the mesenchymal cells formed retain the ability to revert back to an epithelial state through the process of mesenchymal-to-epithelial transition (MET) [19]. Type II EMT occurs in the context of reparation activities such as wound healing, the regeneration of tissue, or organ fibrosis. This type of EMT occurs in response to inflammation and stops when inflammation has subsided [17, 18]. Type III EMT, the type of EMT most pertinent to hepatocellular carcinoma, occurs in the context of carcinoma cells that undergo multiple biochemical and morphological changes, which favor cancer cell invasion, migration, and metastasis, and consequently cancer progression [17, 18].

8.2   Understanding the Complex Orchestration of EMT

To be able to exploit any aspects of EMT for cancer diagnostic or therapeutic purposes, it is essential to fully understand the process, what regulates it, and how EMT—a normal biological process required under certain physiological circumstances—is manipulated by tumorigenic cells. It is important to note that the signals that induce EMT are cell- and tissue-specific and require the orchestration of multiple regulators and signaling pathways [20]. We will discuss some of these molecular regulators and molecular signaling effects of EMT here, with some focus on HCC.

8.2.1   Molecules Responsible for Executing EMT: The Effectors

The expression profile of a number of specific proteins that are characteristics of either the epithelial or mesenchymal cell phenotype has been established. Furthermore, the types of changes in the expression of these specific proteins during the course of EMT have been established [21]. Proteins associated with an epithelial cell identity include the following: E-cadherin, alpha-catenin, and gamma-catenin [22–24]. These are three of the established molecules associated with and important in cell-cell junctions and adhesion. Among these, loss of E-cadherin is the most widely used molecular characteristic to indicate that EMT has occurred. Whether through promoter methylation, transcriptional repression, or protein phosphorylation followed by protein degradation, E-cadherin expression has been shown to be decreased in multiple human and mouse studies of HCC [25–30]. Loss of E-cadherin expression has also been linked to a more metastatic phenotype in a variety of other cancers [31–34].

In addition to the downregulation of epithelial markers, EMT is also characterized by simultaneous upregulation of mesenchymal markers. These mesenchymal markers include N-cadherin, vimentin, fibronectin, CD44, and integrin B6 [21]. During EMT, N-cadherin expression typically increases as E-cadherin expression decreases, thereby leading to a change that both disturb cell adhesion and promote cell migration and invasion [35–37]. Another significant molecular change that typically occurs as epithelial cell transition to a mesenchymal phenotype involves the transition from cytokeratin to more vimentin intermediate filament proteins. Increased vimentin expression results in greater contractibility and stability of cells in response to mechanical activity, thereby supporting greater migration [38–40]. Similarly, fibronectin (an extracellular matrix glycoprotein) [41–43], CD44 [44, 45] (a transmembrane glycoprotein), and integrins (transmembrane receptors controlling cell-cell and cell-matrix adhesion) [46] are all upregulated in cells that have undergone EMT, and they are associated with poor prognosis [7].

8.2.2   Transcription Factors Orchestrating EMT: The Core Regulators

Another set of molecules critically important for EMT are the key regulating transcription factors. These include molecules such as Snail zinc finger family, Zeb homeobox family, and the basic helix-loop-helix (bHLH) family of transcription factors. Each of these EMT-regulating transcription factors has well-established roles in migration, invasion, and proliferation [47, 48].

The Snail transcription factors, for example, include proteins such as Snail and Slug. Both Snail and Slug have been noted to be upregulated in a variety of metastatic cancers. Snail and Slug are also known to have increased expression in cells that have been treated with EMT-inducing agents [49, 50]. Snail and

Slug are also associated with the disassembly of cell-cell and cell-extracellular matrix adhesions, such as desmosomes, tight junctions, and gap junctions. They are also negative regulators of epithelial molecular markers like E-cadherin and accomplish their repression of E-cadherin and other markers of the epithelial phenotype by binding to the enhancer box DNA sequences of these genes to inhibit their transcription [51–54]. In addition, Snail and Slug transcription factors promote the transcription of genes contributing to the mesenchymal phenotype [18, 55, 56].

Similarly, the ZEB transcription factors repress epithelial gene transcription such as transcription of the E-cadherin gene. The ZEB transcription factors also activate gene transcription of mesenchymal markers by binding to the regulatory enhancer box sequences of mesenchymal marker genes. They can be induced by tumor-promoting TGFβ signaling as well as growth factors activating the RAS-MAPK pathway. In addition, they have been shown to be activated by the EMT-regulating Snail 1 transcription factor, and they also inhibit the expression of claudins and ZO-1 which are both important for cell junction adhesion [20, 55, 56].

The basic helix-loop-helix (bHLH) transcription factor family, which includes Twist 1, Twist 2, and E12/47, can induce EMT by acting alone or cooperatively with one another or other molecules. Their activities include inhibition of E-cadherin, induction of N-cadherin, and activation of molecular signaling pathways promoting invasion, among many other tumor-promoting activities. In addition, these transcription factors function as either homodimers or heterodimers to regulate gene expression [20, 57–59].

8.2.3 Extracellular Factors Inducing Cells to Undergo EMT: The Inducers/Activators

In addition to the molecules that characterize mesenchymal and epithelial cellular identity, and the transcription factors that execute the EMT program, the agents that induce EMT to occur are also of critical importance. These are the molecules that serve as "on" and "off" switches and regulate EMT's occurrence during both normal development and tumorigenesis. For example, different major signaling pathways, such as Notch, Wnt, and growth factor signaling cascades (transforming growth factor beta, TGFB; fibroblast growth factor, FGF; hepatocyte growth factor, HGF; epidermal growth factor, EGF; insulin-like growth factor 1, IGF1; and platelet-derived growth factor, PDGF), have all been implicated in EMT induction. These regulatory signals tend to be tissue-specific and involve multiple signaling pathways in order to promote a more mesenchymal cell phenotype, favoring invasion and migration [20]. Table 8.1 summarizes the different signaling pathways that will be discussed in Sects. 8.2.3.1–8.2.3.3, with particular interest in those demonstrated to have a role in HCC. Other EMT inducers will also be discussed, including hypoxia, inflammation, and microRNAs.

Table 8.1 Some signaling pathways regulating EMT in HCC

TGF-β	
Fransvea, E et al. (2008)	Blocking transforming growth factor beta upregulates E-cadherin and reduces migration and invasion of hepatocellular carcinoma cells [74]
Fransvea, E. et al. (2009)	Targeting transforming growth factor (TGF)-betaRI inhibits activation of beta 1 integrin and blocks vascular invasion in hepatocellular carcinoma [75]
Reichl, P. et al. (2012)	TGFβ in epithelial-to-mesenchymal transition and metastasis of hepatocellular carcinoma [76]
Dituri, F et al. (2013)	Differential inhibition of TGFβ signaling pathway in HCC cells using the small molecule inhibitor LY2157299 and the D10 monoclonal antibody against TGFβ receptor type II [77]
Steinway, SN et al. (2014)	Network modeling of TGFβ signaling in hepatocellular carcinoma epithelial-to-mesenchymal transition reveals joint sonic hedgehog and Wnt pathway activation [78]
Qin, G. et al. (2016)	Reciprocal activation between MMP-8 and TGFβ1 stimulates EMT and malignant progression of hepatocellular carcinoma [79]
HGF	
Nagai, T. et al. (2011)	Sorafenib inhibits the hepatocyte growth factor-mediated epithelial-to-mesenchymal transition in hepatocellular carcinoma [80]
Ogunwobi, O and Liu C (2011)	Hepatocyte growth factor upregulation promotes carcinogenesis and epithelial-to-mesenchymal transition in hepatocellular carcinoma via Akt and COX-2 pathways [81]
Ogunwobi, O et al. (2013)	Epigenetic upregulation of HGF and c-Met drives metastasis in hepatocellular carcinoma [82]
PI3K	
Wang, H et al. (2014)	Activation of phosphatidylinositol 3-kinase/Akt signaling mediates sorafenib-induced invasion and metastasis in hepatocellular carcinoma [83]
Zhang, PF, et al. (2016)	Galectin-1 induces hepatocellular carcinoma EMT and sorafenib resistance by activating FAK/PI3K/AKT signaling [84]
WNT	
Zhang, Q, et al. (2013)	Wnt/B-catenin signaling enhances hypoxia-induced epithelial-mesenchymal transition in hepatocellular carcinoma via cross talk with HIF-1alpha signaling [85]
Yang, M. et al. (2013)	A double-negative feedback loop between Wnt/β-catenin signaling and HNF4a regulates epithelial-mesenchymal transition in hepatocellular carcinoma [86]
Jiang, Lei et al. (2014)	CLDN3 inhibits cancer aggressiveness via Wnt-EMT signaling and is a potential prognostic biomarker for hepatocellular carcinoma [87]
Notch	
Wan, X et al. (2016)	CD24 promotes HCC progression via triggering Notch-related EMT and modulation of tumor microenvironment [88]
Jia, Meng et al. (2016)	LincRNA-p21 inhibits invasion and metastasis of hepatocellular carcinoma through Notch signaling-induced epithelial-to-mesenchymal transition [89]
Xiao, S. et al. (2016)	Actin-like 6A predicts poor prognosis of hepatocellular carcinoma and promotes metastasis and epithelial-to-mesenchymal transition [90]

Transforming Growth Factor β (TGFβ)

Of the growth factor signaling cascades, TGFβ is considered to be one of the most potent inducers of EMT. It is a key signaling pathway very important in development that also presents serious consequences when dysregulated. It has been commonly implicated in a variety of cancers. It consists of several family members including the TGFβs, BMPs, and activins. Ligand binding to TGFβ type II receptors will activate TGFβ type I receptors, which will in turn lead to the activation of a cascade of SMAD molecules depending on which particular TGFβ pathway is activated (SMAD2 and/or SMAD3, followed by SMAD4 if the TGFβ/activin mechanism has been activated, SMAD1/5/9 followed by SMAD4 if the BMP mechanism has been activated). These cytoplasmic SMAD complexes will then travel to the nucleus and combine with other transcription factors and co-activators/corepressors to regulate gene expression [60]. Some of the genes induced by the SMAD complexes are genes promoting different aspects of tumorigenesis including suppression of the immune response as well as promotion of cell proliferation, angiogenesis, cancer cell stemness, metastasis, and EMT—the focus of this chapter [60, 61]. Genes induced by TGFβ that contribute to EMT include mesenchymal markers (fibronectin, vimentin, and collagen I) as well as EMT transcriptional regulators (Snail1/2 and ZEB1). SMAD activation has also been shown to repress E-cadherin and occludin gene expression, ultimately reducing cell-cell adhesion [62, 63].

However, TGFβ also promotes EMT regulatory gene expression through other signaling pathways independent of the SMAD protein complexes. These alternative pathways include the phosphatidylinositol 3-kinase (PI3K) and MAPK pathways as well as signaling through the Rho, CDC42, and Rac GTPases [64, 65]. Induction of the PI3K pathway leads to the activation of AKT, followed by activation of the mTORC1 and mTORC2 complexes, leading to stabilization of the Snail 1 transcription factor, the inhibition of E-cadherin, and ultimately the acquisition of more invasive/motile characteristics, all characteristics of EMT [66]. The ERK, p38, and JNK MAPK pathways are distinct MAPK pathways, which have been shown to be necessary for TGFβ-induced transcription of genes promoting EMT [67]. Finally, TGFβ activation of the Rho, Cdc42, and Rac GTPases leads to the reorganization of actin and the formation of filopodia and lamellipodia, favoring mesenchymal and motile activity [64].

Other Growth Factors

In addition to TGFβ, a number of other growth factors serve as inducers of the EMT process: FGF, HGF, EGF, IGF1, and PDGF. Similar to TGFβ, they promote EMT via ligand binding of specific receptors and subsequent induction of signaling cascades [20]. Most of these growth factors, however, work by induction of transmembrane receptor tyrosine kinases (RTKs), which often activate the PI3K/AKT pathway or the ERK or p38 or JNK MAPK pathways for EMT induction [68]. Although most of these growth factors have roles in inducing EMT during normal development, these growth factors can also lead to the promotion of a more mesenchymal phenotype in the context of pathological processes, leading to greater invasiveness, migration, as well as tumorigenesis [69, 70]. This is most often achieved by the transcription and stabilization of mesenchymal markers (such as snail, twist, N-cadherin, and vimentin) as well as repression of markers important for cell adhesion, such as E-cadherin [20].

Additional Signaling Pathways

Other signaling pathways that regulate EMT besides the TGFβ/SMAD, PI3K/AKT, ERK, p38, and JNK MAPK pathways include the Wnt, Hedgehog, and Notch signaling pathways [20].

Usually, when the Wnt signaling pathway is off, GSK3β kinase is active, and together with axin and adenomatous polyposis coli (APC), it phosphorylates β-catenin to keep it in the cytoplasm where it will get tagged and eventually get degraded. However, when Wnt ligand binds to its Frizzled receptor, this receptor inhibits GSK3β kinase from phosphorylating β-catenin. Instead of being ubiquitinylated and labeled for degradation, β-catenin is now free to regulate gene expression to induce EMT by promoting the stability of snail, increasing fibronectin, and lowering levels of E-cadherin [71].

For the hedgehog signaling pathway, when the sonic hedgehog (SHH) ligand is not there, patched (PTC) receptor inhibits the cytoplasmic protein smoothened (SMO) from activating GLI transcription factors. However, the binding of SHH to PTC receptor relieves the inhibition of SMO, which then goes on to activate the GLI transcription factors which travel into the nucleus. Once in the nucleus, these GLI transcription factors increase SNAIL1 transcription, reduce E-cadherin expression, and result in increased cell motility [72].

Another signaling pathway involved in regulating EMT is the notch signaling pathway. The binding of the notch ligand (Delta-like or Jagged) to the notch receptor on another cell will lead to the proteolytic cleavage of the intracellular domain of the notch receptor, which will then enter the nucleus and begin regulating notch target gene expression to promote EMT, for example, SNAIL2 induction and E-cadherin repression [73].

Hypoxia

Besides growth factors and the signaling pathways we have discussed so far, there are additional factors in the tumor microenvironment that can induce EMT. One such factor is hypoxia, a condition of low oxygen tension at tissue level. The hypoxic state is often prevalent in growing tumors and serves to turn on HIF1α transcription factor expression, which promotes EMT by activating twist and SNAIL1 expression [91, 92]. In a study using hepatocellular carcinoma cell lines, it was found that the Wnt/β-catenin pathway may further enhance HIF1α's induction of EMT, demonstrating the intricate cross talk that occurs among the different EMT-inducing signaling pathways in the tumor microenvironment [20, 85].

Inflammatory Cytokines

Another essential component of the tumor microenvironment contributing to EMT is the inflammatory state. Numerous studies have shown that there is a link between chronic inflammation and the progression of cancer [93]. For example, patients who have chronic hepatitis B or C virus infection (both conditions well characterized by chronic inflammation in the liver) are significantly much more likely to develop hepatocellular carcinoma than patients without chronic viral hepatitis [2]. Some of the cells responsible for releasing inflammatory cytokines are immune cells recruited to the cancer microenvironment, cancer-associated fibroblasts (CAFs), and endothelial cells in the surrounding area. Among the cytokines that are often released by such cells and have been implicated in EMT include interleukin-6 (IL-6) [94]. In breast cancer cell lines, for example, this cytokine has been associated with lower E-cadherin expression as well as increased expression of N-cadherin, vimentin, and EMT-promoting transcription factors: twist and SNAIL1 [95]. Similarly, another inflammatory cytokine often released by immune cells such as tumor-associated macrophages (TAMs), which contributes to carcinogenesis, is TNFα. This cytokine has been shown to induce snail expression as well as upregulate TGFβ expression, which is one of the most potent inducers of EMT, as discussed above [20, 96, 97].

MicroRNAs

EMT can also be regulated and induced by microRNAs. MicroRNAs are small noncoding strands of RNA that are highly conserved and control gene expression by either targeting specific mRNA sequences for degradation or inhibiting their translation into proteins. Interestingly, these 19–22-nucleotide-long molecules can function as tumor suppressors or oncogenes, and their dysregulated expression has been noted in several human cancers [98]. Specifically in hepatocellular carcinoma, the following microRNAs (miRNAs) have been observed to have tumor-suppressive properties: the miR-200 family, miR-205 (which inhibits EMT by decreasing vimentin and increasing E-cadherin expression), miR-449a (which suppresses EMT via multiple targets), miR-26a (which suppresses EMT by decreasing EZH2 and increasing E-cadherin), and miR-124 (which inhibits EMT by decreasing cytoskeletal changes brought about by ROCK2 and by inhibiting EZH2). Likewise, there are specific miRNAs that have been observed to be oncogenic and promote EMT in hepatocellular carcinoma, for example, miR-520g (which induces EMT by targeting SMAD7), miR-155 (which induces invasion by targeting RhoA and facilitating TGFβ-induced EMT), and miR-124 (which supports metastasis and EMT via oncogenic RAS signaling) [20, 99, 100].

In summary, multiple factors in the tumor microenvironment likely play a role in the induction or suppression of EMT, including growth factors, hypoxic conditions, multiple signaling pathways, inflammatory cytokines, as well as microRNAs, as indicated in Fig. 8.2. All of these, as well as the effectors and transcription factors needed for EMT to occur, work in a complex and intricate manner to be able to promote tumorigenicity.

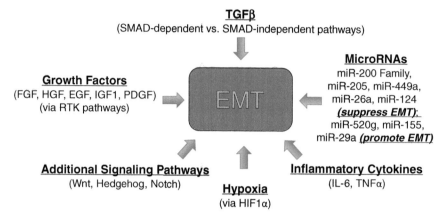

Fig. 8.2 Different extracellular factors that can engage cells to undergo EMT

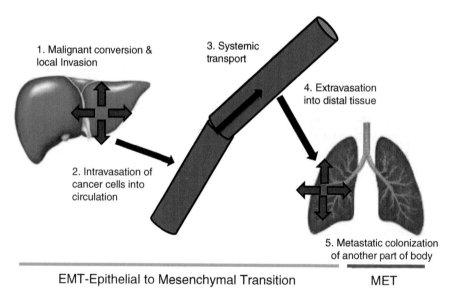

Fig. 8.3 EMT's involvement in the different stages of metastasis

8.3   EMT and Cancer Metastasis

Metastasis is a reason for which patients with HCC succumb to the disease. This is because by the time most people present with noticeable symptoms, the disease has already progressed beyond a focal lesion in the liver. As such, identifying the roles EMT plays in HCC progression is very useful. The importance of this lies in possibly using EMT markers as prognostic biomarkers in HCC or as potential novel therapeutic targets.

Although originally thought to occur during later stages of tumorigenesis, studies have implicated EMT in earlier stages of tumorigenesis (as shown in Fig. 8.3), as early as malignant cell conversion [55, 101–103].

8.3.1 Malignant Cell Conversion and Localized Invasion

This first step of tumorigenesis is characterized by the conversion of a normal healthy cell into a malignant one as well as factors in the tumor microenvironment supporting progression of the disease. EMT transcription factors have been shown to be involved in this early stage by promoting transformation. Apart from its well-defined role of serving as a transcription factor to lower E-cadherin expression, increase N-cadherin expression, and promote invasion, Twist 1 has also been shown to override cellular senescence and apoptosis as well as cooperate with other molecules to promote malignant transformation. In addition, EMT makes cancer cells lose adhesion to one another through downregulation of E-cadherin and other cell junction proteins and upregulation of mesenchymal markers and makes them migrate to and invade into local tissues around the site of primary cancer origin. Some of the EMT transcription factors such as SNAIL1 have also been shown to upregulate enzymes that degrade the extracellular matrix, such as matric metalloproteinases (MMPs). And still other EMT transcription factors such as Twist 1 have been shown to induce invadopodia formation, which leads to the recruitment of various proteases that will degrade the ECM and help facilitate invasion by cancer cells [102–104].

8.3.2 Intravasation of Cancer Cells into Circulation

This step in the metastatic process occurs after local invasion by cancer cells and is otherwise known as intravasation. This is the process by which cancer cells are able to cross the endothelium to enter the bloodstream and lymphatic system for dissemination into other parts of the body [101]. Studies have shown that EMT plays a role in modulating cancer cell migratory properties such that entry of cancer cells into the vasculature will be facilitated. For example, using the transendothelial migration assay, it was found that the EMT transcription factor, Zeb1, is needed for greater ability of cells to pass through the endothelial cell barrier [105]. It was also found in a breast cancer cell model that overexpression of the EMT transcription factor Snail1 was needed for greater intravasation via the activation of certain membrane-bound matrix metalloproteinases (MMPs) [106].

8.3.3 Systemic Transport Through the Bloodstream

When cancer cells have breached the endothelial barrier and enter the bloodstream, the next step is transportation through the circulatory system. At this point, tumor cells are known as circulating tumor cells (CTCs). CTCs have been particularly difficult to study because there are only a few cancer cells that are able to make it and survive the harsh conditions of being outside their normal environment and traveling through the bloodstream [107]. Studies on CTCs have revealed that many CTCs have mesenchymal features indicating that EMT may have taken place [108–111]. Indeed, it has also been observed that expression of the EMT transcription factors

Twist1 and Snail1 significantly increased CTC numbers and promoted microtubule membrane protrusions, which are thought to help CTCs aggregate and attach to the endothelial wall to aid in their survival and in the next step of the metastatic cascade. The fact that several studies also found that mesenchymal CTCs were associated with platelets, which are major secretors of TGFβ (a major inducer of EMT), supports the fact that EMT may be a characteristic feature of CTCs in the bloodstream and may contribute to the promotion of metastasis.

8.3.4   Extravasation of Cancer Cells from the Bloodstream into Distal Tissue

As CTCs travel through the bloodstream and aggregate and attach to the endothelial wall of blood vessels, the cancer cells will cross the endothelial barrier yet again, this time to leave the bloodstream and spread into the surrounding tissue [101]. Extravasation assays using zebra fish showed that the EMT transcription factor Twist 1 was able to form large membrane protrusions in cancer cells ready to cross the endothelial blood vessel barrier and enhance cancer cell extravasation into the surrounding tissue [112]. Others showed that the protrusions formed in tumor cells depended on the mesenchymal state of the cancer cells and could also be induced by the EMT transcription factors Twist1 and Snail1 [113]. Thus, in this way, EMT may facilitate extravasation of cancer cells into the surrounding parenchyma.

8.3.5   Cancer Cell Colonization of Secondary Sites

There is evidence to suggest that when CTCs get to secondary sites, colonization of the secondary site by cancer cells involves gradual transition of cancer cells from a predominantly mesenchymal cell phenotype to a more epithelial state [19, 101, 114–116]. Whereas cancer cells in the primary tumor and CTCs exhibit EMT, there is evidence suggesting that cancer cells colonizing distant tissues display mesenchymal-to-epithelial transition (MET), this being possible since EMT is a readily reversible biological process [19].

This progressive understanding may help us determine which steps during carcinogenesis that EMT detection and targeting may be useful for potential clinical applications [117]. For example, it is conceivable that our knowledge of EMT may have diagnostic applications in HCC and other cancers given that EMT plays an early role in the malignant conversion of a normal cell into a cancerous cell. Thus EMT markers may be useful biomarkers for earlier detection of HCC, if image-guided biopsy is performed early. It is also conceivable that "liquid biopsies" to obtain CTCs from the blood can be used to detect EMT markers in CTCs, thus diagnosing progression of HCC noninvasively. Moreover, the knowledge that increased expression of mesenchymal markers is observed and may contribute to several of the steps of the metastatic cascade opens up the possibility of targeting them to lower their expression, EMT, and possibly to inhibit or eliminate metastasis.

Table 8.2 Epithelial and mesenchymal markers that have been implicated in specific cases of hepatocellular carcinoma

E-Cadherin	Epithelial	Hashiguchi, M, et al. (2013) [26]; Wei Y et al. (2002) [29]; Matsumura, T et al. (2001) [27]; Wang XQ et al. (2012) [28]; Cho SB et al. (2008) [25]
N-Cadherin	Mesenchymal	Cho SB et al. (2008) [25]; Gwak, Geum-Youn et al. (2006) [37]
Vimentin	Mesenchymal	Hu L et al. (2004) [40]
Fibronectin	Mesenchymal	Gupta, N et al. (2006) [118]; Torbenson, M et al. (2002) [119]
Snail	Mesenchymal	Sugimachi, K et al. (2003) [54]; Yang, M et al. (2009) [58]; Wang XQ et al. (2012) [28]
Slug	Mesenchymal	Sun Y et al. (2014) [120]
ZEB	Mesenchymal	Hashiguchi, M, et al. (2013) [26]
Twist	Mesenchymal	Lee TK, et al. (2006) [59]; Yang, M et al. (2009) [58]
Goosecoid	Mesenchymal	Xue TC, et al. (2014) [121]
MMP9	Mesenchymal	Nart D et al. (2010) [122]

8.4 Potential Biomarkers for Diagnosing HCC Earlier

There are several molecular features that have been associated with epithelial-to-mesenchymal transition (EMT) that can serve as biomarkers of HCC. During EMT, for example, cell-to-cell adhesion is lost, and molecules that usually connect cells together such as some cadherins, catenins, and claudins are downregulated. In addition, transcription factors such as Snail, Slug, Twist, Zeb1, and Goosecoid are also activated. And genes associated with the mesenchymal phenotype, such as vimentin, fibronectin, CD44, integrin β6, and matrix metalloproteinases (MMPs), are also commonly upregulated [55, 101–104]. Table 8.2 shows the different epithelial and mesenchymal markers as detected in HCC cell lines or biopsies from patients with HCC.

8.5 Targeting EMT as a Potential HCC Therapeutic Strategy

As discussed above, it is important to be able to diagnose HCC earlier to optimize treatment and be more successful at removing this disease. The difficulty in treating HCC lies in the fact that by the time patients present with definitive symptoms, the cancer has likely advanced, and curative treatment options are either very limited or not available. As mentioned previously, EMT markers have a potential role in earlier HCC diagnosis and in the noninvasive monitoring of HCC progression.

However, EMT markers may also have potential application in HCC as therapeutic targets for inhibiting or eliminating progression and metastasis. There are several ways EMT can be targeted: through its effectors, transcription factors, or inducers. Each of these will be discussed below [123–125].

8.5.1 EMT Effectors as Possible Targets for HCC

EMT effectors are molecules that define the epithelial and mesenchymal state, for example, those mentioned before: E-cadherin, N-cadherin, vimentin, fibronectin, etc. While there are as yet no clinical applications of these EMT effectors as therapeutic targets, in vitro and preclinical studies have shown promising results [123]. For example, peptide ADH1 and quercetin both lower N-cadherin expression and thus prevent migration and tumor progression [126, 127]. Similarly, agents that lower vimentin levels such as withaferin A, silibinin, flavonolignan, and salinomycin exhibit antitumorigenic effects [128–131]. However, despite these observations, many EMT effectors have complex, time-dependent, and context-specific roles. Consequently, targeting them may prove challenging [123].

8.5.2 EMT Transcription Factors as Possible Targets for HCC

EMT transcription factors are the molecules that carry out EMT (such as Snail1, basic HLH family such as Twist1, and Zeb1). While preclinical studies have revealed promising results suggesting that EMT transcription factors are good therapeutic targets [132–134], these transcription factors have proven challenging to target in a clinical context [123]. Nevertheless, agents shown to decrease Twist1 expression (such as sulforaphane and moscatilin) all show a disruption of EMT as well as inhibition of tumorigenicity [135, 136]. Similarly, fucoidan, which decreases Twist1, Snail1, and Slug expression via various signaling pathways and microRNAs, also inhibits EMT [137–139].

8.5.3 EMT Inducers as Possible Therapeutic Targets for HCC

In addition to EMT effectors and transcription factors being possible therapeutic targets, we may also be able to target the factors that induce EMT for potential therapeutic applications [123]. With the recent clinical use of sorafenib for treatment of advanced HCC, high-throughput screening and an ongoing search are underway for other agents that could possibly have antitumorigenic benefits and extend lifespan while demonstrating limited toxicity [140, 141]. Interestingly, most of the relevant clinical trials currently ongoing target EMT inducers rather than target EMT effectors or transcription factors [123]. Indeed, sorafenib, while possessing anti-angiogenic effects, also inhibits tumor progression by suppressing EMT in HCC cases where percutaneous ablation is not an option. Sorafenib also inhibits migration and invasion by suppressing MMPs and HGF-induced EMT via the c-Met and ERK-MAPK pathways. And sorafenib's efficacy in inhibiting TGFβ has been demonstrated in mouse hepatocytes [140–144]. Several other agents inhibiting TGFβ (e.g., LY2157299, a selective inhibitor of TGFβR1) and c-Met (e.g., tivantinib) have also been investigated, with seemingly promising results in HCC [123].

Other agents being examined in clinical trials target other EMT inducers such as EGF, FGF, PI3K/AKT/mTOR, MEK, and IGF signaling and perhaps target microR-NAs that modulate EMT status [123].

Conclusion

Unfortunately, because HCC patients are frequently diagnosed when the cancer has already advanced, their prognosis is often dismal. To date, there is a lack of effective therapeutics for the treatment of advanced HCC [1]. Currently, sorafenib is the only FDA-approved drug for the treatment of advanced HCC, and it prolongs survival of patients with advanced HCC by only a few months [5]. Consequently, we urgently need discovery of molecular mechanisms that can be exploited for early diagnosis of HCC, monitoring of HCC progression, effective treatment of advanced HCC, and monitoring of response to drug treatment of HCC.

Although clinical applications of EMT markers may take a few more years to actualize, current research suggests that EMT markers may hold promise as potential biomarkers for early diagnosis and development of novel targeted therapeutic strategies for HCC (see Table 8.2). Because EMT is a phenomenon observed as early as the malignant conversion of a healthy cell into a cancer cell and present through multiple stages of tumorigenesis, it is likely to have potential applications for early detection and curative treatments of early cancers. Indeed, as mentioned above, there are a number of preclinical and clinical trials that are currently ongoing to determine potential therapeutic applications from targeting specific EMT markers [123]. While dysregulated expression of EMT effectors and transcription factors may one day prove useful as biomarkers for early diagnosis of HCC, it appears that some clinical trials are showing promising results from targeting EMT inducers [145–147]. It is possible that combining sorafenib with one or more of these novel EMT marker-based therapeutics that may yet come through may provide additional beneficial outcomes for patients with advanced HCC [148].

Of course, therapeutic targeting of EMT markers may be associated with currently unknown side effects. These may be related to issues such as intratumor heterogeneous expression of EMT markers. Also, EMT appears to be context- and time-dependent and transient. These issues may create side effects from targeting EMT markers. However, with increasingly greater knowledge being gained from large cancer sequencing projects, it may be that it is possible to combine other novel targeted therapies with therapeutic targeting of EMT markers in such a way as to minimize side effects [145–147]. Moreover, better understanding of the most appropriate timing of when EMT inhibition would be most effective at combating HCC and other cancers could contribute to developing effective new drug treatments. Our current understanding of the role of EMT in HCC certainly suggests that EMT is important in HCC development and progression and that further research into the role of EMT in HCC is required to create beneficial clinical applications in HCC.

References

1. Raza A, et al. Hepatocellular carcinoma review: current treatment, and evidence-based medicine. World J Gastroenterol. 2014;20(15):4115–27. https://doi.org/10.3748/wjg.v20.i15.4115.
2. Schütte K, Balbisi F, Malfertheiner P. Prevention of hepatocellular carcinoma. Gastrointest Tumors. 2016;3(1):37–43. https://doi.org/10.1159/000446680.
3. Villanueva A, Hernandez-Gea V, Llovet J. Medical therapies for hepatocellular carcinoma: a critical view of the evidence. Nat Rev Gastroenterol Hepatol. 2013;10:34–42. https://doi.org/10.1038/nrgastro.2012.199.
4. Colagrande S, Inghilesi AL, Aburas S, Taliani GG, Nardi C, Marra F. Challenges of advanced hepatocellular carcinoma. World J Gastroenterol. 2016;22(34):7645–59. https://doi.org/10.3748/wjg.v22.i34.7645.
5. Di Marco V, De Vita F, Koskinas J, Semela D, Toniutto P, Verslype C. Sorafenib: from literature to clinical practice. Ann Oncol. 2013;24(Suppl 2):ii30–7. https://doi.org/10.1093/annonc/mdt055.
6. American Cancer Society. Cancer facts & figures 2016. Atlanta: American Cancer Society; 2016.
7. Acloque H, et al. Epithelial-mesenchymal transitions: the importance of changing cell state in development and disease. J Clin Invest. 2009;119(6):1438–49.
8. Kalluri R. When epithelial cells decide to become mesenchymal-like cells. J Clin Invest. 2009;119(6):1417–9.
9. Martin-Belmonte F, Perez-Moreno M. Epithelial cell polarity, stem cells and cancer. Nat Rev Cancer. 2012;12:23–8.
10. Krakhmal N, Zavyalova M, et al. Cancer invasion: patterns and mechanisms. Acta Nat. 2015;7(2):17–28.
11. Nakaya Y, Sheng G. Epithelial to mesenchymal transition during gastrulation: an embryological view. Develop Growth Differ. 2008;50(9):755–66.
12. Kerosuo L, Bronner-Fraser M. What is bad in cancer is good in the embryo: importance of EMT in neural crest development. Semin Cell Dev Biol. 2012;23(3):320–32.
13. Risky DC. Epithelial-mesenchymal transition. J Cell Sci. 2005;118(19):4325–6. https://doi.org/10.1242/jcs.02552.
14. Stone RC, Pastar I, et al. Epithelial-mesenchymal transition in tissue repair and fibrosis. Cell Tissue Res. 2016;365(3):495–506.
15. Inman JL, Robertson C, et al. Mammary gland development: cell fate specification, stem cells, and the microenvironment. Development. 2015;142:1028–42.
16. Guislaine B, et al. Epithelial mesenchymal transition: a double-edged sword. Clin Transl Med. 2015;4:14.
17. Kalluri R, Weinberg RA. The basics of epithelial-mesenchymal transition. J Clin Invest. 2009;119(6):1420–8. https://doi.org/10.1172/JCI39104.
18. Zeisberg M, Neilson EG. Biomarkers for epithelial-mesenchymal transitions. J Clin Invest. 2009;119(1558–8238 (Electronic)):1429–37. https://doi.org/10.1172/JCI36183.protected.
19. Yao D, Dai C, Peng S. Mechanism of the mesenchymal-epithelial transition and its relationship with metastatic tumor formation. Mol Cancer Res. 2011;9(12):1608–20.
20. Lamouille S. Molecular mechanisms of epithelial-mesenchymal transition. Nat Rev Mol Cell Biol. 2014;15(3):178–96. https://doi.org/10.1038/nrm3758.
21. Sabbah M, Emami S, Redeuilh G, Julien S, Prévost G, Zimber A, et al. Molecular signature and therapeutic perspective of the epithelial-to-mesenchymal transitions in epithelial cancers. Drug Resist Updat. 2008;11(4–5):123–51. https://doi.org/10.1016/j.drup.2008.07.001.
22. Jeanes A, Gottardi CJ, Yap AS. Cadherins and cancer: how does cadherin dysfunction promote tumor progression? Oncogene. 2008;27(55):6920–9. https://doi.org/10.1038/onc.2008.343.
23. Jankowski JA, Bruton R, Shepherd N, Sanders DS. Cadherin and catenin biology represent a global mechanism for epithelial cancer progression. Mol Pathol. 1997;50(6):289–90. http://www.pubmedcentral.nih.gov/articlerender.fcgi?artid=379661&tool=pmcentrez&rendertype=abstract

24. Pirinen RT, Hirvikoski P, Johansson RT, Hollmén S, Kosma VM. Reduced expression of alpha-catenin, beta-catenin, and gamma-catenin is associated with high cell proliferative activity and poor differentiation in non-small cell lung cancer. J Clin Pathol. 2001;54(5):391–5. https://doi.org/10.1136/jcp.54.5.391.

25. Cho SB. Expression of E- and N-cadherin and clinicopathology in hepatocellular carcinoma. Pathol Int. 2008;58(10):635–42. https://doi.org/10.1111/j.1440-1827.2008.02282.x.

26. Hashiguchi M, Ueno S, Sakoda M, Iino S, Hiwatashi K, Minami K, et al. Clinical implication of ZEB-1 and E-cadherin expression in hepatocellular carcinoma (HCC). BMC Cancer. 2013;13:572. https://doi.org/10.1186/1471-2407-13-572.

27. Matsumura T, Makino R, Mitamura K. Frequent down-regulation of E-cadherin by genetic and epigenetic changes in the malignant progression of HCC. Clin Cancer Res. 2001;7:594–9.

28. Wang XQ, Zhang W, Lui ELH, Zhu Y, Lu P, Yu X, et al. Notch1-Snail1-E-cadherin pathway in metastatic hepatocellular carcinoma. Int J Cancer. 2012;131(3):163–72. https://doi.org/10.1002/ijc.27336.

29. Wei Y, Van Nhieu JT, Prigent S, Srivatanakul P, Tiollais P, Buendia M-A. Altered expression of E-cadherin in hepatocellular carcinoma: correlations with genetic alterations, beta-catenin expression, and clinical features. Hepatology. 2002;36(3):692–701. https://doi.org/10.1053/jhep.2002.35342.

30. Yi K, Kim H, Sim J, Chan Y. Clinicopathologic correlations of E-cadherin and Prrx-1 expression loss in hepatocellular carcinoma. J Pathol Transl Med. 2016;50(5):327–36.

31. Petrova Y, et al. Roles for E-cadherin cell surface regulation in cancer. Mol Biol Cell. 2016;27(21):3233–44.

32. Abou Khouzam R, et al. Digital PCR identifies changes in CDH1 (E-Cadherin) transcription pattern in intestinal-type gastric cancer. Oncotarget. 2017;8(12):18811–20. 10.18632/oncotarget.13401.

33. Cheung SY, et al. Role of epithelial-mesenchymal transition markers in triple negative breast cancer. Breast Cancer Res Treat. 2015;152(3):489–98.

34. Margineanu E, et al. Correlation between E-cadherin abnormal expressions in different types of cancer and the process of metastasis. Rev Med Chir Soc Med Nat Iasi. 2008;112(2):432–6.

35. Cavaliaro U, et al. Cadherins and the tumour progression: is it all in a switch? Cancer Lett. 2002;176(2):123–8.

36. Derycke LD, Bracke ME. N-Cadherin in the spotlight of cell-cell adhesion, differentiation, embryogenesis, invasion, and signaling. Int J Dev Biol. 2004;48(5–6):463–76.

37. Gwak GY, Yoon JH, Yu SJ, Park SC, Jang JJ, Lee KB, et al. Anti-apoptotic N-cadherin signaling and its prognostic implication in human hepatocellular carcinomas. Oncol Rep. 2006;15(5):1117–23.

38. Bernal SD, Stahel RA. Cytoskeleton-associated proteins: their role as cellular integrators in the neoplastic process. Crit Rev Oncol Hematol. 1985;3(3):191–204.

39. Dey P, Togra J, Mitra S. Intermediate filament: structure, function, and applications in cytology. Diagn Cytopathol. 2014;42(7):628–35.

40. Hu L, Lau SH, Tzang C-H, Wen J-M, Wang W, Xie D, et al. Association of Vimentin overexpression and hepatocellular carcinoma metastasis. Oncogene. 2004;23(1):298–302. https://doi.org/10.1038/sj.onc.1206483.

41. Okushin H, et al. Immunohistochemical study of fibronectin, lysozyme, and alpha fetoprotein (AFP) in human hepatocellular carcinoma. Gastroenterol Jpn. 1987;22(1):44–54.

42. Matsui S, Takahashi T, Oyanagi Y, Takahashi S, Boku S, Takahashi K, et al. Expression, localization and alternative splicing pattern of fibronectin messenger RNA in fibrotic human liver and hepatocellular carcinoma. J Hepatol. 1997;27(5):843–53. https://doi.org/10.1016/S0168-8278(97)80322-4.

43. Das D, Naidoo M, Ilboudo A, et al. miR-1207-3p regulates the androgen receptor in prostate cancer via FNDC1/fibronectin. Exp Cell Res. 2016;348(2):190–200. https://doi.org/10.1016/j.yexcr.2016.09.021.

44. Endo K, Terada T. Protein expression of CD44 (standard and variant isoforms) in hepatocellular carcinoma: relationships with tumor grade, clinicopathologic parameters, p53 expression, and patient survival. J Hepatol. 2000;32(1):78–84.
45. Xie Z, et al. Inhibition of CD44 expression in hepatocellular carcinoma cells enhances apoptosis, chemosensitivity, and reduces tumorigenesis and invasion. Cancer Chemother Pharmacol. 2008;62(6):949–57.
46. Wu Y, et al. Targeting integrins in hepatocellular carcinoma. Expert Opin Ther Targets. 2011;15(4):421–37.
47. Diaz VM, Viñas-Castells R, Garcia de Herreros A. Regulation of the protein stability of EMT transcription factors. Cell Adh Migr. 2014;8(4):418–28.
48. Peinado H, Olmeda D, Cano A. Snail, Zeb, and bHLH factors in tumour progression: an alliance against the epithelial phenotype? Nat Rev Cancer. 2007;7(6):415–28.
49. Becker KF, et al. Analysis of the E-cadherin repressor Snail in primary human cancers. Cells Tissues Organs. 2007;185(1–3):204–12.
50. Alves CC, et al. Role of the epithelial-mesenchymal transition regulator Slug in primary human cancers. Front Biosci (Landmark Ed). 2009;14:3035–50.
51. Cano A, et al. The transcription factor snail controls epithelial-mesenchymal transitions by repressing E-cadherin expression. Nat Cell Biol. 2000;2(2):76–83.
52. Castro Alves C, et al. Slug is overexpressed in gastric carcinomas and may act synergistically with SIP1 and Snail in the downregulation of E-cadherin. J Pathol. 2007;211(5):507–15.
53. Ikenouchi J, et al. Regulation of tight junctions during the epithelium-mesenchyme transition: direct repression of the gene expression of claudins/occluding by Snail. J Cell Sci. 2003;116(Pt 10):1959–67.
54. Sugimachi K, Tanaka S, Kameyama T, Taguchi K, Aishima S, Shimada M, et al. Transcriptional repressor snail and progression of human hepatocellular carcinoma. Clin Cancer Res. 2003;9(7):2657–64. http://www.ncbi.nlm.nih.gov/pubmed/12855644
55. Samatov TR, Tonevitsky AG, Schumacher U. Epithelial-mesenchymal transition: focus on metastatic cascade, alternative splicing, non-coding RNAs and modulating compounds. Mol Cancer. 2013;12(1):107. https://doi.org/10.1186/1476-4598-12-107.
56. Voulgari A, Pintzas A. Epithelial-mesenchymal transition in cancer metastasis: mechanisms, markers and strategies to overcome drug resistance in the clinic. Biochim Biophys Acta. 2009;1796(2):75–90. https://doi.org/10.1016/j.bbcan.2009.03.002.
57. Zhang P, Hu P, Shen H, Yu J, Liu Q, Du J. Prognostic role of twist or snail in various carcinomas: a systematic review and meta-analysis. Eur J Clin Invest. 2014;44(11):1072–94. https://doi.org/10.1111/eci.12343.
58. Yang MH, Chen CL, Chau GY, Chiou SH, Su CW, Chou TY, et al. Comprehensive analysis of the independent effect of twist and snail in promoting metastasis of hepatocellular carcinoma. Hepatology. 2009;50(5):1464–74. https://doi.org/10.1002/hep.23221.
59. Lee TK, Poon RTP, Yuen AP, Ling MT, Kwok WK, Wang XH, et al. Twist overexpression correlates with hepatocellular carcinoma metastasis through induction of epithelial-mesenchymal transition. Clin Cancer Res. 2006;12(18):5369–76. https://doi.org/10.1158/1078-0432.CCR-05-2722.
60. Giannelli G, et al. Transforming Growth-B as a therapeutic target in hepatocellular carcinoma. Cancer Res. 2014;74(7):1890–4. https://doi.org/10.1158/0008-5472.CAN-14-0243.
61. Massagué J. TGFβ in cancer. Cell. 2008;134(2):215–30. https://doi.org/10.1016/j.cell.2008.07.001.
62. Morrison CD, Parvani JG, Schiemann WP. The relevance of the TGFβ paradox to EMT-MET programs. Cancer Lett. 2013;341(1):30–40. https://doi.org/10.1016/j.canlet.2013.02.048.
63. Papageorgis P. TGF-beta signaling in tumor initiation, epithelial-to-mesenchymal transition, and metastasis. J Oncol. 2015;2015. doi:https://doi.org/10.1155/2015/587193.
64. Zhang Y. Non-Smad pathways in TGF-beta signaling. Cell Res. 2009;19(1):128–39.
65. Giehl K, Imamichi Y, Menke A. Smad4-indeendent TGF-beta signaling in tumor cell migration. Cells Tissues Organs. 2007;185(1–3):123–30.

66. Zhang L, et al. Signaling interplay between transforming growth factor-B receptor and PI3K/AKT pathways in cancer. Trends Biochem Sci. 2013;38(12):612–20.
67. Gui T, et al. The roles of mitogen-activated protein kinase pathways in TGF-β-induced epithelial-mesenchymal transition. J Signal Transduct. 2012;2012:289243.
68. Paul M, Mukhopadhyay A. Tyrosine kinase—role and significance in cancer. Int J Med Sci. 2004;1(2):101–15.
69. Cross M, Dexter TM. Growth factors in development, transformation, and tumorigenesis. Cell. 1991;64(2):271–80.
70. Witsch E, et al. Roles for growth factors in cancer progression. Physiology. 2010;25(2):85–101.
71. Komiya Y, Habas R. Wnt signal transduction pathways. Organogenesis. 2008;4(2):68–75.
72. Varjosalo M, Taipale J. Hedgehog: functions and mechanisms. Genes Dev. 2008;22:2454–72.
73. Wang Z, et al. The role of Notch signaling pathway in epithelial-mesenchymal transition (EMT) during development and tumor aggressiveness. Curr Drug Targets. 2010;11(6):745–51.
74. Fransvea E, et al. Blocking transforming growth factor-beta up-regulates E-cadherin and reduces migration and invasion of hepatocellular carcinoma cells. Hepatology. 2008;47:1557–66.
75. Fransvea E, et al. Targeting transforming growth factor (TGF)-betaRI inhibits activation of beta 1 integrin and blocks vascular invasion in hepatocellular carcinoma. Hepatology. 2009;49:839–50.
76. Reichl P, et al. TGF-β in epithelial to mesenchymal transition and metastasis of liver carcinoma. Curr Pharm Des. 2012;18(27):4135–47.
77. Dituri F, et al. Differential Inhibition of TGF-beta signaling pathway in HCC cells using the small molecule inhibitor LY2157299 and the D10 monoclonal antibody against TGF-beta receptor type II. PLoS One. 2013;8:e67109.
78. Steinway SN, et al. Network modeling of TGFB signaling in hepatocellular carcinoma epithelial-to-mesenchymal transition reveals joint sonic hedgehog and Wnt pathway activation. Cancer Res. 2014;74(21):5963–77.
79. Qin G, et al. Reciprocal activation between MMP-8 and TGF-b1 stimulates EMT and malignant progression of hepatocellular carcinoma. Cancer Lett. 2016;374:85–95.
80. Nagai T, Arao T, Furuta K, Sakai K, Kudo K, Kaneda H, et al. Sorafenib inhibits the hepatocyte growth factor-mediated epithelial mesenchymal transition in hepatocellular carcinoma. Mol Cancer Ther. 2011;10(1):169–77. https://doi.org/10.1158/1535-7163.MCT-10-0544.
81. Ogunwobi O, Liu C. Hepatocyte growth factor upregulation promotes carcinogenesis and epithelial-mesenchymal transition in hepatocellular carcinoma via Akt and COX-2 pathways. Clin Exp Metastasis. 2011;28(8):721–31.
82. Ogunwobi O, et al. Epigenetic upregulation of HGF and c-Met drives metastasis in hepatocellular carcinoma. PLoS One. 2013;8(5):e63765.
83. Wang H, et al. Activation of phosphatidylinositol 3-kinase/Akt signaling mediates sorafenib-induced invasion and metastasis in hepatocellular carcinoma. Oncol Rep. 2014;32:1465–72. https://doi.org/10.3892/or.2014.3352.
84. Zhang PF, et al. Galectin-1 induces hepatocellular carcinoma EMT and sorafenib resistance by activating FAK/PI3K/AKT signaling. Cell Death Dis. 2016;7:e2201.
85. Zhang Q, et al. Wnt/B-catenin signaling enhances hypoxia-induced epithelial-mesenchymal transition in hepatocellular carcinoma via crosstalk with hif-1a signaling. Carcinogenesis. 2013;34(5):962–73.
86. Yang M, et al. A double-negative feedback loop between Wnt-B-catenin signaling and HNF4a regulates epithelial-mesenchymal transition in hepatocellular carcinoma. J Cell Sci. 2013;126:5692–703.
87. Jiang L, et al. CLDN3 inhibits cancer aggressiveness via Wnt-EMT signaling and is a potential prognostic biomarker for hepatocellular carcinoma. Oncotarget. 2014;5(17):7663–76.
88. Wan X, et al. CD24 promotes HCC progression via triggering Notch-related EMT and modulation of tumor microenvironment. Tumor Biol. 2016;37(5):6073–84.
89. Jia M, et al. LincRNA-p21 inhibits invasion and metastasis of hepatocellular carcinoma through Notch signaling-induced epithelial-mesenchymal transition. Hepatol Res. 2016;46(11):1137–44.

90. Xiao S, et al. Actin-like 6A predicts poor prognosis of hepatocellular carcinoma and promotes metastasis and epithelial-mesenchymal transition. Hepatology. 2016;63(4):1256–71.
91. Vaupel P, Mayer A. Hypoxia in cancer: significance and impact on clinical outcome. Cancer Metastasis Rev. 2007;26(2):225–39.
92. Zhang L, et al. Hypoxia induces epithelial-mesenchymal transition via activation of SNAI1 by hypoxia-inducible factor-1a in hepatocellular carcinoma. BMC Cancer. 2013;13:108.
93. Lu H, et al. Inflammation, a key event in cancer development. Mol Cancer Res. 2006;4(4):221–33.
94. Kubo N, et al. Cancer-associated fibroblasts in hepatocellular carcinoma. World J Gastroenterol. 2016;22(30):6841–50.
95. Sullivan NJ, et al. Interleukin-6 induces an epithelial-mesenchymal transition phenotype in human breast cancer cells. Oncogene. 2009;28:2940–7.
96. Jou J, Diehl AM. Epithelial-mesenchymal transitions and hepatocarcinogenesis. J Clin Invest. 2010;120(4):1031–4. https://doi.org/10.1172/JCI42615.detection.
97. Smith HA, Kang Y. The metastasis-promoting roles of tumor-associated immune cells. J Mol Med. 2013;91(4):411–29. https://doi.org/10.1007/s00109-013-1021-5.
98. Giordano S, Columbano A. MicroRNAs: new tools for diagnosis, prognosis, and therapy in hepatocellular carcinoma? Hepatology. 2013;57(2):840–7. https://doi.org/10.1002/hep.26095.
99. Callegari E, Elamin BK, Sabbioni S, Gramantieri L, Negrini M. Role of microRNAs in hepatocellular carcinoma: a clinical perspective. Onco Targets Ther. 2013;6:1167–78. https://doi.org/10.2147/OTT.S36161.
100. Qin Z, He W, Tang J, Ye Q, Dang W, Lu Y, Ma J. MicroRNAs provide feedback regulation of epithelial-mesenchymal transition induced by growth factors. J Cell Physiol. 2016;231(1):120–9. https://doi.org/10.1002/jcp.25060.
101. Tsai JH, Yang J. Epithelial-mesenchymal plasticity in carcinoma metastasis. Genes Dev. 2013;27:2192–206.
102. Ferrara N. From local invasion to metastatic cancer. Anticancer Res. 2009;29. doi:https://doi.org/10.1007/978-1-60327-087-8.
103. Gavert N, Ben-Ze'ev A. Epithelial–mesenchymal transition and the invasive potential of tumors. Trends Mol Med. 2008;14(5):199–209. https://doi.org/10.1016/j.molmed.2008.03.004.
104. Heerboth S, et al. EMT and tumor metastasis. Clin Transl Med. 2015;4(1):6. https://doi.org/10.1186/s40169-015-0048-3.
105. Drake JM, Strohbehn G, Bair TB, Moreland JG, Henry MD. ZEB1 enhances transendothelial migration and represses the epithelial phenotype of prostate cancer cells. Mol Biol Cell. 2009;20:2207–17.
106. Ota I, Li XY, Hu Y, Weiss SJ. Induction of a MT1-MMP and MT2-MMP-dependent basement membrane transmigration program in cancer cells by Snail1. Proc Natl Acad Sci. 2009;106:20318–23.
107. Yap TA, et al. Circulating tumor cells: a multifunctional biomarker. Clin Cancer Res. 2014;20(10):2553–68.
108. Li Y, et al. Epithelial–mesenchymal transition markers expressed in circulating tumor cells in hepatocellular carcinoma patients with different stages of disease. Cell Death Dis. 2013;4(10):e831. https://doi.org/10.1038/cddis.2013.347.
109. Liu H, Zhang X, Li J, Sun B, Qian H, Yin Z. The biological and clinical importance of epithelial-mesenchymal transition in circulating tumor cells. J Cancer Res Clin Oncol. 2015;141(2):189–201. https://doi.org/10.1007/s00432-014-1752-x.
110. Satelli A, et al. Epithelial-mesenchymal transitioned circulating tumor cells capture for detecting tumor progression. Clin Cancer Res. 2014;21(4):899–906. https://doi.org/10.1158/1078-0432.CCR-14-0894.
111. Huaman J, et al. Circulating tumor cells from a syngeneic mouse model of hepatocellular carcinoma demonstrate epithelial-mesenchymal transition, decreased MHCI expression and increased CCR7 expression; Abstract #1547; American Association for Cancer Research, April 16–20. 2016.

112. Stoletov K, Kato H, Zardouzian E, Kelber J, Yang J, Shattil S, Klemke R. Visualizing extravasation dynamics of metastatic tumor cells. J Cell Sci. 2010;123:2332–41.
113. Shibue T, Brooks MW, Inan MF, Reinhardt F, Weinberg RA. The outgrowth of micrometastases is enabled by the formation of filopodium-like protrusions. Cancer Discov. 2012;2:706–21.
114. Yu M, Bardia A, Wittner BS, Stott SL, Smas ME, Ting DT, et al. Circulating breast tumor cells exhibit dynamic changes in epithelial and mesenchymal composition. Science. 2013;339(6119):580–4.
115. Polioudaki H, Agelaki S, Chiotaki R, Politaki E, Mavroudis D, Matikas A, et al. Variable expression levels of keratin and vimentin reveal differential EMT status of circulating tumor cells and correlation with clinical characteristics and outcome of patients with metastatic breast cancer. BMC Cancer. 2015;15:399.
116. Hong Y, Zhang Q. Phenotype of circulating tumor cell: face-off between epithelial and mesenchymal masks. Tumour Biol. 2015;37(5):5663–74.
117. van Zijl F et al. Epithelial to mesenchymal transition in hepatocellular carcinoma. Future Oncol. 2009;5(8):1169–79. https://doi.org/10.2217/fon.09.91.Epithelial.
118. Gupta N. Pattern of fibronectin in HCC and its significance. Indian J Pathol Microbiol. 2006;49(3):362–4.
119. Torbenson M, Wang J, Choti M, Ashfaq R, Maitra A, Wilentz RE, Boitnott J. Hepatocellular carcinomas show abnormal expression of fibronectin protein. Mod Pathol. 2002;15(8):826–30. https://doi.org/10.1097/01.MP.0000024257.83046.7C.
120. Sun Y, Song GD, Sun N, Chen JQ, Yang SS. Slug overexpression induces stemness and promotes hepatocellular carcinoma cell invasion and metastasis. Oncol Lett. 2014;7(6):1936–40. https://doi.org/10.3892/ol.2014.2037.
121. Xue TC, Ge NL, Zhang L, Cui JF, Chen RX, You Y, et al. Goosecoid promotes the metastasis of hepatocellular carcinoma by modulating the epithelial-mesenchymal transition. PLoS One. 2014;9(10):1–10. https://doi.org/10.1371/journal.pone.0109695.
122. Nart D, et al. Expression of matrix metalloproteinase-9 in predicting prognosis of Hepatocellular carcinoma after liver transplantation. Liver Transpl. 2010;16:621–30.
123. Pasquier J, Abu-Kaoud N, Thani HA, Rafii A. Epithelial to mesenchymal transition in a clinical perspective. J Oncol. 2015;2015:792182. https://doi.org/10.1155/2015/792182.
124. Shen Y-C, Lin Z-Z, Hsu C-H, Hsu C, Shao Y-Y, Cheng A-L. Clinical trials in hepatocellular carcinoma: an update. Liver Cancer. 2013;2(3–4):345–64. https://doi.org/10.1159/000343850.
125. Ogunwobi OO, Liu C. Therapeutic and prognostic importance of epithelial–mesenchymal transition in liver cancers: insights from experimental models. Crit Rev Oncol Hematol. 2012;83(3):319–28. https://doi.org/10.1016/j.critrevonc.2011.11.007.
126. Shintani Y, et al. ADH-1 suppresses N-cadherin-dependent pancreatic cancer progression. Int J Cancer. 2008;122(1):71–7.
127. Chang W, et al. Quercetin in elimination of tumor initiating stem-like and mesenchymal transformation property in head and neck cancer. Head Neck. 2013;35(3):413–9.
128. Lahat G, et al. Vimentin is a novel anti-cancer therapeutic target; insights from *In Vitro* and *In Vivo* mice xenograft studies. PLoS One. 2010;5(4):e10105.
129. Singh RP, et al. Silibinin inhibits established prostate tumor growth, progression, invasion, and metastasis and suppresses tumor angiogenesis and epithelial-mesenchymal transition in transgenic adenocarcinoma of the mouse prostate model mice. Clin Cancer Res. 2008;14(23):7773–80.
130. Wu KJ, et al. Silibinin inhibits prostate cancer invasion, motility and migration by suppressing vimentin and MMP-2 expression. Acta Pharmacol Sin. 2009;30(8):1162–8.
131. Dong T, et al. Salinomycin selectively targets 'CD133+' cell subpopulations and decreases malignant traits in colorectal cancer lines. Ann Surg Oncol. 2011;18(6):1797–804.
132. Chung MT, et al. SFRP1 and SFRP2 suppress the transformation and invasion abilities of cervical cancer cells through Wnt signal pathway. Gynecol Oncol. 2009;112(3):646–53.
133. Zhuo W, et al. Knockdown of Snail, a novel zinc-finger transcription factor, via RNA interference increases A549 cell sensitivity to cisplatin via JNK/mitochondrial pathway. Lung Cancer. 2008;62(1):8–14.

134. Zhuo WL, et al. Short interfering RNA directed against TWIST, a novel zinc finger transcription factor, increases A549 cell sensitivity to cisplatin via MAPK/mitochondrial pathway. Biochem Biophys Res Commun. 2008;369(4):1098–102.

135. Srivastava R, et al. Sulforaphane synergizes with quercetin to inhibit self-renewal capacity of pancreatic cancer stem cells. Front Biosci (Elite Ed). 2011;3(2):515–28.

136. Pai HC, et al. Moscatilin inhibits migration and metastasis of human breast cancer MDA-MB-231 cells through inhibition of Akt and Twist signaling pathway. J Mol Med. 2013;91(3):347–56.

137. Hsu HY, et al. Fucoidan induces changes in the epithelial to mesenchymal transition and decreases metastasis by enhancing ubiquitin-dependent TGF-beta receptor degradation in breast cancer. Carcinogenesis. 2013;34(4):874–84.

138. Cho Y, Yoon J-H, Yoo J, Lee M, Lee DH, Cho EJ, et al. Fucoidan protects hepatocytes from apoptosis and inhibits invasion of hepatocellular carcinoma by up-regulating p42/44 MAPK-dependent NDRG-1/CAP43. Acta Pharm Sin B. 2015;5(6):544–53. https://doi.org/10.1016/j.apsb.2015.09.004.

139. Yan MD, Yao CJ, Chow JM, Chang CL, Hwang PA, Chuang SE, et al. Fucoidan elevates MicroRNA-29b to regulate DNMT3B-MTSS1 axis and inhibit EMT in human hepatocellular carcinoma cells. Mar Drugs. 2015;13(10):6099–116. https://doi.org/10.3390/md13106099.

140. Reka AK, et al. Identifying inhibitors of epithelial-mesenchymal transition by connectivity map-based systems approach. J Thorac Oncol. 2011;6(11):1784–92.

141. Chua KN, et al. A cell-based small molecule screening method for identifying inhibitors of epithelial-mesenchymal transition in carcinoma. PLoS One. 2012;7(3):e33183.

142. Huang XY, Ke AW, Shi GM, Zhang X, Zhang C, Shi YH, et al. αB-crystallin complexes with 14-3-3ζ to induce epithelial-mesenchymal transition and resistance to sorafenib in hepatocellular carcinoma. Hepatology. 2013;57(6):2235–47. https://doi.org/10.1002/hep.26255.

143. Chen J, Jin R, Zhao J, Liu J, Ying H, Yan H, et al. Potential molecular, cellular and microenvironmental mechanism of sorafenib resistance in hepatocellular carcinoma. Cancer Lett. 2015;367(1):1–11. https://doi.org/10.1016/j.canlet.2015.06.019.

144. Chen YL, Lv X, Ye XL, Sun MY, Xu Q, Liu CH, et al. Sorafenib inhibits transforming growth factor β1-Mediated Epithelial-Mesenchymal Transition and apoptosis in mouse hepatocytes. Hepatology. 2011;53(5):1708–18. https://doi.org/10.1002/hep.24254.

145. Franco-Chuaire ML, Magda Carolina SC, Chuaire-Noack L. Epithelial-mesenchymal transition (EMT): principles and clinical impact in cancer therapy. Invest Clin. 2013;54(2):186–205.

146. Nantajit D, Lin D, Li JJ. The network of epithelial–mesenchymal transition: potential new targets for tumor resistance. J Cancer Res Clin Oncol. 2015;141(10):1697–713. https://doi.org/10.1007/s00432-014-1840-y.

147. Steinestel K, Eder S, et al. Clinical significance of epithelial-mesenchymal transition. Clin Transl Med. 2014;3:17. http://www.clintransmed.com/content/3/1/17

148. Dong S, Kong J, Kong F, Gao J, Ji L, Pan B, et al. Sorafenib suppresses the epithelial-mesenchymal transition of hepatocellular carcinoma cells after insufficient radiofrequency ablation. BMC Cancer. 2015;15:939. https://doi.org/10.1186/s12885-015-1949-7.

Hepatocellular Carcinoma Metastasis and Circulating Tumor Cells

9

Kien Pham, Dan Delitto, and Chen Liu

9.1 Introduction

A hallmark of aggressive hepatocellular carcinomas (HCCs) is the ability to metastasize. Metastatic lesions are difficult to manage in clinical practice as the extent of disease typically precludes curative resection and resistance to systemic treatments is common [1, 2]. Metastasis is a multistage process in which cancer cells (1) delaminate from the primary site and locally invade the host stroma (*initiation*), (2) enter into blood and/or lymphatic vasculature (*intravasation*), (3) survive and exit the circulation into distant sites (*extravasation*), and (4) colonize the new microenvironment and proliferate to form a macroscopic secondary tumor (*colonization*) [3, 4]. This simplified model provides a framework for a sequence of biological properties that must be acquired during cancer dissemination. Different malignancies, however, demonstrate unique regulatory events in this process largely governed by the complex microenvironment in which the metastatic cells originate and that of the distant location(s) where the metastasis is established [5]. Given the anatomic and physiologic complexity of the liver, the HCC microenvironment is one of the most difficult to reproduce experimentally and, consequently, understand in its totality. In the context of this chapter, HCC metastasis is discussed, with an emphasis on the role of the hepatic microenvironment and the role of circulating cancer cells in the metastatic process.

K. Pham, Ph.D. (✉) • D. Delitto, M.D. • C. Liu, M.D., Ph.D.
Department of Pathology and Laboratory Medicine, Rutgers New Jersey Medical
School and Robert Wood Johnson Medical School, Newark, NJ, USA
e-mail: ptkien@pathology.ufl.edu

© Springer International Publishing AG 2018
C. Liu (ed.), *Precision Molecular Pathology of Liver Cancer*,
Molecular Pathology Library, https://doi.org/10.1007/978-3-319-68082-8_9

9.2 The Dynamic Interaction Between Tumor Cells and the Tumor Microenvironment in HCC

Hepatocellular carcinoma is typically observed clinically as a consequence of chronic inflammation associated with cirrhosis. The etiology of cirrhosis is commonly due to alcoholism, HBV/HCV infection, or metabolic disorders, all of which create a tumor-permissive milieu [6]. Hepatocellular carcinoma is an extraordinarily unique malignancy, in which tumorigenesis and progression are significantly regulated not only by the intrinsic properties of tumor cells but also by constant communication with a heterogeneous microenvironment. Cumulative evidence suggests that the dynamic interaction between tumor cells and their surrounding milieu plays fundamental roles in the initiation of metastatic phenotypes at the primary site [7–10]. This interaction is dynamic, constantly evolving with tumor development. For example, the microenvironment may exert inhibitory effects in early stages. When tumor cells reach a certain point during their progression, they can circumvent these inhibitory signals and actually exploit surrounding nonmalignant cells to support metastasis [5]. The surrounding milieu within the HCC microenvironment may consist of (1) hepatic stellate cells, stromal cells, endothelial cells, and immune cells and (2) growth factors, inflammatory cytokines, and extracellular matrix proteins [11–14]. In this review, the intermingled contribution of the tumor microenvironment to HCC metastasis is emphasized from the perspective of tumor-associated inflammation and immune responses.

9.2.1 Contribution of Distinct Inflammatory Components to the Progression of HCC Metastasis

Direct evidence of the interplay between the hepatic microenvironment and HCC metastasis is evidenced by a comprehensive analysis of global gene expression profiling from the National Cancer Institute [15–17]. In this investigation, the gene expression profiles of nonmalignant hepatic tissue surrounding HCC tumors from patients with intra- or extrahepatic metastases were compared to those with no detectable metastasis. Peripheral stroma associated with HCC metastasis demonstrated a unique gene expression profile when compared to tissue associated with isolated HCC lesions. Importantly, this profile is also significantly different from the intratumoral signature. More specifically, the pattern of inflammatory cytokine expression was also unique in HCC patients with venous metastasis, suggesting that cytokines may contribute to the metastatic process. These data strongly suggest that the metastatic potential HCC may be influenced by the inflammatory response of the host microenvironment.

Hepatic Stellate Cells
The hepatic stellate cell (HSC), first described by Kupffer in the nineteenth century, has emerged in the past 25 years as a remarkably versatile mesenchymal cell with vital functions not only in liver injury but also in hepatic development, regeneration,

xenobiotic responses, metabolism, and immune regulation [13, 18–20]. Equally intriguing is the remarkable plasticity of stellate cells. Stellate cells can be viewed as the nexus in a complex sinusoidal milieu that requires tightly regulated autocrine and paracrine cross talk, rapid responses to evolving extracellular matrix content, and exquisite responsiveness to the metabolic needs imposed by liver growth and repair [21, 22]. Moreover, stellate cells maintain systemic homeostasis through storage and mobilization of retinoids, antigen presentation and the induction of immune tolerance, as well as an emerging relationship with bone marrow-derived cells [22, 23]. In the tumor milieu, HSCs undergo a transition from the "quiescent" to "activated" state. Upon activation, HSCs infiltrate malignant hepatic tissue and localize around tumor sinusoids, adjacent fibrous parenchyma, and the tumor capsule [24, 25]. Activated HSCs have also been identified in the periphery of dysplastic hepatic nodules [26]. For tumor-associated HSCs, the restricted control of their function in regulating fibrotic matrix decomposition and degradation is disrupted, leading to the uninhibited production of extracellular matrix (ECM) proteins [20, 23, 27]. As a major source of ECM proteins, HSCs may therefore stimulate HCC metastasis via the regulation of tumor-stroma during the epithelial-to-mesenchymal transition, a process required for metastasis.

Although HSCs are considered central to the stimulation of a pro-metastatic microenvironment in HCC, the molecular mechanisms underlying this modulation are poorly understood. Unsupervised genome-wide expression profiling confirmed that the genes associated with cross talk between tumor cells and HSCs were significantly enriched in cirrhotic tissues from patients with metastasis [25]. These gene expression profiles, which are discussed in detail in subsequent sections, have the capability to activate inflammatory programs, which in turn contribute to tumor progression and metastasis.

Transforming growth factor-β (TGF-β) is secreted by both HSCs and hepatocytes and plays a multifunctional role in HCC pathogenesis [28, 29]. Tumor suppressor functions are observed in the early stages of liver damage and regeneration. Alternatively, during cancer progression, TGF-β may stimulate tumor invasiveness and metastatic behavior [30, 31]. TGF-β modulates the malignant properties of HCC not only through its own canonical signaling cascade but also via cross talk with many other growth factor pathways. Data from murine HCC models and three-dimensional, micro-organoid in vitro models reported by van Zijl et al. suggest a crucial role for the TGF-β/PDGF signaling axis in guiding epithelial-to-mesenchymal transition at the invasive front [32]. In a recent study, Park et al. identified tissue inhibitor of metalloproteinases-1 (TIMP-1) as one of the secreted proteins of HSCs and a key component of TGF-β-mediated cross talk between HSC and HCC cells. TGF-β stimulation led to increased expression of TIMP-1, which activated focal adhesion kinase (FAK) signaling via its interaction with CD63. Inhibition of TGF-β signaling using EW-7197, a small-molecule inhibitor of the TGF-β type I receptor kinase, abrogated TGF-β-mediated epithelial-to-mesenchymal transition in vitro using HCC cell lines and attenuated intrahepatic metastasis of HCC in an orthotopic xenograft mouse model using SK-HEP1-Luc cells [33].

Integrins, consisting of an α- and β-subunit, belong to a family of transmembrane receptors that integrate the extracellular and intracellular environment through binding both the ECM and the cytoskeleton [34]. Via transduction of signals between the internal and external cellular domains, integrins regulate cell adhesion, spreading, migration, proliferation, and differentiation as well as ECM deposition and remodeling [35]. In activated HSC, downstream integrin signaling, via the focal adhesion kinase (FAK)-phosphatidylinositol 3-kinase (PI3K)-Akt signaling pathway, promotes ECM deposition [36]. Integrin subunits α6 and β1 expression in human HCC tissue demonstrated a positive correlation metastasis [37]. These integrins can coordinate with other key signaling components, including but not limited to SERPINA5, CD151, PI3K-Akt, and TGF-β, to facilitate tumor invasion and metastasis properly via epithelial-to-mesenchymal transition [38–41].

A significant increase in Th2 cytokines (e.g., IL-4, IL-8, IL-10, and IL-5) and a concomitant decrease in the pro-inflammatory Th1 cytokines (e.g., IL-1α, IL-1β, IL-2, IL-12p35, IL-12p40, IL-15, and non-ILs, e.g., TNF-α and IFN-γ) were also found in livers associated with metastatic HCC, compared to normal samples. Such a profound Th1 to Th2 profile switch is unique to hepatic tissues from patients with HCC metastasis. This change is not related to the degree of viral hepatitis or cirrhosis, but it is a consequence of tumor burden [9, 15]. The findings strongly imply that an anti-inflammatory cascade, which is likely initiated/upregulated by HSCs, presents and promotes HCC metastasis.

Mesenchymal Stem Cells

Mesenchymal stem cells (MSCs) reside predominantly in the bone marrow, although they are not of hematopoietic origin. MSCs are multipotent cells that differentiate into osteoblasts, chondrocytes, adipocytes, and other cells of mesenchymal origin. In response to inflammation, MSCs are recruited to sites of tissue injury to participate in tissue remodeling and wound healing. The chronic inflammation observed in HCC leads to the local accumulation of MSCs in the liver. Current evidence suggests that tumor-infiltrating MSCs may influence the behavior of neighboring cancer cells [14]. The specific role of MSCs in HCC metastasis remains unclear. Upon co-culture with conditioned medium from TGF-β1-overexpressing MSCs with HCC cell lines having high (MHCC97-H) or low (MHCC97-L) metastatic potential, Li et al. showed that MSCs promote the proliferation of HCC cells and TGF-β1 signaling and inhibit cell migration and thus decrease metastatic potential. Inhibition of metastasis in this manner may be explained by the downregulation of osteopontin (OPN) in HCC cells after co-culture with TGF-β1 overexpressing MSC-conditioned medium [42]. Alternatively, MSCs pre-treated with pro-inflammatory cytokines (IFN-γ and TNF-α) facilitate epithelial-to-mesenchymal transition of HCC cells, possibly through upregulation of TGF-β1 [43]. These findings reinforce the complexity associated with tumor-stromal signaling and illustrate the influence stromal signaling can have over tumor metastasis.

Tumor-Associated Fibroblasts

Tumor-associated fibroblasts (TAFs) are the prominent cell type in HCC microenvironment and play a critical role in tumor-stroma interaction. The origin of TAFs remains unclear. TAFs specifically promote tumor growth, angiogenesis, and metastasis, in part through secretion of high levels of stromal cell-derived factor 1 (SDF1 or CXCL12), properties that render these cells unique from normal fibroblasts [44]. Mazzocca and coworkers showed that HCC cell growth, intravasation, and metastatic spread are dependent upon the presence of CAFs, and HCC cells reciprocally stimulate proliferation of CAFs, suggesting a key role for CAFs in tumor-stromal interaction [40]. There is a complex cross talk between TAFs and tumor cells. For instance, both can secrete PDGF and TGF-β, which leads to stellate cell activation and consequently ECM deposition and also enhances the growth and migration of cancer cells [40]. TAFs interact with the microvasculature by secreting VEGF and MMPs as well as several hepatocyte growth factors such as HGF [45]. TAFs also secrete immune-modulatory cytokines (IFN-γ, IL-6, and TNF) that can mobilize lymphocytes, natural killer cells, and tumor-associated myeloid cells [46–48].

9.2.2 The Signature Roles of Immune Components to the Facilitation of HCC Metastasis

It is widely accepted that immune cells are recruited to the tumor site in response to the chronic inflammatory microenvironment of HCC [9, 11, 49]. In response to the local inflammatory response, at some point, cancer cells evolve mechanisms of immune escape. Evidence continues to accumulate implicating the local immune microenvironment of HCC as one of tolerance [50]. Specifically, a defined expression signature containing 17 immune genes (12 cytokines, HLA-DR, HLA-DPA, ANXA1, PRG1, and CSF1) has recently been validated to evaluate local immune suppression [15, 16]. This set of genes serves as a key orchestrator of the intricate dialogue between infiltrating immune cells and cancer cells. Budhu et al. demonstrated that this immune-related gene panel could successfully predict both venous metastases and extrahepatic metastases by follow-up with more than 92% accuracy. The prognostic performance of this signature was superior to and independent of any clinicopathologic variables, including age, tumor size, microvascular invasion, level of α-fetoprotein and/or albumin, Child-Pugh score for cirrhosis mortality, as well as several staging systems (TNM, CLIP, BCLC, and Okuda) [15]. In the following section, the orchestrated action of these inflammatory genes in regulating HCC metastasis is discussed with specific emphasis on tumor-infiltrating lymphocytes.

T Cells
The majority of tumor-infiltrated lymphocytes in solid tumors are of CD3$^+$ T cells. They can be further stratified into CD4$^+$ helper T cells; among this subset is the CD4$^+$ regulatory T cell (Treg) and CD8$^+$ cytotoxic T cells. T cells can exert either or both tumor-suppressive and tumor-promoting properties [51, 52]. Pathologic skewing of T cells in the tumor microenvironment can suppress antitumor immune responses and is defined as another key regulator in HCC progression. Accounting for 5–10% of all CD4$^+$ T cells, Tregs are thought to be protumorigenic via the

suppression of antitumor immune responses [53]. In HCC, tumor-infiltrating CD4+CD25+forkhead box P3+ (FoxP3) Tregs impair the cytotoxic activity of CD8+ T cells while suppressing the proliferation of IFN-γ secretingCD4+CD25- T cells [54]. In other study, Gao et al. showed that the ratio of intratumoral CD45RO+ to peritumoral CD57+ (memory/senescent) T cells serves as a negative predictor of HCC extrahepatic metastasis [55, 56].

Although the role of T cells in HCC metastasis continues to be investigated, a likely contribution is the array of inflammatory mediators secreted by activated lymphocytes. For example, serum levels of IL-6 were high in metastatic HCC [57] and were able to distinguish primary or metastatic liver tumors from benign HCC lesions [58]. Furthermore, serum levels of the pro-inflammatory cytokines TNF-α and IL-1β were high in HCC prior to resection compared with healthy individuals [59, 60]. In another study, higher levels of IL-1β and TNF-α were found in the tissue surrounding hepatic metastases than within the primary HCC tumor [11]. High expression of IL-8 (or CXCL8), a chemokine with angiogenic action, in malignant hepatic tissue was also associated with a higher frequency of portal vein, venous, and bile duct invasion in HCC patients undergoing operative resection and may therefore be important in invasion and metastasis [15]. Interestingly, Wang et al. demonstrated type I interferon-mediated angiogenesis inhibition by downregulating vascular endothelial growth factor (VEGF) and thus inhibiting metastasis in an HCC xenograft model with high metastatic potential [61].

Tumor-Associated Macrophages

In addition to T cells, tumor-associated macrophages (TAMs) are commonly found in the tumor microenvironment of many types of cancer. TAMs play a major role in mediating the cross talk between cancer and stromal cells, promoting tumor cell proliferation, and stimulating angiogenesis, invasion, and metastasis [62]. In HCC, TAMs are recruited to the tumor milieu, residing predominately in the peritumoral region, by a cascade of growth factors and chemokines secreted by cancer cells [63]. Soluble mediators promoting TAM recruitment include vascular endothelial growth factor (VEGF), platelet-derived growth factor (PDGF), transformation growth factor-β (TGF-β), chemokine (C-C motif) ligand (CCL2), and macrophage colony-stimulating factor (M-CSF) [64, 65]. The expression of glypican-3 (GPC-3) on the surface of HCC cells may also promote TAM recruitment [66]. In human HCC, the majority of TAMs are polarized toward an M2 phenotype, characterized by poor antigen-presenting capability and the secretion of a distinct set of cytokines/chemokines (e.g., IL-10, TGF-β, CCL17, CCL22, CCL24, etc.) that interact with their receptors expressed mainly by Th2 and Treg cells, promoting the recruitment of these ineffective T cell subsets [67]. In the context of HCC metastasis, extensive macrophage infiltration and increased levels of M-CSF have been associated with intrahepatic metastasis and recurrence [68, 69]. Moreover, pharmacological approaches to directly target TAMs, via knocking out CCL2 or other TAM-specific chemokines, reduced migration and invasion of HCC cell lines [70].

The cross talk between tumor-associated macrophages and cancer cells in mediating HCC metastasis is conducted through various TAM-secreted factors and signaling pathways. Increased expression of CXCL12 and its corresponding receptor CXCR4, a particularly well-studied chemokine signaling axis, is associated with lymphatic metastasis in HCC patients [71]. This CXCL12/CXCR4 axis stimulates the growth, invasion, and metastasis of HCC cell lines, in part through enhancing the secretion of matrix metalloproteases (MMPs) 2 and 9 [72]. Upregulation of TAM-secreted IL-8 and its receptor CXCR2 have also been associated with intrahepatic metastasis of HCC [73]. In addition to chemokine signaling, TAM-derived growth factors also play a role in metastasis. Among these, TGF-β is well known for its role in tumor growth and metastasis. In HCC, TGF-β induces epithelial-to-mesenchymal transition through stimulation of the E- to N-cadherin switch, a signature event required for EMT, by upregulating Snail, an E-cadherin repressor, and PDGF signaling pathway [32, 74]. TGF-β can also affect α3β1 integrin, SMAD-2, and focal adhesion kinase (FAK), all of which are known to regulate tumor invasiveness [75]. All of these functions are regulated through TGF-β cross talk with other signaling cascades, such as FAK, PDGFR, STAT, HIF, etc. In addition to TGF-β signaling, osteopontin (OPN), a phosphorylated acidic glycoprotein which was found to be expressed in macrophages after liver injury [76], also contributes to HCC invasion and metastasis via the interaction with integrins [76]. OPN plasma levels were found increased in HCC patients and were associated with reduced liver function and worse prognosis [77]. Neutralizing OPN by anti-OPN antibodies resulted in strong inhibition of invasion and metastasis of HCC cells in vitro and in vivo [78].

9.3 Circulating Tumor Cells: The Foundation of Cancer Dissemination in HCC Metastasis

A highly heterogeneous subpopulation of cancer cells, termed circulating tumor cells (CTCs), is able to physically translocate from the primary tumor site to the peripheral circulation [79–81]. Historically, the presence of tumor cells in the peripheral circulation of cancer patients was first reported by Thomas Ashworth in 1869 [82]. Not long after, in 1889, Stephen Paget proposed the "seed and soil" hypothesis to explain the nonrandom pattern of metastasis to visceral organs and bones [83]. The presence of CTCs in the bloodstream of patients with epithelial cancers fits very well with this theory and has contributed to our understanding of cancer pathogenesis and metastasis [81]. Circulating tumor cells have frequently been observed in patients undergoing surgical resection or liver transplantation for HCC [84]. Although it remains unclear as to where these cells fall on the spectrum of primary to metastatic tumor cells, CTCs do appear to represent the link between a localized primary tumor and metastatic lesion. During the metastatic process, cancer cells must acquire traits to degrade and invade through the extracellular matrix of the surrounding tissue toward blood and lymphatic vessels [4]. The presence of CTCs correlates with the extent of metastatic burden, aggressive disease, and reduced time to progression [85]. An investigation by Vona et al. in 2004 detected CTCs in 52% of blood samples using the ISET (Isolation by Size of Epithelial/Throphoblastic Tumor cells) platform, from 44 HCC [86]. In other independent study, Xu et al. showed that CTCs were detected in more than 80% of HCC patients but not in healthy person or patients with benign liver diseases [87]. Fan et al. further demonstrated that CTCs were reduced in the peripheral blood of HCC patients after resection. Moreover, patients with greater than 0.01% CTCs in their blood were at a significantly elevated risk of disease progression and metastasis [88]. Taken together, these findings suggest that CTCs serve as a major contributor to HCC recurrence and metastasis.

Physically, circulating tumor cells 20–30 µm in diameter are far too large to pass through pulmonary capillary beds [86]. Theoretically, within minutes of being released by primary tumors into the venous circulation, CTCs should be trapped in these capillaries during their first pass through the heart. In addition, CTCs have a limited half-life (1–2.4 h) in the circulation, possibly due to circulatory shear stress or the loss of matrix-derived survival signals (anoikis) [89]. Based on these points, it would be logical to assume that only exceptionally small or physically plastic CTCs can transition through pulmonary microvasculature, thereby successfully surviving in the circulation to colonize a particular organ [3, 90]. Molecular analyses of CTCs demonstrate a heterogeneous gene expression pattern. CTCs have been generally recognized as negative for CD45 (a hematopoietic marker) and positive for extracellular epithelial cell adhesion molecule (EpCAM) and intracellular cytokeratins specific to epithelial cells (CK8/18/19), all of which have become "gold standard" markers for the detection of CTCs with an epithelial phenotype in patients with cancer [91, 92]. The reliance on epithelial markers to detect CTCs poses another challenge, in that tumor cells tend to lose epithelial characteristics and acquire mesenchymal features in order to metastasize [93]. Indeed, recent studies have shown that CTCs also expressed mesenchymal markers, such as Vimentin and N-cadherin [94–96]. The discrepancy in CTC marker expression suggests that CTCs represent a heterogeneous population that includes cells that have lost or are losing epithelial markers and that have undergone or are undergoing the EMT. It is reasonable to suggest that this is a dynamic event during which cells gradually lose their epithelial features to acquire other features that enable them to extravasate into circulation and then undergo the reverse process, which allows the cells to travel to the site of metastasis [81].

The lack of specific surface hepatic markers challenges CTC detection in HCC, which in turn limits investigation of this cell type. To date, there are only a few studies that have been conducted to identify and characterize these cells. Similar to CTCs derived from other tumors, HCC-derived CTCs were detected with mesenchymal as well as epithelial markers [97–99]. Compared with epithelial CTCs detected by the conventional markers EpCAM and cytokeratin, the high rates of EMT-associated CTCs correlated with poor prognosis in patients with hepatocellular carcinoma [84, 100–102]. A prospective study of 46 patients with liver cancer showed the EMT markers TWIST1 and Vimentin in 84.8% and 80.4% of those patients' CTC samples, respectively [103]; tumor progression correlated with the presence of mesenchymal CTCs in those patients. In addition, some markers for cancer stem cells, such as CD44, CD133, CD90, or ICAM, were also detected in HCC CTCs [104]. Altogether these findings raise the possibility that significant overlap may exist between CTCs, cancer stem cells, and HCC cells that underwent EMT. Despite these complexities in the molecular expression of CTCs, a thorough understanding of the biology of CTCs in the metastatic process nonetheless offers the prospect of creating a highly useful diagnostic and prognostic surrogate measure. In this review, the discussion of CTCs emphasizes two major aspects: (1) the relationship between circulating tumor and cancer stem cells and (2) the molecular linkage between these subpopulations – the epithelial-to-mesenchymal transition.

9.3.1 Relationship Between Circulating Tumor Cells and Cancer Stem Cells

Found in many types of cancer, cancer stem cells (CSCs) are a rare subpopulation that possesses the ability to generate new tumors that consistently recapitulate the morphology of original tumors. Following the hierarchical hypothesis of CSC clonal evolution, these cells are able to self-renew and generate differentiated in a similar manner to normal stem cells [105–107]. CTCs appear to have a critical role in metastasis. The motility, invasiveness, and heightened resistance to apoptosis are instrumental for metastatic initiation, while the self-renewal and tumor-initiating ability are critical for successful metastatic establishment [108].

The Expression of CSC Markers in CTCs
Although it may not be specific for CSCs of HCC origin, commonly reported markers include EpCAM, CD133, CD90, CD44, and CD24 [84, 102, 109–111]. Most of these markers are expressed in normal hepatic progenitors and are known as oncofetal markers [107]. Tumor cells expressing these markers have demonstrated heightened tumorigenicity and metastasis using HCC cell lines and primary HCC models [98, 112]. These common CSC markers were also detected in the CTC subpopulation within the peripheral blood of HCC patients [87]. A recent prospective study by Fan et al. revealed a strong correlation between the number of cancer stem cells (CD45−/CD90+/CD44+) in the blood and post-hepatectomy intrahepatic recurrence and lower recurrence-free survival of HCC. Further, circulating CSCs >0.01%, tumor stage, and tumor size were all independent risk factors in predicting recurrence-free survival [88]. In another investigation, the Cell Search System was developed to examine preoperative blood samples from 123 HCC patients. Here, Sun et al. detected at least one EpCAM$^+$ CTC in 66.7% of the samples, among which 41.5% had at least two EpCAM$^+$ CTCs, and further determined that preoperative detection of at least two CTCs was an independent risk factor for postoperative recurrence [101]. The same group also reported expression of the CSC biomarkers CD133 and ABCG2 in EpCAM$^+$ CTCs from 82 patients with HCC. A study by Schulze et al. reported at least one EpCAM$^+$ CTC in 30.5% of HCC patients and in 5.3% of patients with cirrhosis, demonstrating a strong correlation between EpCAM$^+$ CTCs and survival [100]. Furthermore, Liu et al. identified 30 out of 60 patients with greater than 0.157% circulating CD45$^-$ ICAM-1$^+$ tumor cells. Again, these patients demonstrated significantly shorter disease-free and overall survival

[113]. These investigations suggest that CTCs with stem cell-like phenotypes may represent a subset of CTCs with a more aggressive phenotype, leading to early recurrence, metastasis, and reduced overall survival.

Tumor Self-Seeding: A CSC Trait of CTCs

CTCs can be detected within the bloodstream of the overwhelming majority of carcinoma patients, including those who develop few, if any, overt metastases; however, less than 0.01% of tumor cells that enter into systemic circulation ultimately develop into macroscopic metastases [114, 115]. It has been suggested that CTCs may exist in the latent form in a state of pre-metastasis, defined as the time between primary tumor diagnosis and clinically detectable metastasis [116]. In breast cancer, malignant cells that disseminate early can reside as single cells or as micro-metastatic clusters, as shown in studies of bone marrow samples from patients without overt metastatic disease [117, 118]. These CTCs either lack the ability to colonize or are successful colonization is prevented, possibly by host environmental factors. In order to acquire a micro- to macro-metastatic switch, latent CTCs must have the capability to reinitiate a tumor. The development of macro-metastases is a manifestation of a so-called tumor self-seeding process. This unique cancer stem cell phenotype has been well demonstrated by Kim et al. in experimental mouse models of breast carcinoma, colon carcinoma, and malignant melanoma [119]. In these models, tumor masses become readily seeded by CTCs derived from separate tumors, metastatic lesions, or direct inoculation. Tumor self-seeding selects for highly aggressive CTCs, as evidenced by the consistent observation that metastatic cells are more efficient as seeders than their parental populations. Interestingly, tumor self-seeding in mice carrying high numbers of CTCs was not associated with de novo tumor formation in orthotopic sites, suggesting that self-seeding requires tumor-derived signals. Kim et al. further implicate IL-6 and IL-8 as tumor-derived attractants of CTCs in breast carcinoma and melanoma models, in agreement with other models of tumor cell chemotaxis and metastasis. High serum levels of IL-6 correlate with poor prognosis in breast, colon, and lung cancer [120–122], and high expression of IL-8 in metastatic melanoma is associated with tumor burden [123, 124]. Inflammatory cells recruited to the tumor site can also be sources IL-6 [125, 126]. Thus, stromal and cancer cell-derived factors may contribute to tumor self-seeding process of circulating tumor cells [119].

The Origin of CTCs

Despite advances in our understanding of the relationship between circulating tumor cells and clinical outcomes, the mechanistic role CTCs play in metastatic dissemination remains unclear. This is due, in part, to the limited sensitivity associated with current technical approaches as well as the lack of efficient in vitro and/or in vivo models to detect and characterize this rare subpopulation. One of the most fundamental, yet unanswered, questions relates to the origin of CTCs. Both molecular expressing patterns and functional properties of CSCs within CTC subpopulations point to possible overlap, implying that CTCs may actually represent CSCs in the circulation. Functionally, however, not all CTCs are able to form ectopic metastatic lesions, as would be expected of CSCs. In mouse models involving portal vein cell injections, only 2.5% of CTCs were able to establish metastatic foci, and 1% of micro-metastases progressed to a macro-metastatic tumor at day 13 after injection [127]. Therefore, among the heterogeneous population of CTCs, only a small subset is capable of successfully metastasizing. This subpopulation of CTCs associated with CSC properties has recently been defined as "circulating tumor stem cells" (CTSCs). The origin of circulating tumor stem cells has not been established to date. In a recent review, Yang et al. proposed two non-exclusive hypotheses for the derivation of CTSCs. First, circulating and thus metastatic cancer stem cells already arise in the primary tumor as cancer stem cells with additional features rendering them capable of evading the primary tumor, surviving in the bloodstream, and subsequently initiating metastasis. Second, circulating cancer stem cells may actually arise from previously disseminated tumor cells, e.g., out of a state of dormancy at a distant site after escape from the primary tumor. Importantly, CTCs must survive the hostile environment of the peripheral blood, evade immune surveillance, and extravasate at a distant location. These features are certainly not present in all CTCs [128]. While both hypotheses are reasonable, neither has been validated conclusively to date. Consistent with the hypothesis that circulating cancer stem cells are already present in primary tumors, primary tumor cells bearing CSC markers are able to form distant metastases when transplanted into a secondary host [129, 130]. As cancer stem cells are also associated with the functional plasticity required to transition between mesenchymal-like and epithelial-like states, these cells are a likely source of metastasis.

9.3.2 Epithelial-to-Mesenchymal Transition: A Hallmark of Metastasis That Links Circulating Tumor Cells and Cancer Stem Cells

Recent investigations have suggested that circulating tumor cells (CTCs) manifest phenotypes associated with both CSCs and epithelial-mesenchymal transition (EMT). Compelling evidence indicates that cancer cells are endowed with invasive characteristics through the EMT, which is a complex process leading to the loss of epithelial features and gain of mesenchymal traits via cellular rearrangement of junctional proteins and eventually the loss of cell adhesion. This transition enables the tumor cells to acquire migratory and invasive abilities, which facilitates metastasis through intravasation from the primary tumor site to the vascular system and extravasation to the secondary location [3, 43, 131]. However, EMT is often transient and reversible. Reestablishment of micro-metastasis in the distant sites requires a reversal process, termed the mesenchymal-to-epithelial transition (MET), by which cells regain epithelial characteristics necessary for further colonization [3]. Thus, the EMT-MET transition processes are critical to metastasis in all cancer cells.

The Evidences of EMT Phenotype in CTCs

The expression of EMT-related proteins (Vimentin, N-cadherin, and TWIST1) has been documented in CTCs obtained from patients with breast, lung, colon cancer as well as hepatocellular carcinoma [97, 132–135]. Li et al. isolated CTCs from 46 of 60 (76.7%) HCC patients, and immunofluorescence staining detected TWIST1 and Vimentin expression in CTCs obtained from 39 (84.8%) and 37 (80.4%) of the 46 patients, respectively. The expression of both TWIST1 and Vimentin in CTCs significantly correlated with portal vein tumor thrombus. Co-expression of TWIST1 and Vimentin in CTCs could be detected in 32 (69.6%) of the 46 patients and correlated strongly with portal vein tumor thrombus, TNM classification, and tumor size. Western blot analysis revealed that the expression levels of E-cadherin, Vimentin, and TWIST1 in primary HCC tumors were correlated with marker positivity in isolated CTCs ($P = 0.013$, $P = 0.012$, $P = 0.009$, respectively). However, there was no significant difference in ZEB1, ZEB2, snail, and slug expression levels in CTCs, primary HCC tumors, and adjacent hepatic tissue across samples with regard to clinicopathological parameters [136].

The contribution of EMT to CTC properties may be regulated through inducers of EMT and/or the mechanisms of signal transduction that facilitate this process. For example, TGF-β1 induces EMT in HCC by activating a cascade of signaling mechanisms including the platelet-derived growth factor (PDGF), cyclooxygenase-2, and phosphatidylinositol-2/Akt (PI3K/Akt) signaling pathways [30, 38, 131, 137]. Additionally, Ogunwobi et al. demonstrated that CTCs display phenotypic evidence of having undergone EMT, which appears to be inducible by HGF, using murine CTC cell lines established from an HCC model of BNL 1MEA.7R.1. CTCs are highly enriched for the expression of HGF and its receptor c-Met compared to the parental 1MEA cells. Moreover, upregulation of HGF and c-Met may be the consequence of a loss of DNA methylation in six CpG islands at the c-Met promoter [138].

Lee et al. reported an interesting role for TM4SF5, a transmembrane 4 L six family member 5, which is highly expressed in hepatic cancers and stimulates metastasis by enhancing cellular migration. Here, a novel TM4SF5/CD44 interaction mediated self-renewal and circulating tumor cell (CTC) capacities. TM4SF5-dependent sphere growth correlated with CD133+, CD24−, and ALDH activity and a physical association between CD44 and TM4SF5. In serial xenografts of less than 5000 cells per injection, TM4SF5-positive tumors exhibited increased CD44 expression, suggesting tumor cell differentiation. TM4SF5-positive cells were identified circulating in the blood 4–6 weeks after orthotopic liver injection. Anti-TM4SF reagents reduced metastasis. Such TM4SF5-mediated properties were supported by CD133/TM4SF5/CD44 (bound to TM4SF5)/c-Src/STAT3/TWIST1/Bmi-1 signaling pathways. Suppression of CD133, TM4SF5, or CD44 or disruption of the interaction between TM4SF5 and CD44 abolished the self-renewal and circulating tumor cell properties [139]. This study therefore elucidated a critical link between EMT, CSCs, and CTCs in hepatocellular carcinoma.

Dynamic Role of EMT in Postulating Cancer Stem Cell Phenotype of CTCs

Recent clinicopathologic and experimental evidence support the coexistence of both EMT and CSC phenotypes in CTC subpopulations of patients with metastasis [132]. The reciprocal action of these three components, however, is still not fully understood. EMT has been suggested to play a key role in the formation of CTCs, which can eventually form metastatic tumors. EMT may propagate or, in some instances, even generate neoplastic epithelial cells through the acquisition of stem-like characteristics [129, 136, 140–142]. Indeed, Mani et al. first demonstrated that EMT was sufficient to induce a population of cells with characteristics of stem cells bearing migratory and invasive capabilities [142]. Moreover, the overexpression of EMT markers on CTCs was often accompanied by the presence of the stem cell markers, including but not limited to ALDH1, CD133, and CD44 [95, 132]. Given the fact that EMT can induce non-CSCs to enter a CSC-like state, tumor cells may resemble CSCs through this process and transition to circulating tumor stem cells with high metastatic potential. On the other hand, several studies suggested that CTCs that are "frozen" in a mesenchymal phenotype seem to be unable to form metastases [143], as tumor cell lines that are arrested in a mesenchymal state by expression of EMT-inducing proteins such as Snail, TWIST1, or ZEB1 are more invasive and easily enter the bloodstream, but they are unable to form overt metastases after homing to distant organs [93, 144–146]. These cells may not be able to undergo the reverse process of mesenchymal-to-epithelial transition to establish micro-metastasis.

These observations are not contradictory. They indeed provide evidence for a dynamic regulation of EMT toward CTCs in a reversible manner. Early in the metastatic cascade, EMT is responsible for inducing mesenchymal and cancer stem cell phenotypes. These are obligatory properties required for intravasation from the primary tumor and extravasation to the metastatic site of CTSCs. At a late metastatic phase after CTSC homing, EMT may be switched to MET, by which cells regain epithelial characteristics necessary for colonization and establish macro-metastasis. Despite a profound contribution to the success of metastasis, the master controller(s) of the switch between EMT and MET is not yet understood. It is possible that this EMT/MET balance is driven by intrinsic properties of tumor cells as well as extrinsic components from both primary and secondary microenvironments.

Conclusion

Metastasis formation represents the dominant rate-limiting step of the invasion-metastasis cascade. In spite of this gross inefficiency of metastatic establishment, a small minority of disseminated carcinoma cells undergoes gradual genetic and/or epigenetic evolution to acquire the adaptive traits required for metastatic colonization. The tumor cells could not execute this complicated transformation alone but through their extensive communication with the microenvironment of the primary tumor and the metastatic site. Concomitant to anatomical and hemodynamical features of the liver, hepatocellular carcinoma represents one of the most complicated tumor microenvironments with a high degree of heterogeneity in cellular and molecular components, which contributes another layer of complexity to the metastatic process. The milieu of HCC is composed of a wide variety of inflammatory cell types, all of which interact with each other and tumor cells, directly or indirectly through factors that they secrete, in order to acquire a pathologic phenotype and alter the function of tumor cells. This mutual interaction between cancer cells and host components is dynamic, constantly evolving with tumor progression. Under microenvironmental signals, tumor cells can be transformed into metastatic circulating tumor cells through the process of epithelial-to-mesenchymal transition. This intriguing group of so-called circulating tumor stem cells can acquire unique stemlike characteristics simultaneously, a prerequisite for the success of metastasis. Better understanding of the biology behind these processes is critical to develop effective strategies for early cancer detection and novel treatment approaches that can be translated into clinical practice.

References

1. Yeung YP, Lo CM, Liu CL, Wong BC, Fan ST, Wong J. Natural history of untreated nonsurgical hepatocellular carcinoma. Am J Gastroenterol. 2005;100(9):1995–2004.
2. Paschos KA, Bird NC. Liver regeneration and its impact on post-hepatectomy metastatic tumour recurrence. Anticancer Res. 2010;30(6):2161–70.
3. Chaffer CL, Weinberg RA. A perspective on cancer cell metastasis. Science. 2011;331(6024):1559–64.
4. Nguyen DX, Bos PD, Massague J. Metastasis: from dissemination to organ-specific colonization. Nat Rev Cancer. 2009;9(4):274–84.
5. Joyce JA, Pollard JW. Microenvironmental regulation of metastasis. Nat Rev Cancer. 2009;9(4):239–52.
6. Schutte K, Bornschein J, Malfertheiner P. Hepatocellular carcinoma—epidemiological trends and risk factors. Dig Dis. 2009;27(2):80–92.
7. Hernandez-Gea V, Toffanin S, Friedman SL, Llovet JM. Role of the microenvironment in the pathogenesis and treatment of hepatocellular carcinoma. Gastroenterology. 2013;144(3):512–27.
8. Van den Eynden GG, Majeed AW, Illemann M, Vermeulen PB, Bird NC, Hoyer-Hansen G, et al. The multifaceted role of the microenvironment in liver metastasis: biology and clinical implications. Cancer Res. 2013;73(7):2031–43.
9. Qin LX. Inflammatory immune responses in tumor microenvironment and metastasis of hepatocellular carcinoma. Cancer Microenviron. 2012;5(3):203–9.
10. Tu T, Budzinska MA, Maczurek AE, Cheng R, Di Bartolomeo A, Warner FJ, et al. Novel aspects of the liver microenvironment in hepatocellular carcinoma pathogenesis and development. Int J Mol Sci. 2014;15:9422–58.
11. Wang H, Chen L. Tumor microenvironment and hepatocellular carcinoma metastasis. J Gastroenterol Hepatol. 2013;28(Suppl 1):43–8.
12. Schrader J, Iredale JP. The inflammatory microenvironment of HCC—the plot becomes complex. J Hepatol. 2011;54:853–5. England.
13. Yang JD, Nakamura I, Roberts LR. The tumor microenvironment in hepatocellular carcinoma: current status and therapeutic targets. Semin Cancer Biol. 2011;21(1):35–43.
14. Heindryckx F, Gerwins P. Targeting the tumor stroma in hepatocellular carcinoma. World J Hepatol. 2015;7(2):165–76.

15. Budhu A, Forgues M, Ye QH, Jia HL, He P, Zanetti KA, et al. Prediction of venous metastases, recurrence, and prognosis in hepatocellular carcinoma based on a unique immune response signature of the liver microenvironment. Cancer Cell. 2006;10(2):99–111.
16. Budhu AS, Zipser B, Forgues M, Ye QH, Sun Z, Wang XW. The molecular signature of metastases of human hepatocellular carcinoma. Oncology. 2005;69(Suppl 1):23–7.
17. Roessler S, Jia H-L, Budhu A, Forgues M, Ye Q-H, Lee J-S, et al. A unique metastasis gene signature enables prediction of tumor relapse in early-stage hepatocellular carcinoma patients. Cancer Res. 2010;70(24):10202–12.
18. Kalluri R, Zeisberg M. Fibroblasts in cancer. Nat Rev Cancer. 2006;6(5):392–401.
19. Vidal-Vanaclocha F. The prometastatic microenvironment of the liver. Cancer Microenviron. 2008;1(1):113–29.
20. Friedman SL. Hepatic stellate cells: protean, multifunctional, and enigmatic cells of the liver. Physiol Rev. 2008;88(1):125–72.
21. Faouzi S, Le Bail B, Neaud V, Boussarie L, Saric J, Bioulac-Sage P, et al. Myofibroblasts are responsible for collagen synthesis in the stroma of human hepatocellular carcinoma: an in vivo and in vitro study. J Hepatol. 1999;30(2):275–84.
22. Dubuisson L, Lepreux S, Bioulac-Sage P, Balabaud C, Costa AM, Rosenbaum J, et al. Expression and cellular localization of fibrillin-1 in normal and pathological human liver. J Hepatol. 2001;34(4):514–22.
23. Friedman SL. Molecular regulation of hepatic fibrosis, an integrated cellular response to tissue injury. J Biol Chem. 2000;275(4):2247–50.
24. Thompson AI, Conroy KP, Henderson NC. Hepatic stellate cells: central modulators of hepatic carcinogenesis. BMC Gastroenterol. 2015;15:63.
25. Coulouarn C, Corlu A, Glaise D, Guénon I, Thorgeirsson SS, Clément B. Hepatocyte–stellate cell cross-talk in the liver engenders a permissive inflammatory microenvironment that drives progression in hepatocellular carcinoma. Cancer Res. 2012;72(10):2533–42.
26. Park YN, Yang CP, Cubukcu O, Thung SN, Theise ND. Hepatic stellate cell activation in dysplastic nodules: evidence for an alternate hypothesis concerning human hepatocarcinogenesis. Liver. 1997;17(6):271–4.
27. Carloni V, Luong TV, Rombouts K. Hepatic stellate cells and extracellular matrix in hepatocellular carcinoma: more complicated than ever. Liver Int. 2014;34(6):834–43.
28. Yoshida K, Murata M, Yamaguchi T, Matsuzaki K. TGF-beta/Smad signaling during hepatic fibro-carcinogenesis (review). Int J Oncol. 2014;45(4):1363–71.
29. Dooley S, Weng H, Mertens PR. Hypotheses on the role of transforming growth factor-beta in the onset and progression of hepatocellular carcinoma. Dig Dis. 2009;27(2):93–101.
30. Papageorgis P. TGFbeta signaling in tumor initiation, epithelial-to-mesenchymal transition, and metastasis. J Oncol. 2015;2015:587193.
31. Geng ZM, Li QH, Li WZ, Zheng JB, Shah V. Activated human hepatic stellate cells promote growth of human hepatocellular carcinoma in a subcutaneous xenograft nude mouse model. Cell Biochem Biophys. 2014;70(1):337–47.
32. van Zijl F, Mair M, Csiszar A, Schneller D, Zulehner G, Huber H, et al. Hepatic tumor-stroma crosstalk guides epithelial to mesenchymal transition at the tumor edge. Oncogene. 2009;28(45):4022–33.
33. Park SA, Kim MJ, Park SY, Kim JS, Lim W, Nam JS, et al. TIMP-1 mediates TGF-beta-dependent crosstalk between hepatic stellate and cancer cells via FAK signaling. Sci Rep. 2015;5:16492.
34. Legate KR, Wickstrom SA, Fassler R. Genetic and cell biological analysis of integrin outside-in signaling. Genes Dev. 2009;23(4):397–418.
35. Desgrosellier JS, Cheresh DA. Integrins in cancer: biological implications and therapeutic opportunities. Nat Rev Cancer. 2010;10(1):9–22.
36. Reif S, Lang A, Lindquist JN, Yata Y, Gabele E, Scanga A, et al. The role of focal adhesion kinase-phosphatidylinositol 3-kinase-akt signaling in hepatic stellate cell proliferation and type I collagen expression. J Biol Chem. 2003;278(10):8083–90.

37. Zhao G, Cui J, Qin Q, Zhang J, Liu L, Deng S, et al. Mechanical stiffness of liver tissues in relation to integrin beta1 expression may influence the development of hepatic cirrhosis and hepatocellular carcinoma. J Surg Oncol. 2010;102(5):482–9.
38. Ke AW, Shi GM, Zhou J, Huang XY, Shi YH, Ding ZB, et al. CD151 amplifies signaling by integrin alpha6beta1 to PI3K and induces the epithelial-mesenchymal transition in HCC cells. Gastroenterology. 2011;140(5):1629–41.e15.
39. Giannelli G, Fransvea E, Marinosci F, Bergamini C, Colucci S, Schiraldi O, et al. Transforming growth factor-beta1 triggers hepatocellular carcinoma invasiveness via alpha3beta1 integrin. Am J Pathol. 2002;161(1):183–93.
40. Fransvea E, Mazzocca A, Antonaci S, Giannelli G. Targeting transforming growth factor (TGF)-betaRI inhibits activation of beta1 integrin and blocks vascular invasion in hepatocellular carcinoma. Hepatology. 2009;49(3):839–50.
41. Jing Y, Jia D, Wong CM, Oi-Lin Ng I, Zhang Z, Liu L, et al. SERPINA5 inhibits tumor cell migration by modulating the fibronectin-integrin beta1 signaling pathway in hepatocellular carcinoma. Mol Oncol. 2014;8(2):366–77.
42. Li GC, Ye QH, Xue YH, Sun HJ, Zhou HJ, Ren N, et al. Human mesenchymal stem cells inhibit metastasis of a hepatocellular carcinoma model using the MHCC97-H cell line. Cancer Sci. 2010;101(12):2546–53.
43. Jing Y, Han Z, Liu Y, Sun K, Zhang S, Jiang G, et al. Mesenchymal stem cells in inflammation microenvironment accelerates hepatocellular carcinoma metastasis by inducing epithelial-mesenchymal transition. PLoS One. 2012;7(8):e43272.
44. Song T, Dou C, Jia Y, Tu K, Zheng X. TIMP-1 activated carcinoma-associated fibroblasts inhibit tumor apoptosis by activating SDF1/CXCR4 signaling in hepatocellular carcinoma. Oncotarget. 2015;6(14):12061–79.
45. Kaminski A, Hahne JC, Haddouti e-M, Florin A, Wellmann A, Wernert N. Tumour-stroma interactions between metastatic prostate cancer cells and fibroblasts. Int J Mol Med. 2006;18(5):941–50.
46. Lin ZY, Chuang WL. Hepatocellular carcinoma cells cause different responses in expressions of cancer-promoting genes in different cancer-associated fibroblasts. Kaohsiung J Med Sci. 2013;29(6):312–8.
47. Pietras K, Ostman A. Hallmarks of cancer: interactions with the tumor stroma. Exp Cell Res. 2010;316(8):1324–31.
48. Bhowmick NA, Neilson EG, Moses HL. Stromal fibroblasts in cancer initiation and progression. Nature. 2004;432(7015):332–7.
49. Farazi PA, DePinho RA. Hepatocellular carcinoma pathogenesis: from genes to environment. Nat Rev Cancer. 2006;6(9):674–87.
50. Gajewski TF, Schreiber H, Fu YX. Innate and adaptive immune cells in the tumor microenvironment. Nat Immunol. 2013;14(10):1014–22.
51. DeNardo DG, Barreto JB, Andreu P, Vasquez L, Tawfik D, Kolhatkar N, et al. CD4(+) T cells regulate pulmonary metastasis of mammary carcinomas by enhancing protumor properties of macrophages. Cancer Cell. 2009;16(2):91–102.
52. Smyth MJ, Dunn GP, Schreiber RD. Cancer immunosurveillance and immunoediting: the roles of immunity in suppressing tumor development and shaping tumor immunogenicity. Adv Immunol. 2006;90:1–50.
53. Yakirevich E, Resnick MB. Regulatory T lymphocytes: pivotal components of the host anti-tumor response. J Clin Oncol. 2007;25:2506–8. United States.
54. Chen KJ, Lin SZ, Zhou L, Xie HY, Zhou WH, Taki-Eldin A, et al. Selective recruitment of regulatory T cell through CCR6-CCL20 in hepatocellular carcinoma fosters tumor progression and predicts poor prognosis. PLoS One. 2011;6(9):e24671.
55. Gao Q, Zhou J, Wang XY, Qiu SJ, Song K, Huang XW, et al. Infiltrating memory/senescent T cell ratio predicts extrahepatic metastasis of hepatocellular carcinoma. Ann Surg Oncol. 2012;19(2):455–66.
56. Gao Q, Qiu SJ, Fan J, Zhou J, Wang XY, Xiao YS, et al. Intratumoral balance of regulatory and cytotoxic T cells is associated with prognosis of hepatocellular carcinoma after resection. J Clin Oncol. 2007;25(18):2586–93.

57. Tilg H, Wilmer A, Vogel W, Herold M, Nolchen B, Judmaier G, et al. Serum levels of cytokines in chronic liver diseases. Gastroenterology. 1992;103(1):264–74.
58. Zhu AX, Sahani DV, Duda DG, di Tomaso E, Ancukiewicz M, Catalano OA, et al. Efficacy, safety, and potential biomarkers of sunitinib monotherapy in advanced hepatocellular carcinoma: a phase II study. J Clin Oncol. 2009;27(18):3027–35.
59. Fausto N, Campbell JS, Riehle KJ. Liver regeneration. Hepatology. 2006;43(2 Suppl 1):S45–53.
60. Akira S, Uematsu S, Takeuchi O. Pathogen recognition and innate immunity. Cell. 2006;124(4):783–801.
61. Wang L, Wu WZ, Sun HC, Wu XF, Qin LX, Liu YK, et al. Mechanism of interferon alpha on inhibition of metastasis and angiogenesis of hepatocellular carcinoma after curative resection in nude mice. J Gastrointest Surg. 2003;7(5):587–94.
62. Ostuni R, Kratochvill F, Murray PJ, Natoli G. Macrophages and cancer: from mechanisms to therapeutic implications. Trends Immunol. 2015;36(4):229–39.
63. Shirabe K, Mano Y, Muto J, Matono R, Motomura T, Toshima T, et al. Role of tumor-associated macrophages in the progression of hepatocellular carcinoma. Surg Today. 2012;42(1):1–7.
64. Porta C, Larghi P, Rimoldi M, Totaro MG, Allavena P, Mantovani A, et al. Cellular and molecular pathways linking inflammation and cancer. Immunobiology. 2009;214(9–10):761–77.
65. Capece D, Fischietti M, Verzella D, Gaggiano A, Cicciarelli G, Tessitore A, et al. The inflammatory microenvironment in hepatocellular carcinoma: a pivotal role for tumor-associated macrophages. Biomed Res Int. 2013;2013.
66. Takai H, Kato A, Kato C, Watanabe T, Matsubara K, Suzuki M, et al. The expression profile of glypican-3 and its relation to macrophage population in human hepatocellular carcinoma. Liver Int. 2009;29(7):1056–64.
67. Biswas SK, Mantovani A. Macrophage plasticity and interaction with lymphocyte subsets: cancer as a paradigm. Nat Immunol. 2010;11:889–96.
68. Zhu XD, Zhang JB, Zhuang PY, Zhu HG, Zhang W, Xiong YQ, et al. High expression of macrophage colony-stimulating factor in peritumoral liver tissue is associated with poor survival after curative resection of hepatocellular carcinoma. J Clin Oncol. 2008;26(16):2707–16.
69. Jia JB, Wang WQ, Sun HC, Zhu XD, Liu L, Zhuang PY, et al. High expression of macrophage colony-stimulating factor-1 receptor in peritumoral liver tissue is associated with poor outcome in hepatocellular carcinoma after curative resection. Oncologist. 2010;15(7):732–43.
70. Chen TA, Wang JL, Hung SW, Chu CL, Cheng YC, Liang SM. Recombinant VP1, an Akt inhibitor, suppresses progression of hepatocellular carcinoma by inducing apoptosis and modulation of CCL2 production. PLoS One. 2011;6(8):e23317.
71. Schimanski CC, Bahre R, Gockel I, Muller A, Frerichs K, Horner V, et al. Dissemination of hepatocellular carcinoma is mediated via chemokine receptor CXCR4. Br J Cancer. 2006;95(2):210–7.
72. Chu H, Zhou H, Liu Y, Liu X, Hu Y, Zhang J. Functional expression of CXC chemokine receptor-4 mediates the secretion of matrix metalloproteinases from mouse hepatocarcinoma cell lines with different lymphatic metastasis ability. Int J Biochem Cell Biol. 2007;39(1):197–205.
73. Liu Z, Yang L, Xu J, Zhang X, Wang B. Enhanced expression and clinical significance of chemokine receptor CXCR2 in hepatocellular carcinoma. J Surg Res. 2011;166(2):241–6.
74. Giannelli G, Bergamini C, Fransvea E, Sgarra C, Antonaci S. Laminin-5 with transforming growth factor-beta1 induces epithelial to mesenchymal transition in hepatocellular carcinoma. Gastroenterology. 2005;129(5):1375–83.
75. Fransvea E, Mazzocca A, Santamato A, Azzariti A, Antonaci S, Giannelli G. Kinase activation profile associated with TGF-beta-dependent migration of HCC cells: a preclinical study. Cancer Chemother Pharmacol. 2011;68(1):79–86.
76. Ramaiah SK, Rittling S. Pathophysiological role of osteopontin in hepatic inflammation, toxicity, and cancer. Toxicol Sci. 2008;103(1):4–13.
77. Kim J, Ki SS, Lee SD, Han CJ, Kim YC, Park SH, et al. Elevated plasma osteopontin levels in patients with hepatocellular carcinoma. Am J Gastroenterol. 2006;101(9):2051–9.

78. Ye Q-H, Qin L-X, Forgues M, He P, Kim JW, Peng AC, et al. Predicting hepatitis B virus-positive metastatic hepatocellular carcinomas using gene expression profiling and supervised machine learning. Nat Med. 2003;9(4):416–23.

79. Fidler IJ. The pathogenesis of cancer metastasis: the 'seed and soil' hypothesis revisited. Nat Rev Cancer. 2003;3(6):453–8.

80. Lin EH, Jiang Y, Deng Y, Lapsiwala R, Lin T, Blau CA. Cancer stem cells, endothelial progenitors, and mesenchymal stem cells: "seed and soil" theory revisited. Gastrointest Cancer Res. 2008;2(4):169–74.

81. Scatena R, Bottoni P, Giardina B. Circulating tumour cells and cancer stem cells: a role for proteomics in defining the interrelationships between function, phenotype and differentiation with potential clinical applications. Biochim Biophys Acta. 2013;1835(2):129–43.

82. Ashworth T. A case of cancer in which cells similar to those in the tumours were seen in the blood after death. Aust Med J. 1869;14:146.

83. Paget S. The distribution of secondary growths in cancer of the breast. Lancet. 1889;1:571–3.

84. Zhang Y, Shi ZL, Yang X, Yin ZF. Targeting of circulating hepatocellular carcinoma cells to prevent postoperative recurrence and metastasis. World J Gastroenterol. 2014;20(1):142–7.

85. Yap TA, Lorente D, Omlin A, Olmos D, de Bono JS. Circulating tumor cells: a multifunctional biomarker. Clin Cancer Res. 2014;20(10):2553–68.

86. Vona G, Sabile A, Louha M, Sitruk V, Romana S, Schutze K, et al. Isolation by size of epithelial tumor cells: a new method for the immunomorphological and molecular characterization of circulating tumor cells. Am J Pathol. 2000;156(1):57–63.

87. Xu W, Cao L, Chen L, Li J, Zhang XF, Qian HH, et al. Isolation of circulating tumor cells in patients with hepatocellular carcinoma using a novel cell separation strategy. Clin Cancer Res. 2011;17(11):3783–93.

88. Fan ST, Yang ZF, Ho DW, Ng MN, Yu WC, Wong J. Prediction of posthepatectomy recurrence of hepatocellular carcinoma by circulating cancer stem cells: a prospective study. Ann Surg. 2011;254(4):569–76.

89. Stott SL, Lee RJ, Nagrath S, Yu M, Miyamoto DT, Ulkus L, et al. Isolation and characterization of circulating tumor cells from patients with localized and metastatic prostate cancer. Sci Transl Med. 2010;2(25):25ra3.

90. Tseng JY, Yang CY, Liang SC, Liu RS, Jiang JK, Lin CH. Dynamic changes in numbers and properties of circulating tumor cells and their potential applications. Cancers (Basel). 2014;6:2369–86.

91. Punnoose EA, Atwal SK, Spoerke JM, Savage H, Pandita A, Yeh RF, et al. Molecular biomarker analyses using circulating tumor cells. PLoS One. 2010;5(9):e12517.

92. Yu M, Stott S, Toner M, Maheswaran S, Haber DA. Circulating tumor cells: approaches to isolation and characterization. J Cell Biol. 2011;192(3):373–82.

93. Alix-Panabières C, Pantel K. Challenges in circulating tumour cell research. Nat Rev Cancer. 2014;14:623–31.

94. Velpula KK, Dasari VR, Tsung AJ, Dinh DH, Rao JS. Cord blood stem cells revert glioma stem cell EMT by down regulating transcriptional activation of Sox2 and Twist1. Oncotarget. 2011;2(12):1028–42.

95. Armstrong AJ, Marengo MS, Oltean S, Kemeny G, Bitting RL, Turnbull JD, et al. Circulating tumor cells from patients with advanced prostate and breast cancer display both epithelial and mesenchymal markers. Mol Cancer Res. 2011;9(8):997–1007.

96. Yang J, Eddy JA, Pan Y, Hategan A, Tabus I, Wang Y, et al. Integrated proteomics and genomics analysis reveals a novel mesenchymal to epithelial reverting transition in leiomyosarcoma through regulation of slug*. Mol Cell Proteomics. 2010;9:2405–13.

97. Burak KW, Kneteman NM. An evidence-based miltidisciplinary approach to the management of hepatocellular carcinoma (HCC): The Alberta HCC algorithm. Can J Gastroenterol. 2010;24(11):643–50.

98. Chow AK, Ng L, Lam CS, Wong SK, Wan TM, Cheng NS, et al. The enhanced metastatic potential of hepatocellular carcinoma (HCC) cells with sorafenib resistance. PLoS One. 2013;8(11):e78675.

99. Li YM, Xu SC, Li J, Han KQ, Pi HF, Zheng L, et al. Epithelial-mesenchymal transition markers expressed in circulating tumor cells in hepatocellular carcinoma patients with different stages of disease. Cell Death Dis. 2013;4:e831.
100. Schulze K, Gasch C, Staufer K, Nashan B, Lohse AW, Pantel K, et al. Presence of EpCAM-positive circulating tumor cells as biomarker for systemic disease strongly correlates to survival in patients with hepatocellular carcinoma. Int J Cancer. 2013;133(9):2165–71.
101. Sun YF, Xu Y, Yang XR, Guo W, Zhang X, Qiu SJ, et al. Circulating stem cell-like epithelial cell adhesion molecule-positive tumor cells indicate poor prognosis of hepatocellular carcinoma after curative resection. Hepatology. 2013;57(4):1458–68.
102. Zhang Y, Li J, Cao L, Xu W, Yin Z. Circulating tumor cells in hepatocellular carcinoma: detection techniques, clinical implications, and future perspectives. Semin Oncol. 2012;39(4):449–60.
103. Christofori G. New signals from the invasive front. Nature. 2006;441(7092):444–50.
104. Nel I, David P, Gerken GG, Schlaak JF, Hoffmann AC. Role of circulating tumor cells and cancer stem cells in hepatocellular carcinoma. Hepatol Int. 2014;8(3):321–9.
105. Jordan CT, Guzman ML, Noble M. Cancer stem cells. N Engl J Med. 2006;355(12):1253–61.
106. Trumpp A, Wiestler OD. Mechanisms of Disease: cancer stem cells—targeting the evil twin. Nat Clin Pract Oncol. 2008;5(6):337–47.
107. Reya T, Morrison SJ, Clarke MF, Weissman IL. Stem cells, cancer, and cancer stem cells. Nature. 2001;414(6859):105–11.
108. Pantel K, Brakenhoff RH, Brandt B. Detection, clinical relevance and specific biological properties of disseminating tumour cells. Nat Rev Cancer. 2008;8(5):329–40.
109. Polyak K, Weinberg RA. Transitions between epithelial and mesenchymal states: acquisition of malignant and stem cell traits. Nat Rev Cancer. 2009;9(4):265–73.
110. Woodward WA, Sulman EP. Cancer stem cells: markers or biomarkers? Cancer Metastasis Rev. 2008;27(3):459–70.
111. Zhu CP, Wang AQ, Zhang HH, Wan XS, Yang XB, Chen SG, et al. Research progress and prospects of markers for liver cancer stem cells. World J Gastroenterol. 2015;21(42):12190–6.
112. Ma S. Biology and clinical implications of CD133(+) liver cancer stem cells. Exp Cell Res. 2013;319(2):126–32.
113. Liu S, Li N, Yu X, Xiao X, Cheng K, Hu J, et al. Expression of intercellular adhesion molecule 1 by hepatocellular carcinoma stem cells and circulating tumor cells. Gastroenterology. 2013;144(5):1031–41.e10.
114. Valastyan S, Weinberg RA. Tumor metastasis: molecular insights and evolving paradigms. Cell. 2011;147(2):275–92.
115. Chambers AF, Groom AC, MacDonald IC. Dissemination and growth of cancer cells in metastatic sites. Nat Rev Cancer. 2002;2(8):563–72.
116. Pantel K, Brakenhoff RH. Dissecting the metastatic cascade. Nat Rev Cancer. 2004;4(6):448–56.
117. Husemann Y, Geigl JB, Schubert F, Musiani P, Meyer M, Burghart E, et al. Systemic spread is an early step in breast cancer. Cancer Cell. 2008;13(1):58–68.
118. Braun S, Vogl FD, Naume B, Janni W, Osborne MP, Coombes RC, et al. A pooled analysis of bone marrow micrometastasis in breast cancer. N Engl J Med. 2005;353(8):793–802.
119. Kim MY, Oskarsson T, Acharyya S, Nguyen DX, Zhang XHF, Norton L, et al. Tumor self-seeding by circulating cancer cells. Cell. 2009;139(7):1315–26.
120. Esfandi F, Mohammadzadeh Ghobadloo S, Basati G. Interleukin-6 level in patients with colorectal cancer. Cancer Lett. 2006;244(1):76–8.
121. Knupfer H, Preiss R. Significance of interleukin-6 (IL-6) in breast cancer (review). Breast Cancer Res Treat. 2007;102(2):129–35.
122. Schafer ZT, Brugge JS. IL-6 involvement in epithelial cancers. J Clin Invest. 2007;117(12):3660–3.
123. Scheibenbogen C, Mohler T, Haefele J, Hunstein W, Keilholz U. Serum interleukin-8 (IL-8) is elevated in patients with metastatic melanoma and correlates with tumour load. Melanoma Res. 1995;5(3):179–81.

124. Ugurel S, Rappl G, Tilgen W, Reinhold U. Increased serum concentration of angiogenic factors in malignant melanoma patients correlates with tumor progression and survival. J Clin Oncol. 2001;19(2):577–83.

125. Balkwill F, Charles KA, Mantovani A. Smoldering and polarized inflammation in the initiation and promotion of malignant disease. Cancer Cell. 2005;7(3):211–7.

126. Grivennikov S, Karin E, Terzic J, Mucida D, Yu GY, Vallabhapurapu S, et al. IL-6 and Stat3 are required for survival of intestinal epithelial cells and development of colitis-associated cancer. Cancer Cell. 2009;15(2):103–13.

127. Luzzi KJ, MacDonald IC, Schmidt EE, Kerkvliet N, Morris VL, Chambers AF, et al. Multistep nature of metastatic inefficiency: dormancy of solitary cells after successful extravasation and limited survival of early micrometastases. Am J Pathol. 1998;153(3):865–73.

128. Yang MH, Imrali A, Heeschen C. Circulating cancer stem cells: the importance to select. Chin J Cancer Res. 2015;27(5):437–49.

129. Hollier BG, Evans K, Mani SA. The epithelial-to-mesenchymal transition and cancer stem cells: a coalition against cancer therapies. J Mammary Gland Biol Neoplasia. 2009;14(1):29–43.

130. Brabletz T, Jung A, Spaderna S, Hlubek F, Kirchner T. Opinion: migrating cancer stem cells—an integrated concept of malignant tumour progression. Nat Rev Cancer. 2005;5(9):744–9.

131. Ogunwobi OO, Liu C. Therapeutic and prognostic importance of epithelial-mesenchymal transition in liver cancers: insights from experimental models. Crit Rev Oncol Hematol. 2012;83(3):319–28.

132. Aktas B, Tewes M, Fehm T, Hauch S, Kimmig R, Kasimir-Bauer S. Stem cell and epithelial-mesenchymal transition markers are frequently overexpressed in circulating tumor cells of metastatic breast cancer patients. Breast Cancer Res. 2009;11(4):R46.

133. Kasimir-Bauer S, Hoffmann O, Wallwiener D, Kimmig R, Fehm T. Expression of stem cell and epithelial-mesenchymal transition markers in primary breast cancer patients with circulating tumor cells. Breast Cancer Res. 2012;14(1):R15.

134. Krawczyk N, Meier-Stiegen F, Banys M, Neubauer H, Ruckhaeberle E, Fehm T, et al. Expression of stem cell and epithelial-mesenchymal transition markers in circulating tumor cells of breast cancer patients. Biomed Res Int. 2014;2014:415721.

135. Raimondi C, Gradilone A, Naso G, Vincenzi B, Petracca A, Nicolazzo C, et al. Epithelial-mesenchymal transition and stemness features in circulating tumor cells from breast cancer patients. Breast Cancer Res Treat. 2011;130(2):449–55.

136. Gunasinghe NP, Wells A, Thompson EW, Hugo HJ. Mesenchymal-epithelial transition (MET) as a mechanism for metastatic colonisation in breast cancer. Cancer Metastasis Rev. 2012;31(3–4):469–78.

137. Olorunseun OO, Wang T, Zhang L, Liu C. COX-2 and Akt mediate multiple growth factor-induced epithelial-mesenchymal transition in human hepatocellular carcinoma. J Gastroenterol Hepatol. 2012;27(3):566–78.

138. Ogunwobi OO, Puszyk W, Dong HJ, Liu C. Epigenetic upregulation of HGF and c-Met drives metastasis in hepatocellular carcinoma. PLoS One. 2013;8(5):e63765.

139. Lee D, Lee JW. Self-renewal and circulating capacities of metastatic hepatocarcinoma cells required for collaboration between TM4SF5 and CD44. BMB Rep. 2015;48(3):127–8.

140. Mani SA, Guo W, Liao MJ, Eaton EN, Ayyanan A, Zhou AY, Brooks M, Reinhard F, Zhang CC, Shipitsin M, Campbell LL, Polyak K, Brisken C, Yang J, Weinberg RA. The epithelial-mesenchymal transition generates cells with properties of stem cells. Cell. 2008;133(4):704–15.

141. Książkiewicz M, Markiewicz A, Zaczek AJ. Epithelial-mesenchymal transition: a hallmark in metastasis formation linking circulating tumor cells and cancer stem cells. Pathobiology. 2012;79(4):195–208.

142. Mani SA, Guo W, Liao MJ, Eaton EN, Ayyanan A, Zhou AY, et al. The epithelial-mesenchymal transition generates cells with properties of stem cells. Cell. 2008;133(4):704–15.

143. Kang Y, Pantel K. Tumor cell dissemination: emerging biological insights from animal models and cancer patients. Cancer Cell. 2013;23(5):573–81.

144. Ocana OH, Corcoles R, Fabra A, Moreno-Bueno G, Acloque H, Vega S, et al. Metastatic colonization requires the repression of the epithelial-mesenchymal transition inducer Prrx1. Cancer Cell. 2012;22(6):709–24.
145. Tsai JH, Donaher JL, Murphy DA, Chau S, Yang J. Spatiotemporal regulation of epithelial-mesenchymal transition is essential for squamous cell carcinoma metastasis. Cancer Cell. 2012;22(6):725–36.
146. Tsuji T, Ibaragi S, Shima K, Hu MG, Katsurano M, Sasaki A, et al. Epithelial-mesenchymal transition induced by growth suppressor p12CDK2-AP1 promotes tumor cell local invasion but suppresses distant colony growth. Cancer Res. 2008;68(24):10377–86.

Immune Regulation in HCC and the Prospect of Immunotherapy

10

Joydeep Chakraborty, Eric Hilgenfeldt, and Roniel Cabrera

Abbreviations

AFP	Alpha-fetoprotein
APC	Antigen-presenting cell
CD	Cluster of differentiation
CTA	Cancer testis antigen
CTL	Cytotoxic T lymphocyte
CTLA	Cytotoxic T lymphocyte-associated antigen
DC	Dendritic cell
FGF	Fibroblast growth factor
GM-CSF	Granulocyte-macrophage colony-stimulating factor
GPC3	Glypican-3
HCC	Hepatocellular carcinoma
hTERT	Human telomerase reverse transcriptase
ICAM	Intercellular adhesion molecule
IDO	Indoleamine dioxygenase
IFN	Interferon
IL	Interleukin

J. Chakraborty, M.D.
Division of Gastroenterology, Hepatology, and Nutrition, University of Florida,
1600 SW Archer Road, Gainesville, FL 32610, USA
e-mail: joydeep.chakraborty@medicine.ufl.edu

E. Hilgenfeldt, M.D.
Division of Gastroenterology, Department of Internal Medicine,
Carolinas Medical Center, Charlotte, NC, USA
e-mail: eric.hilgenfeldt@gmail.com

R. Cabrera, M.D. (✉)
Division of Gastroenterology, Hepatology, and Nutrition, University of Florida,
1600 SW Archer Road, Gainesville, FL 32610, USA
e-mail: roniel.cabrera@medicine.ufl.edu

© Springer International Publishing AG 2018
C. Liu (ed.), *Precision Molecular Pathology of Liver Cancer*,
Molecular Pathology Library, https://doi.org/10.1007/978-3-319-68082-8_10

LFA   Lymphocyte function-associated antigen
LSEC   Liver sinusoidal endothelial cells
MDSC   Myeloid-derived suppressor cells
MHC   Major histocompatibility complex
NK   Natural killer
PBMC   Peripheral blood mononuclear cells
PD-1   Programmed death receptor 1
PD-L1   Programmed death-1 ligand
PG   Prostaglandin
RFA   Radiofrequency ablation
TAA   Tumor-associated antigen
TACE   Transarterial chemoembolization
TGF   Transforming growth factor
TIL   Tumor-infiltrating lymphocytes
TLR   Toll-like receptor
TNF   Tumor necrosis factor
Treg   T regulatory cells
VEGF   Vascular endothelial growth factor

10.1 Introduction

Hepatocellular carcinoma (HCC) is becoming an ever-increasing cause for mortality from cancer-related deaths in the United States. Currently it is the third leading cause of cancer-related death worldwide, approaching this in the United States, and remains one of the leading causes of death in patients with cirrhosis [1]. With rates of nonalcoholic fatty liver disease on the rise, hepatocellular carcinoma is also expected to increase. Effective therapy exists if hepatocellular carcinoma is caught in the early stages; however, when the disease progresses beyond the point at which surgical approaches or endovascular approaches can be utilized, very little options have been proven as effective forms of treatment. Current standard of care for advanced HCC with sorafenib has only been shown to provide a 2-month increase in life expectancy. Even with this marginal improvement, the estimated survival in patients with advanced HCC is only 1 year. It is for these reasons that many have gone back to the benchtop to understand the exact molecular and immunological pathophysiology so that it can be exploited and hopefully provide more a meaningful treatment for patients with HCC. In this chapter, we will discuss the immunological mechanisms underpinning the development of HCC and currently tested therapies using these mechanisms.

10.2 Current Medical Therapy for HCC

Predisposing conditions that lead to the development of HCC include all factors that lead to hepatic fibrosis and cirrhosis. It should be no surprise then that specific associations have been identified between hepatitis B virus infection, hepatitis C virus infection, alcoholic liver disease, hemochromatosis, primary biliary cirrhosis, alpha-1 antitrypsin deficiency, and nonalcoholic steatohepatitis [2–4]. Individual indices of development of hepatocellular carcinoma varies anywhere from 0.5 to 2.4% annually. Additionally, 5-year cumulative incidence data is known and ranges from 8 to 30% for several of these conditions [2, 5]. Recent increases in rates of HCC have been attributed to the worldwide increase in the prevalence of HCV infection [6]. With the expectation of increasing rates of metabolic syndrome, nonalcoholic steatohepatitis is expected to lead to even further increases in the rate of HCC [7].

Liver transplantation can be offered to otherwise healthy individuals who have localized HCC based on the Milan criteria of either a solitary tumor <5 cm in diameter or up to three lesions, each <3 cm in diameter, without evidence of vascular invasion or extrahepatic spread and who are not otherwise resection candidates [8]. Liver transplantation can eliminate HCC and is thought to represent the best chance for cure. Unfortunately, the availability of liver transplantation limits the widespread use of this approach.

Due to the limited availability and long wait times, the current treatment of choice remains hepatic resection. Strict selection criteria are employed in order to prevent postoperative complications and mortality [9]. Unfortunately, even with resection, HCC recurs at an estimated 70% over the next 5 years [10]. Additionally, only 20% of HCC is found at an early enough stage that curative procedures such as resection or total liver transplantation can be utilized.

Abbreviated recovery periods, minimally invasive approach, and comparable results have led some to consider the typically well-tolerated approach of percutaneous ablation for treatment of early-stage HCC lesions. Many have not yet adopted this approach, but large randomized controlled trials are currently ongoing [11–15]. For now, these procedures are reserved for intermediate-stage disease or in patients with underlying cirrhosis and who are otherwise not surgical candidates [16–18]. The use of radiofrequency ablation, cryoablation, or transarterial embolization can often slow the growth of HCC and essentially debulk the tumor. Due to the unique pathophysiology of HCC and the unique anatomy of the liver vasculature, embolization has been increasingly effective at treating HCC. Although generally better tolerated than surgery, transarterial embolization is not without its share of side effects [18–21].

For those with an advanced disease, palliative therapy with sorafenib, an oral multi-kinase inhibitor, can be used. Approved by the FDA in 2007, sorafenib acts by inhibiting cell growth, causing induction of apoptosis, and downregulating anti-apoptotic protein Mcl-1 [22]. Additionally, it was also found to reduce tumor angiogenesis, tumor cell signaling, and tumor growth in a dose-dependent manner in mouse xenograft models of HCC by blocking Raf/MEK/ERK pathway and other extracellular receptor tyrosine kinases [23–25]. Despite these promising molecular mechanisms, actual results of sorafenib therapy have unfortunately only been shown to increase average life span by 2 months beyond the median survival of around 12–24 months [26].

10.3   Immunosuppressive Factors for HCC

The liver's ability to evade the immune system is inherent and necessary; however, by doing so, it has detrimental effects when it comes to being able to monitor the liver for cancer. The liver's natural tolerogenicity allows liver transplant candidates the ability to be maintained on minimal doses of immunosuppressants. Despite this positive effect, the innate and adaptive immune tolerance also leads to increased risk for metastasis and makes carcinogenesis from hepatocellular carcinoma possible [27]. It is postulated that due to the numerous antigens that are presented to the liver from the gut on a routine basis via the portal circulation, the liver has evolved various immune tolerance mechanisms in order to inhibit unnecessary immune responses. These mechanisms include recruitment of immunosuppressive regulatory cells as well as alteration of cytokine pathways and other immunomodulators. Numerous reports have shown that hepatocytes, normally not thought to contribute to antigen presentation, under the influence of viral or autoimmune hepatitis aberrantly express major histocompatibility complex (MHC) class II [27, 28]. Normally, the expression of MHC class II causes activation of naïve CD4+ T cells; however, in cases of hepatocellular carcinoma, diseased hepatocytes lack the appropriate costimulatory signals needed for this interaction and instead cause naïve CD4+ T cells to become inactive and thus evade endogenous immune responses (Table 10.1). In the paragraphs that follow, we will discuss these mechanisms and the relevant data, which indicate the integral role they have in allowing carcinogenesis in HCC (immunosuppressive mechanisms of immune cells are illustrated in Fig. 10.1).

The exposure to exogenous antigens, both blood-derived and microbial byproducts from intestinal flora, places the liver in a constant state of immune activation. Without mechanisms to quell the immune response, these foreign molecules and antigens would elicit states of severe inflammation and damage. The liver's ability to avoid immune response is accomplished through several mechanisms via interactions of cytokines and between antigen-presenting cells and T cells.

Supplied by sinusoidal vessels, hepatic lobules are units comprised of both hepatocytes and non-parenchymal liver cells that interact with nutrient-rich portal venous blood and hepatic arterial blood before flowing into the central vein and finally into the hepatic vein. In general, non-parenchymal cells interact first with the nutrient-rich sinusoidal blood. By doing so, the hepatocytes avoid direct interaction with the bloodstream. Instead, non-parenchymal cells such as stellate cells, liver sinusoidal endothelial cells, dendritic cells, Kupffer cells, natural killer (NK) cells, and other lymphocytes have first contact with sinusoidal blood.

Table 10.1 Immune subsets involved in tumor-related immune suppression

Immune cell subset	Known effects on immune function
Liver sinusoidal endothelial cell	– Produces IL-10 and thus forms Tregs
	– Apoptosis of T cells in interaction of PD-L1 on LSEC with PD-1 on T cells
Kupffer cells	– Downregulate immune response via TNF-α, TGF-β, IL-10, PGE2, CD95 ligand, galectin-1, and indoleamine dioxygenase (IDO)
	– Primary cells for apoptosis of activated T cells in the liver
Dendritic cells	Produce IL-10 and thus CD4+ T-cell polarization into Tregs
Myeloid-derived suppressor cell	– Induces IL-10 and Foxp3 expression in CD4+ T cells
NK cell	– Functional impairment of NK cells and decreased IFN-gamma production
T regulatory cell	Major role in inhibition of tumor-specific T-cell response

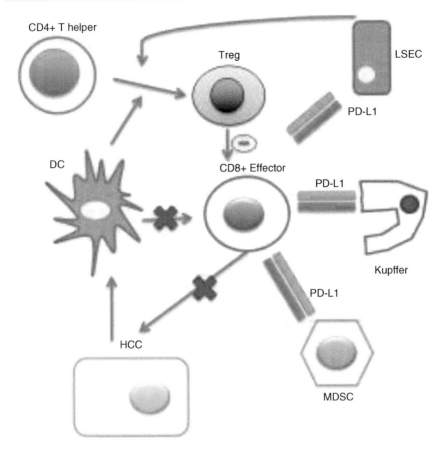

Fig. 10.1 Immunosuppressive mechanisms of HCC: The various immune cells like LSEC, Kupffer cells, MDSC, and Treg cells together with the immune checkpoint pathway (PD1/PD-L1) play a major role in the immune escape mechanism of HCC. *DC* dendritic cell, *Tregs* T regulatory cells, *LSEC* liver sinusoidal endothelial cells, *MDSC* myeloid-derived suppressor cells, *HCC* hepatocellular carcinoma cell, *PD-L1* programmed death-1 ligand

10.4   LSEC

Liver sinusoidal endothelial cells (LSEC) are commonly the first to interact with exogenous antigens and proteins from the bloodstream because, as their name implies, they line the hepatic sinusoids. Once exposed, LSEC process these particles and present them via MHC class I and II molecules to CD8+ and CD4+ T cells. Upon interaction with LSEC, naïve CD4+ T cells differentiate preferentially into the T regulatory phenotype. This is thought to be from LSEC-produced IL-10 [29]. With interaction between LSEC and naïve CD8+ T cells, only partial activation occurs. This interaction is thought to be secondary to PD-1 on the T cells and B7-H1/PD-L1 on the LSEC [30–32]. These partially activated CD8+ T cells later go on to passive apoptosis and eventual phagocytosis by Kupffer cells. Interleukin (IL)-2 has been postulated to reverse the liver sinusoidal-mediated CD8+ T-cell partial activation.

10.5   Kupffer

Both indirectly and directly, liver-specific macrophages known as Kupffer cells play an important role in immune regulation of HCC. Kupffer cells are known to produce anti-inflammatory cytokines and pro-apoptotic signals. Of these, tumor necrosis factor-alpha (TNF-alpha), TGF-beta, IL-10, PGE2, CD95 ligand, galectin-1, and indoleamine dioxygenase (IDO) have been implicated in downregulating the immune response and thus increasing tolerogenicity [31]. Direct relationships between other cytokines also play a part. For instance, interferon gamma (IFN-gamma), produced by activated CD8+ T cells, is known to increase the concentration of CD95 ligand and TNF-alpha produced by Kupffer cells, thereby leading to more apoptosis [33, 34]. Directly, Kupffer cells appear to be the primary cells implicated in the apoptosis of activated CD8+ T cells that enter the liver [35]. After the presentation of antigen via MHC class I molecules by Kupffer cells, the increased affinity of ICAM-1 on Kupffer cells and LFA-1 binding on CD8+ T cell results in apoptosis. Given this, some postulate inhibition of antigen presentation to be a possible mechanism for allowing expansion of effector CD8+ T cells and thus increasing immune surveillance.

10.6   Stellate and MDSC

Both hepatocytes and non-parenchymal cells serve a regulatory immune role. Activated hepatic stellate cells, which reside in the subendothelial space of Disse [36], are thought to play an integral role in the development of hepatocellular carcinoma [37]. Exact mechanisms remain unclear; however, it is thought that activated stellate cells cause a preferential increase in myeloid-derived suppressor cells (MDSC) [38]. These cells go on to develop into neutrophils, monocytes, and macrophages. Induction of MDSC in the liver leads to suppression of the antitumor immune responses and therefore creates a favorable environment for the spread and development of HCC. MDSC induction occurs not only in HCC but also in acute and chronic hepatitis.

10.7   DC

The majority of dendritic cells (DC) within the liver reside in the areas adjacent to the portal triad and in healthy conditions are primarily in their immature form [39]. Once matured from their myeloid state after toll-like receptor 4 (TLR4) ligation, these DC have been found to produce large amounts of IL-10 and similar to LSEC cause CD4+ T-cell polarization into T regulatory induction and poor antigen recall response. Decrease in the number of circulating DCs and reduction in their cytokine production have been demonstrated by Ormandy et al. This may indicate impaired TAA presentation by DCs [40]. Therefore, they shift the state of inflammation to one of immunosuppression and thus allowing a pro-tumorigenic environment for the spread and development of hepatocellular carcinoma. Marked dendritic cell infiltration in HCC nodules correlated well with better prognosis of HCC after resection [41].

10.8   NK

In addition to the decreased NK cell function that is induced by the HCV envelope protein E2, expanded population of MDSC also wreaks havoc [42, 43]. MDSC have been found to cause inhibition of NK cell function thus leading to hyporesponsive NK cells. Aside from functional impairment in patients with HCC, decreased NK cell frequency as well as diminished production of IFN-gamma was noted [44]. The decreased IFN-gamma is known to be associated with increased CD4+ T regulatory cells. NK cells are also being used as one of the adoptive cell therapies (other cells that are also being studied include DCs, chimeric antigen receptor T cells, cytokine-induced killer cells) in HCC [45]. A study (NCT01147380) to evaluate feasibility and safety of the adoptive transfer of IL-2-activated NK cells (extracted from cadaveric donor liver graft perfusate) for liver transplant recipients with hepatocellular carcinoma (HCC) has been completed in December 2014 [46].

10.9   T Cells

For patients with underlying hepatitis B or C virus, both innate and adaptive immune system alterations are known to occur as a result of viral-mediated effects. HBV, in particular, has been observed to increase the circulating levels of IL-10 [47]. The increased levels of regulatory T cells (Tregs) have been correlated with viral load and ultimately impair CD8+ T-cell-mediated clearance of the virus [48].

HCV also leads to adaptive immune cell dysfunction. This T effector cell dysfunction that occurs is thought to be secondary to uptitration of PD-1 and Tim-3 receptors [49–51]. In a recent study, IFN-alpha, previously known to be a component of standard of care for treatment of HCV infection [52], leads to decreased memory T cells and telomere loss in naïve CD8+ T cells [53]. Innate immunity is also impaired by HCV. As a consequence of viral proteins, monocyte-derived dendritic cells remain in their immature forms despite maturation stimuli, and NK cells lose their effector function [43, 54].

CD4+ CD25+ T regulatory cells (Tregs) play a major role in inhibiting tumor-specific T-cell response in HCC. Increased frequency of CD4+ CD25+ Tregs has been reported in tumor-infiltrating lymphocytes (TILs) and peripheral blood mononuclear cells (PBMCs) [55]. The increased Tregs then express Foxp3 and inhibit CD3/CD28-stimulated CD8+ T-cell proliferation [40]. Depletion or inhibition of

Tregs using anti-CD25 mAbs or cyclophosphamide has shown enhanced antitumor effects in preclinical models [56].

10.10 HCC-Specific Antigens/Tumor-Associated Antigens (TAAs)

An understanding of TAAs is prime in the development of tumor-specific immune therapy (summarized in Table 10.2).

10.10.1 AFP

Alpha-fetoprotein is an oncofetal antigen which is expressed during fetal development. It is the most abundant protein in the serum of a fetus [57]. It is produced in large amounts by the yolk sac and fetal liver and is transcriptionally repressed shortly after birth. AFP is reexpressed in 40–80% of HCC, and germ cell tumors and serum assays of AFP help in diagnosing and monitoring response to therapy [31]. AFP is currently the most well-studied target antigen for hepatocellular carcinoma immunotherapy.

AFP is a self-protein, and therefore it was thought that AFP-specific T-cell responses are suppressed and thus difficult to activate. But now studies have shown that more AFP-specific epitopes exist, which can mount AFP-specific CD-8$^+$ T-cell responses. In one such study [40], HLA-A2-restricted AFP-specific CD-8$^+$ T-cell epitope was identified, and its ability to mount CD-8$^+$ T-cell responses in human

Table 10.2 Targetable tumor-associated antigens

Tumor-associated antigen (TAA)	Type of TAA	Frequency of expression in HCC	Potential for immunotherapy
AFP	Oncofetal protein	40–80%	– AFP peptide vaccination [58] – DC pulsed with AFP peptides [56]
Glypican-3	Cell surface heparin sulfate and oncofetal protein	84%	– In development for HLA-A2 individuals – Anti-GPC3 chimeric antigen receptor (CAR) T-cell therapy (NCT02395250)
NY-ESO-1	Cancer testis antigen (CTA)	13–51%	– A DC205-NY-ESO-1 vaccine with or without sirolimus in solid tumors expressing NY-ESO-1 is ongoing (NCT01522820)
TERT	Enzyme for telomere elongation	80–90%	– hTERT-derived peptide (hTERT461) vaccine for HCC [79]
HCA519/TPX2	Microtubule-associated protein	100%	– Potential for immunotherapy as it is highly expressed in HCC tissue

lymphocyte cultures as well as HLA-A2 transgenic mice was demonstrated. In the same study, four dominant and ten subdominant AFP-specific epitopes were identified which generated low to moderate CD-8$^+$ T-cell responses in peripheral blood mononuclear cells (PBMCs) of HCC patients [58, 59]. AFP-specific T cells were found in patients with HCC as well as in patients with chronic HCV infection, some other liver diseases, and less commonly in healthy subjects [60]. Depletion of T regulatory cells (CD4CD25Foxp regulatory T cells) has resulted in the unmasking of AFP-specific T-cell responses in HCC patients and could be used with other immunotherapeutic approaches for HCC [61]. AFP is also one of the candidates for peptide-based vaccines against HCC (tumor vaccines for HCC will be discussed separately).

10.10.2 Glypican-3 (GPC3)

GPC3 is a cell surface heparan sulfate proteoglycan which is also a fetal oncoprotein. It can bind growth factors like Wnt, Hedgehog (Hh) signaling protein, VEGF, and FGF (fibroblast growth factor) 1/2 and help in growth of the tumor [40, 62]. It is expressed by 84% of HCC and was found to be immunogenic in murine models and human cell culture [62]. On one hand, GPC3 overexpression indicates a poor prognosis in HCC patients—with significant association with high tumor grade, late TNM stage, and vascular invasion [63, 64]. On the other hand, it is not expressed in normal adult tissue and benign liver lesions, thus making it an ideal tumor antigen for HCC Immunotherapy [65].

Previous studies had shown that GPC3 (144–152) and GPC (298–306) peptides induced specific CD8$^+$ CTLs in HCC patients with HLA-A2 and HLA-A24 restriction, respectively [66]. Inoculation of these CTLs reduced the mass of the human HCC tumor implanted into nonobese diabetic/severe combined immunodeficiency mice. In a recent study published by Dargel et al., peptide GPC3367 was identified as a predominant peptide on HLA-A2. To overcome the problem of immune tolerance due to fetal expression of GPC3, dendritic cells from HLA-A2-negative donors were co-transfected with GPC3 and HLA-A2 RNA to stimulate the GPC3-specific T cells. Expression of GPC3367-specific T-cell receptor by T cells allowed them to eliminate GPC3-positive xenograft tumor grown from human HCC cells in mice [67].

GPC3 cDNA vaccine has also been studied for cellular antitumor activity of specific CTLs for treatment of HCC in a C57BL/6 mouse model [65].

10.10.3 NY-ESO-1

NY-ESO-1 is one of the antigens of the cancer testis antigen (CTA) family (includes NY-ESO-1, members of SSX family, MAGE family, SCP-1, CTP11) which is expressed in multiple cancers including HCC (in 13–51% of HCC) but not in a normal tissue except for the testis [56, 68]. Therefore, it is a potential target for immunotherapy in HCC [69]. Combined expression of CTA (MAGE-A3, MAGE-A4, and NY-ESO-1) mRNA enhances the prediction of recurrence of HCC, therefore acting as a potential prognostic marker.

In an initial study, spontaneous NY-ESO-1-specific antibody response and functional CD4+ and CD8+ T-cell responses were seen in NY-ESO-1-expressing HCC [70]. Another study demonstrated increased frequency of specific CD8+ T-cell responses to HLA-A2-restricted NY-ESO-1b (p 157–165) in NY-ESO-1 mRNA(+)HLA-A2(+) HCC patients [68]. As opposed to stimulating T-cell response to NY-ESO-1 antigen, it was seen that we could significantly enhance the antitumor cytotoxic T lymphocyte response to HCC by depleting Treg cells followed by stimulation by NY-ESO-1b peptide [71].

10.10.4 Telomerase Reverse Transcriptase (TERT)

Human TERT (hTERT) is a catalytic enzyme required for telomere elongation. Tumors have to maintain the telomeric ends of their linear chromosomes, and this is accomplished with the help of TERT. Most tumor cells express TERT, but most adult human cells do not express it. Eighty to ninety percent of HCC express hTERT, thus making it a possible target for immunotherapy in HCC [74]. In a recent study by Huang et al., mutations of the TERT promoter region (which correlated with telomerase activity) were frequently seen in many tumors including HCC (31.4% of HCC) [75]. This emphasizes the importance of telomere maintenance in the development of a tumor.

Mizukoshi et al. identified hTERT-derived, HLA-A*2402-restricted cytotoxic T-cell (CTL) epitopes and found hTERT-specific CTL responses in the peripheral blood of HCC patients [74]. This was also observed in a patient with early stages of HCC.

10.10.5 HCA519/TPX2

HCA519 is a microtubule-associated protein which plays an integral role in the HCC replication cycle. It is also known as the targeting protein for Xklp-2 (TPX2). Significantly higher expression of HCA519/TPX2 is seen within HCC tissue (expressed in 100% of HCC as per Greten et al.) compared to a normal liver tissue [56, 76, 77]. Increased TPX2 production has also been seen in lung and pancreatic cancers [78]. Peptides $HCA519_{464–472}$ and $HCA519_{351–359}$ derived from HCA519/TPX2 were effective in generating HLA-A*0201-restricted CTLs. Therefore, HCA519/TPX2 can be a promising target for immunotherapy in HCC.

10.10.6 Other CTAs: SSX-2 and Melanoma Antigen Gene-A (MAGE-A) Family

SSX-2 and MAGE-A are other cancer testis antigens which are overexpressed in <50% and <80% of HCC patients, respectively [40]. In addition to melanoma, cytotoxic T cells response specifically to MAGE-A10, and SSX-2 was also demonstrated in vivo in HCC patients [72]. Similar CD8+ T-cell response was also seen against MAGE-A1 and MAGE-A3 epitopes in tumor-infiltrating lymphocytes (TILs) but not peripheral blood lymphocytes of HCC patients [73]. These studies point toward a potential use of these TAAs for immunotherapy in HCC.

10.11   Immune Checkpoint Blockade

Immune checkpoint inhibitors are one of the mechanisms to enhance antitumor immunity. The most studied immune checkpoint receptors are CTLA-4, PD-1, TIM-3, BTLA, VISTA, LAG-3, and OX40 [80]. Three checkpoint inhibitors have been approved by US FDA for the treatment of melanoma (ipilimumab, anti-CTLA-4; pembrolizumab, antiPD1; and nivolumab, anti-PD-1) [81]. Ipilimumab was the first to be approved in 2011. The roles of immune checkpoint inhibitors are being studied in the treatment of various solid tumors including HCC.

10.11.1   PD-1/PD-L1 Immune Checkpoint

Programmed death-ligand-1 (PD-L1 also known as B7-H1 or CD274) is expressed by many immune cells as well as cancer cells. The PD-L1 can bind to T-cell receptors—programmed death-1 (PD-1) and B7.1 (CD80)—which suppress T-cell function (T-cell migration, proliferation, secretion of cytotoxic mediators) and therefore block the cancer-immunity cycle [82]. Blockade of the PD-1/PD-L1 pathway has shown significant efficacy in patients with advanced non-small cell lung cancer, melanoma, renal cell cancer, and Hodgkin's lymphoma including upon failure to several lines of therapy [83]. A study of 46 metastatic melanoma patients by Tumeh P. C. and colleagues demonstrated that regression of tumor after PD-1 blockade therapy (pembrolizumab) required preexisting CD8+ T cells which are suppressed by PD-1/PD-L1 antitumor effect [83]. Similar results were shown by Herbst et al. where engineered humanized anti-PD-L1 antibody therapy was used in multiple cancer types [82]. HCC patients were found to have increased PD-1 expression in circulating and intratumor CD8+ T cells [84]. Kupffer cells and cells with MDSC phenotype upregulate PD-1-expressing CD8+ T cells in HCC patients [85, 86]. Anti-PD-1 antibody treatment had additional antitumor effect when combined with AMD3100 (a CXCR-4 inhibitor which targets sorafenib induced hypoxic and immunosuppressive microenvironment) in sorafenib-treated HCC in mice [87].

PD-1 antibodies that are being developed include nivolumab (BMS-936558, Bristol-Myers Squibb, USA), CT-011 (CureTech, Israel), lambrolizumab (MK-3475, Merck, USA), and AMP-224 (Amplimmune, USA). The PD-L1 antibodies currently being developed include MPDL3280A/RG7446 (Genentech, USA, and Roche, Switzerland) and MEDI4376 (MedImmune, USA, and AstraZeneca, UK) [88].

Anti-PD-1 Antibody in Clinical Trials for HCC

The phase I/II clinical trial (NCT00966251) of CT-011 (pidilizumab) in HCC patients not eligible for surgery, TACE, or other systemic therapies was started in 2009 but was terminated due to slow accrual.

Another phase I/II clinical trial (NCT01658878) of nivolumab (fully human IgG4 monoclonal antibody PD-1 inhibitor) in advanced HCC patients by El-Khoueiry et al. with a primary endpoint of safety and a secondary endpoint of antitumor activity [89] is ongoing. The results were presented at the American Society of Clinical Oncology (ASCO) in 2015. The study population included 3 cohorts of patients (total of 41 patients) stratified based on viral infection with HBV (11 patients), HCV (12 patients), or no viral infection. All patients had a Child-Pugh Class B scores of 5 or 6 (indicating relatively good liver function) and Eastern Cooperative Oncology Group (ECOG) performance scores of 0 or 1. Most had metastasis beyond the liver or portal vein tumor invasion. Approximately 75% had previously been treated for HCC, including prior treatment with sorafenib in 68% patients. All patients were treated with intravenous infusions of nivolumab every other week for up to 2 years. The results revealed that this therapy had a manageable safety profile and durable response in all the three patient cohorts. Five percent had complete response, 14% had partial response, and the overall survival rate was 62% at 12 months. These results compared favorably with a complete response rate of around 2% and a 1-year overall survival rate of about 30% with sorafenib.

10.11.2 Cytotoxic T Lymphocyte-Associated Antigen-4 (CTLA-4) Blockade

CTLA-4 (also known as CD152) is an inhibitory co-receptor expressed on T cells and Tregs and can bind CD80 and CD86 on APCs with a much higher affinity than CD28 (CD28 is a costimulatory molecule which also binds CD80 and CD86) and therefore inhibits T-cell activation [80]. Blockade of CTLA-4 suppresses antitumor immune response mediated by T cells.

From the studies of CTLA-4 blockade in other malignancies (breast, colon, lung, prostate, and brain cancers, melanoma, lymphoma, and sarcomas), it has been seen that the efficacy of CTLA-4 correlates with immunogenicity of the tumor and immunotherapy may have better results in smaller tumors [90]. Ipilimumab (MDX-010, Bristol-Myers Squibb, USA) and tremelimumab (formerly referred to as ticilimumab, CP-675,206, MedImmune, USA, and Pfizer, USA) are the two CTLA-4 antibodies which are currently in advanced stages of development.

Anti-CTLA-4 Antibody in Clinical Trials for HCC

Tremelimumab was studied in a phase I clinical trial of 21 patients with advanced HCC not amenable to percutaneous ablation or TACE, and all patients had chronic hepatitis C genotype 1b. Partial response was found in 17.6% of patients, and disease control rate was 76.4%. The time to progression was 6.48 months (95% CI 3.95–9.14) [88]. Another phase I clinical trial of tremelimumab combined with RFA or TACE is ongoing (NCT01853618) [45].

10.12 Anticancer Vaccination Strategies

The main goal of all the vaccination strategies that are being currently studied is to induce a tumor-specific immune response and overcome the inherent immune tolerance of HCC. This is being tried in the following three broad categories.

10.12.1 Peptide-Based Vaccine

It involves the administration of recombinant full-length TAAs or its peptide to cancer patients to stimulate immune response against the tumor. AFP and GPC3 are two frequently used TAAs for this purpose. One of the initial studies was performed by Butterfield et al. in which six AFP-positive HCC patients were vaccinated (intradermal injection) with four immunodominant HLA-A*0201-restricted peptides. This generated measurable AFP-specific T-cell response [58]. GPC3 has also been used for cancer immunotherapy and has been described under Sect. 10.10.2. Recently, an hTERT-derived peptide (hTERT461) was studied as a vaccine in 14 HCC patients. It was administered subcutaneously three times biweekly. This vaccination generated hTERT-specific immunity in 71.4% of patients, and 57.1% of patients who were administered hTERT461 peptide-specific T cells could prevent HCC recurrence after vaccination [79].

10.12.2 Dendritic Cell (DC)-Based Vaccine

Dendritic cells are the most potent APC with the capability to process and present tumor antigens to T cells and stimulate an antitumor immune response. DC-based vaccines are developed by collecting monocytes in peripheral circulation from cancer patients. In the presence of a source of TAAs (autologous tumor tissue or peptides of TAAs or cell line lysate) and maturation stimuli (like interleukins, GM-CSF), these cells are expanded ex vivo and reinfused into the patient to mount a tumor-specific immune response.

A phase I clinical trial was done in which tumor lysate-pulsed autologous DCs were generated ex vivo after stimulation with GM-CSF and IL-4. This was found to be feasible and without any toxicity in patients with unresectable HCC [91]. Intratumoral injection of DC in HCC nodules was also found to be safe in another study [92]. A phase II clinical trial showed that intravenous administration of autologous dendritic cells (DCs) pulsed ex vivo with a liver tumor cell line lysate (HepG2) in patients with advanced HCC was found to be safe, and the radiologically determined disease control rate was 28% [93]. DC infusion performed during TACE was shown to enhance tumor-specific immune response but was not sufficient to prevent HCC recurrence [94].

10.12.3 DNA-Based Vaccine

DNA encoding one or multiple TAAs can be delivered to patients as naked plasmids or within vectors (*Vaccinia virus* [95], adenovirus [96], *Listeria monocytogenes* [97] have been used in preclinical studies). The DNA is expected to undergo transcription and translation to express the TAA peptide and induce immune response. In a study by Butterfield et al., two HCC patients who had received prior locoregional therapy were administered full-length AFP in a plasmid DNA construct together with an AFP-expressing replication-deficient adenovirus (AdV) in a prime-boost vaccine strategy. This strategy generated AFP-specific T-cell response, but both patient had recurrence of HCC (within 9 and 18 months, respectively) [98].

10.12.4 Oncolytic Virus Therapy

Oncolytic viruses are made to selectively replicate within cancer cells and subsequently lyse them. Pexa-Vec (pexastimogene devacirepvec, JX-594) is a thymidine kinase (TK) gene-inactivated oncolytic vaccinia virus which expresses GM-CSF and lac-Z transgenes that causes replication-dependent cell lysis and stimulation of antitumoral immunity [99]. Intratumoral injection of this virus in advanced HCC patients was shown to be safe and feasible [95]. In a pilot study, Hoe et al. studied sequential JX-594 therapy followed by sorafenib in three HCC patients and found this to be well tolerated, having a significantly decreased tumor perfusion and associated with objective tumor response (Choi criteria; up to 100% necrosis) [100].

A multicenter, randomized phase III clinical trial (NCT02562755) to determine whether treatment with Pexa-Vec followed by sorafenib increases survival compared to treatment with sorafenib alone in patients with advanced HCC (mentioned in Table 10.3) who have not received prior systemic therapy is expected to open recruitment in October 2015 [101].

Table 10.3 Ongoing and future clinical trials of immunotherapeutic approaches in hepatocellular carcinoma

Intervention	Registration no.	Study phase	Start date	Primary outcome	Status
Nivolumab (anti-PD-1 monoclonal antibody)	NCT01658878	Phase I	September 2012	Safety	Recruiting
Tremelimumab with TACE or RFA	NCT01853618	Phase I	April 2013	Safety and feasibility	Recruiting
Pexa-Vec (JX-594) followed by sorafenib versus sorafenib (PHOCUS)	NCT02562755	Phase III	Planned for October 2015	Overall survival	Not yet recruiting
Intratumoral COMBIG-DC (allogenic DC) vaccine	NCT01974661	Phase I	October 2013	Adverse events	Recruiting
MG4101(ex vivo expanded allogeneic NK cell) after curative liver resection	NCT02008929	Phase II	August 2014	Disease-free survival for 1 year	Recruiting

Conclusion

We have now looked at the various ways in which immune regulation can affect HCC. The main goal in the future would be to translate all these preclinical and clinical research into a strategy which would be a successful immune therapy for HCC patients.

There have been reports of spontaneous regression of HCC, and in fact, HCC was found to be one of the most common types of cancer with spontaneous regression [102]. The most common causes were thought to be immunologic and decrease blood flow to the tumor. This reemphasizes the potential of immunotherapy in HCC.

One important approach would be to individualize immune therapy for each patient based on the immune arm which is overactive in that patient. This would include using either activation of TAA-specific T cells via vaccination methods or inhibition of the immune evasion mechanisms (immune checkpoint blockade, inhibition of immunoregulatory cell like MDSC/Treg) or a combination of both. Studies have demonstrated increased AFP-specific CD4+ T cells and increased circulating NK cells following TACE and RFA, respectively [103, 104]. This immune response following ablative therapies points toward another therapeutic strategy combining conventional HCC therapy (TACE/RFA, chemotherapy) with immunotherapy.

Though significant development has been made in understanding the immune mechanisms involved in HCC, further well-designed, randomized, controlled clinical trials with appropriate patient population and thorough immunomonitoring are required to develop efficient immunotherapies for HCC.

References

1. Singal AG, El-Serag HB. Hepatocellular carcinoma from epidemiology to prevention: translating knowledge into practice. Clin Gastroenterol Hepatol. 2015;13:2140.
2. Elmberg M, Hultcrantz R, Ekbom A, Brandt L, Olsson S, Olsson R, et al. Cancer risk in patients with hereditary hemochromatosis and in their first-degree relatives. Gastroenterology. 2003;125(6):1733–41.
3. Sherman M. Hepatocellular carcinoma: epidemiology, risk factors, and screening. Semin Liver Dis. 2005;25(2):143–54.
4. Hassan MM, Hwang LY, Hatten CJ, Swaim M, Li D, Abbruzzese JL, et al. Risk factors for hepatocellular carcinoma: synergism of alcohol with viral hepatitis and diabetes mellitus. Hepatology. 2002;36(5):1206–13.
5. Degos F, Christidis C, Ganne-Carrie N, Farmachidi JP, Degott C, Guettier C, et al. Hepatitis C virus related cirrhosis: time to occurrence of hepatocellular carcinoma and death. Gut. 2000;47(1):131–6.
6. El-Serag HB, Rudolph KL. Hepatocellular carcinoma: epidemiology and molecular carcinogenesis. Gastroenterology. 2007;132(7):2557–76.
7. Nordenstedt H, White DL, El-Serag HB. The changing pattern of epidemiology in hepatocellular carcinoma. Dig Liver Dis. 2010;42(Suppl 3):S206–14.
8. Mazzaferro V, Regalia E, Doci R, Andreola S, Pulvirenti A, Bozzetti F, et al. Liver transplantation for the treatment of small hepatocellular carcinomas in patients with cirrhosis. N Engl J Med. 1996;334(11):693–9.

9. Bismuth H, Majno PE. Hepatobiliary surgery. J Hepatol. 2000;32(1 Suppl):208–24.
10. Management of Hepatocellular Carcinoma (HCC) - Viral Hepatitis. 2015. http://www.hepatitis.va.gov/provider/guidelines/2009HCC.asp#note18
11. Chen MS, Li JQ, Zheng Y, Guo RP, Liang HH, Zhang YQ, et al. A prospective randomized trial comparing percutaneous local ablative therapy and partial hepatectomy for small hepatocellular carcinoma. Ann Surg. 2006;243(3):321–8.
12. Brunello F, Veltri A, Carucci P, Pagano E, Ciccone G, Moretto P, et al. Radiofrequency ablation versus ethanol injection for early hepatocellular carcinoma: a randomized controlled trial. Scand J Gastroenterol. 2008;43(6):727–35.
13. Lencioni RA, Allgaier HP, Cioni D, Olschewski M, Deibert P, Crocetti L, et al. Small hepatocellular carcinoma in cirrhosis: randomized comparison of radio-frequency thermal ablation versus percutaneous ethanol injection. Radiology. 2003;228(1):235–40.
14. Shiina S, Teratani T, Obi S, Sato S, Tateishi R, Fujishima T, et al. A randomized controlled trial of radiofrequency ablation with ethanol injection for small hepatocellular carcinoma. Gastroenterology. 2005;129(1):122–30.
15. Hasegawa K, Kokudo N, Shiina S, Tateishi R, Makuuchi M. Surgery versus radiofrequency ablation for small hepatocellular carcinoma: start of a randomized controlled trial (SURF trial). Hepatol Res. 2010;40(8):851–2.
16. Liver EAFTSOT, Cancer EOFRATO. EASL-EORTC clinical practice guidelines: management of hepatocellular carcinoma. J Hepatol. 2012;56(4):908–43.
17. Bruix J, Sherman M, Diseases AAftSoL. Management of hepatocellular carcinoma: an update. Hepatology. 2011;53(3):1020–2.
18. Clark TWI. Complications of hepatic chemoembolization. Semin Intervent Radiol. 2006;23(2):119–25.
19. Lin MT, Kuo PH. Pulmonary lipiodol embolism after transcatheter arterial chemoembolization for hepatocellular carcinoma. J R Soc Med Short Rep. 2010;1:6.
20. Chung JW, Park JH, Han JK, Choi BI, Han MC, Lee HS, et al. Hepatic tumors: predisposing factors for complications of transcatheter oily chemoembolization. Radiology. 1996;198(1):33–40.
21. Berger DH, Carrasco CH, Hohn DC, Curley SA. Hepatic artery chemoembolization or embolization for primary and metastatic liver tumors: post-treatment management and complications. J Surg Oncol. 1995;60(2):116–21.
22. Finn RS. Drug therapy: sorafenib. Hepatology. 2010;51(5):1843–9.
23. Wilhelm SM, Carter C, Tang L, Wilkie D, McNabola A, Rong H, et al. BAY 43-9006 exhibits broad spectrum oral antitumor activity and targets the RAF/MEK/ERK pathway and receptor tyrosine kinases involved in tumor progression and angiogenesis. Cancer Res. 2004;64(19):7099–109.
24. Chang YS, Adnane J, Trail PA, Levy J, Henderson A, Xue D, et al. Sorafenib (BAY 43-9006) inhibits tumor growth and vascularization and induces tumor apoptosis and hypoxia in RCC xenograft models. Cancer Chemother Pharmacol. 2007;59(5):561–74.
25. Liu L, Cao Y, Chen C, Zhang X, McNabola A, Wilkie D, et al. Sorafenib blocks the RAF/MEK/ERK pathway, inhibits tumor angiogenesis, and induces tumor cell apoptosis in hepatocellular carcinoma model PLC/PRF/5. Cancer Res. 2006;66(24):11851–8.
26. Schlachterman A, Craft WW, Hilgenfeldt E, Mitra A, Cabrera R. Current and future treatments for hepatocellular carcinoma. World J Gastroenterol. 2015;21(28):8478–91.
27. Miamen AG, Dong H, Roberts LR. Immunotherapeutic approaches to hepatocellular carcinoma treatment. Liver Cancer. 2012;1(3–4):226–37.
28. Herkel J, Jagemann B, Wiegard C, Lazaro JF, Lueth S, Kanzler S, et al. MHC class II-expressing hepatocytes function as antigen-presenting cells and activate specific CD4 T lymphocytes. Hepatology. 2003;37(5):1079–85.
29. Crispe IN. Hepatic T cells and liver tolerance. Nat Rev Immunol. 2003;3(1):51–62.
30. Schurich A, Berg M, Stabenow D, Böttcher J, Kern M, Schild HJ, et al. Dynamic regulation of CD8 T cell tolerance induction by liver sinusoidal endothelial cells. J Immunol. 2010;184(8):4107–14.

31. Pardee AD, Butterfield LH. Immunotherapy of hepatocellular carcinoma: unique challenges and clinical opportunities. Oncoimmunology. 2012;1(1):48–55.
32. Thomson AW, Knolle PA. Antigen-presenting cell function in the tolerogenic liver environment. Nat Rev Immunol. 2010;10(11):753–66.
33. Müschen M, Warskulat U, Peters-Regehr T, Bode JG, Kubitz R, Häussinger D. Involvement of CD95 (Apo-1/Fas) ligand expressed by rat Kupffer cells in hepatic immunoregulation. Gastroenterology. 1999;116(3):666–77.
34. Bradham CA, Plümpe J, Manns MP, Brenner DA, Trautwein C. Mechanisms of hepatic toxicity. I. TNF-induced liver injury. Am J Physiol. 1998;275(3 Pt 1):G387–92.
35. Kuniyasu Y, Marfani SM, Inayat IB, Sheikh SZ, Mehal WZ. Kupffer cells required for high affinity peptide-induced deletion, not retention, of activated CD8+ T cells by mouse liver. Hepatology. 2004;39(4):1017–27.
36. Crispe IN. The liver as a lymphoid organ. Annu Rev Immunol. 2009;27:147–63.
37. Ji J, Eggert T, Budhu A, Forgues M, Takai A, Dang H, et al. Hepatic stellate cell and monocyte interaction contributes to poor prognosis in hepatocellular carcinoma. Hepatology. 2015;62(2):481–95.
38. Hammerich L, Tacke F. Emerging roles of myeloid derived suppressor cells in hepatic inflammation and fibrosis. World J Gastroint Pathophysiol. 2015;6(3):43–50.
39. Ionescu AG, Streba LA, Vere CC, Ciurea ME, Streba CT, Ionescu M, et al. Histopathological and immunohistochemical study of hepatic stellate cells in patients with viral C chronic liver disease. Rom J Morphol Embryol. 2013;54(4):983–91.
40. Breous E, Thimme R. Potential of immunotherapy for hepatocellular carcinoma. J Hepatol. 2011;54(4):830–4.
41. Cai XY, Gao Q, Qiu SJ, Ye SL, Wu ZQ, Fan J, et al. Dendritic cell infiltration and prognosis of human hepatocellular carcinoma. J Cancer Res Clin Oncol. 2006;132(5):293–301.
42. Hoechst B, Voigtlaender T, Ormandy L, Gamrekelashvili J, Zhao F, Wedemeyer H, et al. Myeloid derived suppressor cells inhibit natural killer cells in patients with hepatocellular carcinoma via the NKp30 receptor. Hepatology. 2009;50(3):799–807.
43. Tseng CT, Klimpel GR. Binding of the hepatitis C virus envelope protein E2 to CD81 inhibits natural killer cell functions. J Exp Med. 2002;195(1):43–9.
44. Cai L, Zhang Z, Zhou L, Wang H, Fu J, Zhang S, et al. Functional impairment in circulating and intrahepatic NK cells and relative mechanism in hepatocellular carcinoma patients. Clin Immunol. 2008;129(3):428–37.
45. Hong YP, Li ZD, Prasoon P, Zhang Q. Immunotherapy for hepatocellular carcinoma: from basic research to clinical use. World J Hepatol. 2015;7(7):980–92.
46. Safety Study of Liver Natural Killer Cell Therapy for Hepatoma Liver Transplantation - Full Text View - ClinicalTrials.gov. 2015. https://www.clinicaltrials.gov/ct2/show/NCT01147380?term=Hepatocellular+carcinoma+immunotherapy&rank=6
47. Hyodo N, Nakamura I, Imawari M. Hepatitis B core antigen stimulates interleukin-10 secretion by both T cells and monocytes from peripheral blood of patients with chronic hepatitis B virus infection. Clin Exp Immunol. 2004;135(3):462–6.
48. Miroux C, Vausselin T, Delhem N. Regulatory T cells in HBV and HCV liver diseases: implication of regulatory T lymphocytes in the control of immune response. Expert Opin Biol Ther. 2010;10(11):1563–72.
49. Golden-Mason L, Palmer B, Klarquist J, Mengshol JA, Castelblanco N, Rosen HR. Upregulation of PD-1 expression on circulating and intrahepatic hepatitis C virus-specific CD8+ T cells associated with reversible immune dysfunction. J Virol. 2007;81(17):9249–58.
50. Golden-Mason L, Palmer BE, Kassam N, Townshend-Bulson L, Livingston S, McMahon BJ, et al. Negative immune regulator Tim-3 is overexpressed on T cells in hepatitis C virus infection and its blockade rescues dysfunctional CD4+ and CD8+ T cells. J Virol. 2009;83(18):9122–30.
51. Shirabe K, Motomura T, Muto J, Toshima T, Matono R, Mano Y, et al. Tumor-infiltrating lymphocytes and hepatocellular carcinoma: pathology and clinical management. Int J Clin Oncol. 2010;15(6):552–8.

52. Hilgenfeldt EG, Schlachterman A, Firpi RJ. Hepatitis C: treatment of difficult to treat patients. World J Hepatol. 2015;7(15):1953–63.
53. O'Bryan JM, Potts JA, Bonkovsky HL, Mathew A, Rothman AL, Group H-CT. Extended interferon-alpha therapy accelerates telomere length loss in human peripheral blood T lymphocytes. PLoS One. 2011;6(8):e20922.
54. Saito K, Ait-Goughoulte M, Truscott SM, Meyer K, Blazevic A, Abate G, et al. Hepatitis C virus inhibits cell surface expression of HLA-DR, prevents dendritic cell maturation, and induces interleukin-10 production. J Virol. 2008;82(7):3320–8.
55. Ormandy LA, Hillemann T, Wedemeyer H, Manns MP, Greten TF, Korangy F. Increased populations of regulatory T cells in peripheral blood of patients with hepatocellular carcinoma. Cancer Res. 2005;65(6):2457–64.
56. Greten TF, Manns MP, Korangy F. Immunotherapy of hepatocellular carcinoma. J Hepatol. 2006;45(6):868–78.
57. Mizejewski GJ. Alpha-fetoprotein structure and function: relevance to isoforms, epitopes, and conformational variants. Exp Biol Med (Maywood). 2001;226(5):377–408.
58. Butterfield LH, Ribas A, Meng WS, Dissette VB, Amarnani S, Vu HT, et al. T-cell responses to HLA-A*0201 immunodominant peptides derived from alpha-fetoprotein in patients with hepatocellular cancer. Clin Cancer Res. 2003;9(16 Pt 1):5902–8.
59. Liu Y, Daley S, Evdokimova VN, Zdobinski DD, Potter DM, Butterfield LH. Hierarchy of alpha fetoprotein (AFP)-specific T cell responses in subjects with AFP-positive hepatocellular cancer. J Immunol. 2006;177(1):712–21.
60. Thimme R, Neagu M, Boettler T, Neumann-Haefelin C, Kersting N, Geissler M, et al. Comprehensive analysis of the alpha-fetoprotein-specific CD8+ T cell responses in patients with hepatocellular carcinoma. Hepatology. 2008;48(6):1821–33.
61. Greten TF, Ormandy LA, Fikuart A, Hochst B, Henschen S, Horning M, et al. Low-dose cyclophosphamide treatment impairs regulatory T cells and unmasks AFP-specific CD4+ T-cell responses in patients with advanced HCC. J Immunother. 2010;33(2):211–8.
62. Ho M, Kim H. Glypican-3: a new target for cancer immunotherapy. Eur J Cancer. 2011;47(3):333–8.
63. Xiao W-K, Qi C-Y, Chen D, Li S-Q, Fu S-J, Peng B-G, et al. Prognostic significance of glypican-3 in hepatocellular carcinoma: a meta-analysis. BMC Cancer. 2014;14(1):104.
64. Wang YL, Zhu ZJ, Teng DH, Yao Z, Gao W, Shen ZY. Glypican-3 expression and its relationship with recurrence of HCC after liver transplantation. World J Gastroenterol. 2012;18(19):2408–14.
65. Li SQ, Lin J, Qi CY, Fu SJ, Xiao WK, Peng BG, et al. GPC3 DNA vaccine elicits potent cellular antitumor immunity against HCC in mice. Hepatogastroenterology. 2014;61(130):278–84.
66. Komori H, Nakatsura T, Senju S, Yoshitake Y, Motomura Y, Ikuta Y, et al. Identification of HLA-A2- or HLA-A24-restricted CTL epitopes possibly useful for glypican-3-specific immunotherapy of hepatocellular carcinoma. Clin Cancer Res. 2006;12(9):2689–97.
67. Dargel C, Bassani-Sternberg M, Hasreiter J, Zani F, Bockmann JH, Thiele F, et al. T cells engineered to express a T-cell receptor specific for Glypican-3 to recognize and kill hepatoma cells in vitro and in mice. Gastroenterology. 2015;149(4):1042–52.
68. Shang XY, Chen HS, Zhang HG, Pang XW, Qiao H, Peng JR, et al. The spontaneous CD8+ T-cell response to HLA-A2-restricted NY-ESO-1b peptide in hepatocellular carcinoma patients. Clin Cancer Res. 2004;10(20):6946–55.
69. Luo G, Huang S, Xie X, Stockert E, Chen YT, Kubuschok B, et al. Expression of cancer-testis genes in human hepatocellular carcinomas. Cancer Immun. 2002;2:11.
70. Korangy F, Ormandy LA, Bleck JS, Klempnauer J, Wilkens L, Manns MP, et al. Spontaneous tumor-specific humoral and cellular immune responses to NY-ESO-1 in hepatocellular carcinoma. Clin Cancer Res. 2004;10(13):4332–41.
71. Zhang HH, Mei MH, Fei R, Liao WJ, Wang XY, Qin LL, et al. Regulatory T cell depletion enhances tumor specific CD8 T-cell responses, elicited by tumor antigen NY-ESO-1b in hepatocellular carcinoma patients, in vitro. Int J Oncol. 2010;36(4):841–8.

72. Bricard G, Bouzourene H, Martinet O, Rimoldi D, Halkic N, Gillet M, et al. Naturally acquired MAGE-A10- and SSX-2-specific CD8+ T cell responses in patients with hepatocellular carcinoma. J Immunol. 2005;174(3):1709–16.
73. Zerbini A, Pilli M, Soliani P, Ziegler S, Pelosi G, Orlandini A, et al. Ex vivo characterization of tumor-derived melanoma antigen encoding gene-specific CD8+cells in patients with hepatocellular carcinoma. J Hepatol. 2004;40(1):102–9.
74. Mizukoshi E, Nakamoto Y, Marukawa Y, Arai K, Yamashita T, Tsuji H, et al. Cytotoxic T cell responses to human telomerase reverse transcriptase in patients with hepatocellular carcinoma. Hepatology. 2006;43(6):1284–94.
75. Huang DS, Wang Z, He XJ, Diplas BH, Yang R, Killela PJ, et al. Recurrent TERT promoter mutations identified in a large-scale study of multiple tumour types are associated with increased TERT expression and telomerase activation. Eur J Cancer. 2015;51(8):969–76.
76. Satow R, Shitashige M, Kanai Y, Takeshita F, Ojima H, Jigami T, et al. Combined functional genome survey of therapeutic targets for hepatocellular carcinoma. Clin Cancer Res. 2010;16(9):2518–28.
77. Aref AM, Hoa NT, Ge L, Agrawal A, Dacosta-Iyer M, Lambrecht N, et al. HCA519/TPX2: a potential T-cell tumor-associated antigen for human hepatocellular carcinoma. Onco Targets Ther. 2014;7:1061–70.
78. Ma Y, Lin D, Sun W, Xiao T, Yuan J, Han N, et al. Expression of targeting protein for xklp2 associated with both malignant transformation of respiratory epithelium and progression of squamous cell lung cancer. Clin Cancer Res. 2006;12(4):1121–7.
79. Mizukoshi E, Nakagawa H, Kitahara M, Yamashita T, Arai K, Sunagozaka H, et al. Immunological features of T cells induced by human telomerase reverse transcriptase-derived peptides in patients with hepatocellular carcinoma. Cancer Lett. 2015;364(2):98–105.
80. Hato T, Goyal L, Greten TF, Duda DG, Zhu AX. Immune checkpoint blockade in hepatocellular carcinoma: current progress and future directions. Hepatology. 2014;60(5):1776–82.
81. Greten TF, Wang XW, Korangy F. Current concepts of immune based treatments for patients with HCC: from basic science to novel treatment approaches. Gut. 2015;64(5):842–8.
82. Herbst RS, Soria JC, Kowanetz M, Fine GD, Hamid O, Gordon MS, et al. Predictive correlates of response to the anti-PD-L1 antibody MPDL3280A in cancer patients. Nature. 2014;515(7528):563–7.
83. Romano E, Romero P. The therapeutic promise of disrupting the PD-1/PD-L1 immune checkpoint in cancer: unleashing the CD8 T cell mediated anti-tumor activity results in significant, unprecedented clinical efficacy in various solid tumors. J Immunother Cancer. 2015;3:15.
84. Shi F, Shi M, Zeng Z, Qi RZ, Liu ZW, Zhang JY, et al. PD-1 and PD-L1 upregulation promotes CD8(+) T-cell apoptosis and postoperative recurrence in hepatocellular carcinoma patients. Int J Cancer. 2011;128(4):887–96.
85. Wu K, Kryczek I, Chen L, Zou W, Welling TH. Kupffer cell suppression of CD8+ T cells in human hepatocellular carcinoma is mediated by B7-H1/programmed death-1 interactions. Cancer Res. 2009;69(20):8067–75.
86. Kuang DM, Zhao Q, Peng C, Xu J, Zhang JP, Wu C, et al. Activated monocytes in peritumoral stroma of hepatocellular carcinoma foster immune privilege and disease progression through PD-L1. J Exp Med. 2009;206(6):1327–37.
87. Chen Y, Ramjiawan RR, Reiberger T, Ng MR, Hato T, Huang Y, et al. CXCR4 inhibition in tumor microenvironment facilitates anti-programmed death receptor-1 immunotherapy in sorafenib-treated hepatocellular carcinoma in mice. Hepatology. 2015;61(5):1591–602.
88. Sangro B, Gomez-Martin C, de la Mata M, Iñarrairaegui M, Garralda E, Barrera P, et al. A clinical trial of CTLA-4 blockade with tremelimumab in patients with hepatocellular carcinoma and chronic hepatitis C. J Hepatol. 2013;59(1):81–8.
89. Phase I/II safety and antitumor activity of nivolumab in patients with advanced hepatocellular carcinoma (HCC): CA209–040. I 2015 ASCO Annual Meeting I Abstracts I Meeting Library. 2015. http://meetinglibrary.asco.org/content/146146-156
90. Grosso JF, Jure-Kunkel MN. CTLA-4 blockade in tumor models: an overview of preclinical and translational research. Cancer Immun. 2013;13:5.

91. Iwashita Y, Tahara K, Goto S, Sasaki A, Kai S, Seike M, et al. A phase I study of autologous dendritic cell-based immunotherapy for patients with unresectable primary liver cancer. Cancer Immunol Immunother. 2003;52(3):155–61.
92. Kumagi T, Akbar SM, Horiike N, Kurose K, Hirooka M, Hiraoka A, et al. Administration of dendritic cells in cancer nodules in hepatocellular carcinoma. Oncol Rep. 2005;14(4):969–73.
93. Palmer DH, Midgley RS, Mirza N, Torr EE, Ahmed F, Steele JC, et al. A phase II study of adoptive immunotherapy using dendritic cells pulsed with tumor lysate in patients with hepatocellular carcinoma. Hepatology. 2009;49(1):124–32.
94. Mizukoshi E, Nakamoto Y, Arai K, Yamashita T, Mukaida N, Matsushima K, et al. Enhancement of tumor-specific T-cell responses by transcatheter arterial embolization with dendritic cell infusion for hepatocellular carcinoma. Int J Cancer. 2010;126(9):2164–74.
95. Heo J, Reid T, Ruo L, Breitbach CJ, Rose S, Bloomston M, et al. Randomized dose-finding clinical trial of oncolytic immunotherapeutic vaccinia JX-594 in liver cancer. Nat Med. 2013;19(3):329–36.
96. Woller N, Knocke S, Mundt B, Gürlevik E, Strüver N, Kloos A, et al. Virus-induced tumor inflammation facilitates effective DC cancer immunotherapy in a Treg-dependent manner in mice. J Clin Invest. 2011;121(7):2570–82.
97. Chen Y, Yang D, Li S, Gao Y, Jiang R, Deng L, et al. Development of a listeria monocytogenes-based vaccine against hepatocellular carcinoma. Oncogene. 2012;31(17):2140–52.
98. Butterfield LH, Economou JS, Gamblin TC, Geller DA. Alpha fetoprotein DNA prime and adenovirus boost immunization of two hepatocellular cancer patients. J Transl Med. 2014;12:86.
99. Parato KA, Breitbach CJ, Le Boeuf F, Wang J, Storbeck C, Ilkow C, et al. The oncolytic poxvirus JX-594 selectively replicates in and destroys cancer cells driven by genetic pathways commonly activated in cancers. Mol Ther. 2012;20(4):749–58.
100. Heo J, Breitbach CJ, Moon A, Kim CW, Patt R, Kim MK, et al. Sequential therapy with JX-594, a targeted oncolytic poxvirus, followed by sorafenib in hepatocellular carcinoma: preclinical and clinical demonstration of combination efficacy. Mol Ther. 2011;19(6):1170–9.
101. Hepatocellular Carcinoma Study Comparing Vaccinia Virus Based Immunotherapy Plus Sorafenib vs Sorafenib Alone - Full Text View - ClinicalTrials.gov. 2015. https://www.clinicaltrials.gov/ct2/show/NCT02562755?term=Hepatocellular+carcinoma+immunotherapy&rank=3
102. Iwanaga T. [Studies on cases of spontaneous regression of cancer in Japan in 2011, and of hepatic carcinoma, lung cancer and pulmonary metastases in the world between 2006 and 2011]. Gan To Kagaku Ryoho. 2013;40(11):1475–87.
103. Ayaru L, Pereira SP, Alisa A, Pathan AA, Williams R, Davidson B, et al. Unmasking of alpha-fetoprotein-specific CD4(+) T cell responses in hepatocellular carcinoma patients undergoing embolization. J Immunol. 2007;178(3):1914–22.
104. Zerbini A, Pilli M, Fagnoni F, Pelosi G, Pizzi MG, Schivazappa S, et al. Increased immunostimulatory activity conferred to antigen-presenting cells by exposure to antigen extract from hepatocellular carcinoma after radiofrequency thermal ablation. J Immunother. 2008;31(3):271–82.

Liver Cell Dysplasia and the Development of HCC

11

Jesse Kresak and Naziheh Assarzadegan

11.1 Introduction

Hepatocellular carcinoma (HCC) is the fifth most common cancer and second leading cause of cancer-related death worldwide [1–4]. Due to a lack of specific symptomatology, HCC is most often diagnosed at an advanced stage leading to limited treatment options and a dismal prognosis [5]. Studies have shown that, when compared to smaller tumors, cure rates for HCC larger than 2 cm decrease and curative treatment become even less likely for lesions larger than 3 cm [6]. Therefore, the ability to identify the precursor lesions at an earlier stage in which resection and cure are still possible has received increased attention in recent years [2, 5, 7].

In several tissue types, namely, the gastrointestinal and genitourinary tracts, epithelial dysplasia is well recognized as a precancerous lesion. The histologic criteria to diagnose such epithelial dysplasia are well-established and show good interobserver agreement. However, the role of dysplasia in the development of hepatocellular carcinoma is neither as well accepted in theory nor as concretely histologically defined.

Early surveillance programs, along with advances in imaging modalities, have led to the detection of small hepatic nodules in livers of high-risk populations, particularly those with cirrhosis. There is increasing evidence that strongly supports a multistep sequence of events in the pathogenesis of hepatocellular carcinoma. It is believed that HCC evolves from precancerous lesions and well-differentiated HCC further progresses to a less differentiated form [3, 8]. By consensus, the lesions in this sequence of events have been termed low-grade dysplastic nodule (LGDN), high-grade dysplastic nodule (HGDN), early HCC (eHCC), and small and progressed HCC [9]. The distinction between the varying

J. Kresak, M.D. (✉) • N. Assarzadegan, M.D.
Department of Pathology, Immunology, and Laboratory Medicine,
University of Florida, Gainesville, FL, USA
e-mail: jkresak@ufl.edu

© Springer International Publishing AG 2018
C. Liu (ed.), *Precision Molecular Pathology of Liver Cancer*,
Molecular Pathology Library, https://doi.org/10.1007/978-3-319-68082-8_11

lesions relies primarily on histologic criteria, although there remains considerable challenge in distinguishing high-grade dysplasia from early HCC even among the most seasoned pathologists.

This chapter will serve primarily as a histologic review of liver cell dysplasia with a brief overview of the current understanding of the pathogenesis into HCC.

11.2   Pathogenesis

Early detection of HCC requires a better understanding of its pathogenesis. There is increasing evidence supporting a stepwise progression of molecular events in hepatocarcinogenesis. Studies have shown that while dysplastic nodules harbor only few genetic mutations, as they progress to an advanced HCC, they can acquire up to 180 genetic mutations [9]. However, this acquisition of genetic mutations does not appear to follow a common pattern for all HCCs, rather the exact genetic alterations may vary greatly between one HCC and another. In fact, studies of multicentric HCCs have shown no common variants via whole-genome sequencing within different concomitant tumors of the same patient [4]. The extensive heterogeneity among genetic alterations in HCCs may be attributable to the various etiologic conditions (e.g., hepatocellular carcinoma rising in a background of viral hepatitis versus nonalcoholic fatty liver disease). A recent study analyzing whole coding sequencing of 243 tumors found mutational processes that congregated into 8 molecular "signatures," which is in turn correlated with 6 demographic and etiologic groups [9], though further studies are needed for refinement of these associations.

11.2.1 Cirrhotic Background

It is well established that cirrhosis is a major predisposing factor to the development of HCC, as more than 85% of HCCs arise in a cirrhotic background [4]. In an overly simplistic viewpoint, chronic hepatic inflammatory processes lead to cellular damage and high cellular turnover which induces a state of constant repair and an environment prone to mutational alterations within an oncogenic microenvironment. Alternatively, the remainder of HCCs can arise without advanced liver damage and fibrosis, suggesting various pathways of liver carcinogenesis. The details of these mutational alterations and tumor microenvironment responsible for the tumorigenesis of HCC are not yet entirely elucidated.

Telomere shortening via mutations in telomerase reverse transcriptase (TERT) promoter appears to be a common and early mechanism of hepatocarcinogenesis on the cirrhotic setting [4]. A recent study of 96 tumors showed a positive correlation between the frequency of TERT promoter mutations and the degree of dysplasia. The frequency of TERT mutations rose from 6% in LGDN to 19% in HGDN to 61% in eHCC. Interestingly, once at the level of HCC, the TERT mutation frequency plateaued, and no significant difference was found between eHCC and advanced

HCC [4]. This finding suggests that TERT mutations, found in up to 68% of HCCs of varying etiologies [4], are an early event and are involved in the transformation from dysplasia to malignancy.

Recurrent inactivating mutations of AT-rich interactive domain (ARID)1A and ARID2 have been reported in about 15% of HCC cases each [4, 10]. ARID1A and ARID2 are components of the SWI/SNF complex implicated in chromatin remodeling and transcription regulation. Chromatin modification is also altered by mutations involving histone methyltransferases, including mutations of *MLL*, *MLL2*, *MLL3*, and *MLL4*, as well as HBV insertions in *MLL4*, with varying reported frequencies of up to 20% [4, 9]. Despite various etiologic causes, a commonality shared among the alterations found in cirrhotic HCCs is their affinity for targeting chromatin remodeling, DNA repair mechanisms, and PI3K-Akt-mTOR pathways.

Direct and local effects of the various underlying liver disease may also be implicated in the development of HCC in cirrhosis. Steatosis, found in nonalcoholic fatty liver disease (NAFLD), alcohol-induced liver injury, and hepatitis C (specifically genotype 3), incites inflammation via cytokines and may also have direct toxic effects. Hepatitis C does not incorporate directly into the host genome (unlike hepatitis B), yet, at least in murine models, Hep C core protein may have direct oncogenic effects upon the liver. Alcohol has not been shown to have specific hepatocarcinogenic properties, though ethanol can be converted into reactive oxygen species leading to chronic stress [11].

11.2.2 Non-cirrhotic Background

HCC can also arise in non-cirrhotic livers, most often in the setting of a pre-existing hepatocellular adenoma or in associated with hepatitis B, and the pathogenesis of these HCCs can follow a different molecular course. For HCC arising in a hepatic adenoma, the most frequent genetic alteration is mutation of beta-catenin (CTNNB1). Similar to TERT mutations in cirrhotic-based liver nodules, the frequency of CTNNB1 mutations increases from 15% in adenomas to 50% in borderline lesions (atypical adenomas inconclusive of HCC) to 60% in HCCs transformed from adenomas [4]. Hepatocellular carcinoma associated with hepatitis B (HBV) infection has decreased in the USA and other developed countries since the inception of the viral specific vaccine; however HBV remains a leading cause of HCC worldwide. A feature which may allow the virus to bypass the chronic inflammation-cirrhotic pathway is direct insertion into the human genome, which can be found in up to 80% of HBV-associated HCC [11, 12]. HBV can insert itself randomly into the genome, yet most frequently is found in promoter regions of genes such as TERT, CCNE1 (cyclin E1), and MLL4, promoting carcinogenesis. In addition, some authors have reported direct oncogenic properties, such as mitotic/apoptotic regulation and chromosomal instability, of the viral protein, HBx. HBx protein and variant truncated forms are produced by HBV and necessary for viral replication. The most frequent genetic mutation found in HBV-associated HCC is somatic TP53 mutation, with a frequency of 12–48% [9, 13].

Aflatoxin B1 (AFB1) exposure leads to the development of HCC with a highly specific R249S mutation of TP53 in codon 249 [14]. Aside from this mutation, AFB1 predisposes to HCC with a similar mutational landscape as hepatitis B due to a particularly high degree of combined exposure particularly in some regions of the world, namely, subtropical Asia and Africa.

11.3 Histologic Classifications

The preneoplastic role of liver cell dysplasia (LCD) was first described in 1973 by Anthony et al. who found a strong association between LCD and HCC in a study of 552 Ugandan African patients. Anthony et al. defined LCD, which is now designated as large LCD/change (LLCD), as cellular enlargement, nuclear pleomorphism, and multinucleation of liver cells occurring in groups or occupying whole cirrhotic nodules [15].

In 1983, Watanabe et al. described a term, small LCD/change (SCLD), characterized by foci of crowded small hepatocytes with high nuclear/cytoplasmic ratio. These lesions have then been recognized to be the precursor lesion to HCC due to their increased proliferative activity and morphologic resemblance to HCC [16, 17]. Over the last two decades, there has been considerable confusion concerning nomenclature and diagnostic approaches to these hepatic nodules and precursor lesions. In 1995, an International Working Party (IWP) of the World Congresses of Gastroenterology proposed a consensus nomenclature and diagnostic criteria for hepatocellular nodular lesions to clarify some of the confusion [18].

The IWP classification categorized nodular lesions in chronic liver disease into large regenerative nodule, low-grade dysplastic nodule (L-DN), high-grade dysplastic nodule (H-DN), and small HCC; this nomenclature has been widely adopted. The IWP consensus also introduced the concept of dysplastic focus as a cluster of hepatocytes with features of early neoplasia (in particular small cell change or iron-free foci in a siderotic background) measuring less than 0.1 cm and defined small HCC as a tumor measuring less than 2 cm [18, 19].

Although IWP criteria have even widely adopted, assessment of small lesions with malignant potential lacks reproducibility as there are differences in application of diagnostic criteria among pathologists. In 2009, an international consensus group for hepatocellular neoplasia (ICGHN), in order to obtain a refined and up-to-date international consensus on the histopathologic diagnosis of nodular lesions, proposed an updated nomenclature for the classification of small hepatocellular lesions (<2 cm) as summarized in Fig. 11.1 [18, 19].

Lesions that are recognizable morphologically during hepatocarcinogenesis include dysplastic lesions (dysplastic foci and dysplastic nodules [DNs]) and small cancerous lesions (=<2 cm in diameter) which itself includes early HCC and small progressed HCC [1, 18, 19].

The pathologic features of each of these lesions, as well as the use of immunohistochemical markers, are discussed.

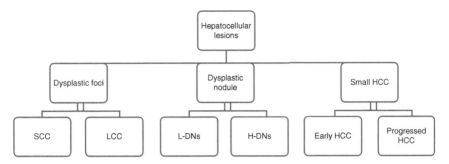

Fig. 11.1 International Consensus Group for Hepatocellular Neoplasia (ICGHN) classification of small hepatocellular lesions. Key: *SCC* small cell changes, *LCC* large cell changes, *L-DNs* low-grade dysplastic nodules, *H-DNs* high-grade dysplastic nodules

11.3.1 Dysplastic Foci

Dysplastic foci are defined as microscopic lesions, occurring in a background of cirrhosis, composed of dysplastic hepatocytes measuring less than 1 mm in size. These foci are not detectable macroscopically, and thus, in most cases, they are incidentally identified in liver biopsies or resected liver specimens [1, 18].

Dysplastic foci are further characterized by small (SCC) or large cell (LCC) changes [1, 15, 16].

SCC is the most common cytologic finding seen in dysplastic foci [16]. SCC was originally described as small cell dysplasia and is defined as hepatocytes showing decreased cell volume, increased nuclear to cytoplasmic ratio, mild nuclear pleomorphism and hyperchromasia, and cytoplasmic basophilia. These features give the impression of nuclear crowding [1] (Fig. 11.2).

Areas with small cell change show a higher proliferative index than the surrounding normal-appearing hepatocytes [1, 20, 21]. Marchio et al. in their study showed that small cell change has similar chromosomal changes to adjacent HCC suggesting the preneoplastic nature of these changes [1, 22]. These chromosomal changes include telomere shortening, p21 checkpoint inactivation, chromosomal instability, and chromosomal gains and losses [1, 21]. SCC can have an expansile or diffuse pattern which can be difficult and challenging to distinguish. It has been shown that the expansile foci are more likely to be associated with the development of HCC [20, 21]. Therefore, in the international working party classification, the expansile foci are considered to correspond to dysplastic foci, whereas the diffuse pattern may be representative of regeneration rather than true dysplasia [1, 18, 20].

Large cell change (LCC), initially termed "liver cell dysplasia" by Anthony et al., is defined as an increase in both nuclear and cytoplasmic size, hence a preserved nuclear to cytoplasmic ratio. Nuclei are hyperchromatic, pleomorphic, and frequently multinucleated [21] (Fig. 11.3).

Data regarding the biologic nature of LCC is conflicting and uncertain. Some data support LCC as being a reactive process related to chronic injury with a low

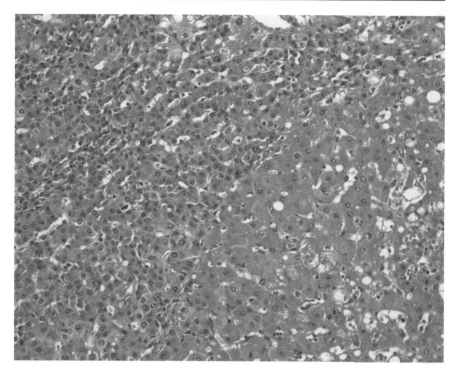

Fig. 11.2 Small cell change, characterized by increased nuclear to cytoplasmic ratio and increased cell density, is present in the left side of histologic picture compared to background hepatocytes on the right

proliferative activity and absence of genetic alterations present in the adjacent HCC. Other data supports LCC as being a prerequisite for hepatocarcinogenesis by showing chromosomal abnormalities and gains and losses [1, 21–25].

This conflicting data suggests the possibility of a heterogeneous nature for LCC with two types: one type is benign, reactive, and non-tumor related, while the other type is true dysplasia and thus tumor related [26]. Despite this conflicting data, the presence of LCC has been reported to be an important independent risk factor for subsequent development of HCC in patients with cirrhosis due to hepatitis B or C by multiple studies [1, 3, 7, 27].

Some studies have shown a progressive increase in chromosomal abnormalities, including telomere shortening, chromosomal instabilities, cell cycle checkpoint inactivation, and DNA damage from LCC to SCC. This data suggest that LCC may be a very early precursor of HCC and that SCC may be a more advanced precursor lesion in chronic hepatitis B or C [1, 28, 29]. In addition to SCC and LCC, iron-free foci in patients with hereditary hemochromatosis have been reported to be associated with a higher incidence of HCC during follow-up [30].

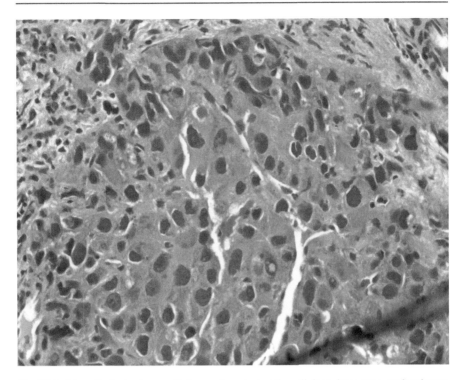

Fig. 11.3 Liver displaying large cell change characterized by cellular enlargement, nuclear hyperchromasia, and pleomorphism

11.3.2 Dysplastic Nodules

A dysplastic nodule is a grossly distinct nodular lesion, usually measure about 1 cm in diameter [1], which differs from the surrounding liver parenchyma in regard to size, color, texture, and degree of bulging of the cut surface [1, 5, 19]. International consensus has divided these nodules to low-grade dysplastic nodules (L-DNs) and high-grade dysplastic nodules (H-DNs) based on the degree of atypia [19].

L-DNs are often distinctly nodular (can sometimes be vaguely nodular) because of the rimming by the peripheral fibrous scar. This is not a true capsule but rather a condensed scar similar to what is seen in cirrhotic nodules [5, 19]. Microscopically, L-DNs show a monotonous cell population lacking architectural atypia with a mild increase in cellularity in comparison to the surrounding cirrhotic liver. Portal tracts can be identified within the nodules. Nodule in nodule formation, where a subnodule is growing within a nodule, is absent in L-DNs. Features of HCC such as pseudoglands and increased trabecular thickness are not present in these lesions [1, 5, 19] (Fig. 11.4).

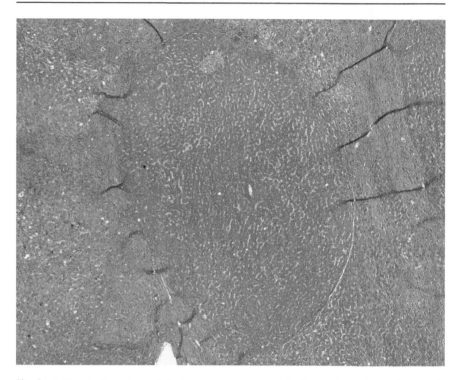

Fig. 11.4 Dysplastic nodule, distinct from surrounding cirrhotic nodules, with predominantly small cell change and intact trabecular thickness

H-DNs can be a distinct nodule or vaguely nodular; however, they are more likely to be vaguely nodular compared to L-DNs. Similar to L-DNs, they lack a true capsule. Microscopically, H-DNs are characterized by architectural and cytological atypia when compared to the surrounding liver yet insufficient to make the diagnosis of HCC. They commonly show increased cellularity that can be more than two times higher than the adjacent non-tumoral liver. SCC is the most frequently seen form of cytologic atypia in H-DNs. LCC may or may not be seen. Similar to L-DNs, portal tracts can be present within the nodules. Nodule in nodule appearance may be seen in H-DNs with the subnodule growing within the H-DNs usually being a well-differentiated HCC [19] (Fig. 11.5).

In regard to vascular supply, high- and low-grade dysplastic nodules can receive their blood supply from portal vessels as well as from "unpaired or non-triadal arteries." The "unpaired arteries" are absent in cirrhosis [1, 19, 31]. The findings of unpaired arteries and sinusoidal capillarization are minimal in cirrhosis and increase from low-grade to high-grade DN and approach the peak in HCC [32].

Stromal invasion is a diagnostic criterion used for the differentiation of H-DNs from early HCC. Cytokeratin 7 and/or 19 immunohistochemical stains can be helpful in areas of questionable invasion, whereby ductular reaction will be immunoreactive for these stains representing pseudoinvasion rather than HCC [32].

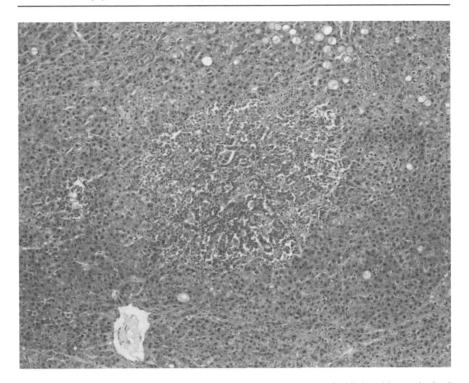

Fig. 11.5 Nodule within a nodule. Microscopic focus of high-grade dysplasia with pseudogland formation and high nuclear/cytoplasmic ratio arising in a dysplastic nodule with small cell change

Radiology is also helpful in distinguishing DNs from HCC. DNs are typically isovascular or hypovascular compared with the surrounding parenchyma, while HCC appears to be hypervascular in contrast-enhanced imaging [19, 33, 34].

Several follow-up studies of cirrhotic patients have evaluated the natural history of hepatic nodules, including large regenerative nodules and low-grade and high-grade DNs. These studies have reported that dysplastic nodules are associated with a higher risk for development of HCC [1, 21, 35]. In addition, similarities in molecular alterations have been detected in DNs and the adjacent HCC supporting the premalignant nature of DNs [36]. It has been shown that these lesions, especially high-grade DNs, had similar chromosomal gains and losses [37] and loss of heterogeneity in microsatellite foci with the adjacent HCC [21, 37, 38]. Dysplastic nodules, especially high-grade DNs, have also shown telomere shortening, increased telomerase activity, and strong expression of hTERT mRNA at levels similar to HCC [1, 39]. Moreover, DNs show inactivation of p21 checkpoint in contrary to cirrhotic nodules where they show activation [40]. The chromosomal changes in dysplastic nodules, especially high grade, make them more susceptible to further genetic changes required for malignant transformation [1].

11.3.3 Small HCC

Small HCC is defined as a low-grade carcinoma that measures less than 2.0 cm in diameter. Small HCC is subdivided into two groups based on gross and microscopic features: early HCC and (small) progressed HCC [1]. Subdividing small HCCs into early and progressed HCC have also been supported by recent studies with the clinical implication that early HCC has a longer time to recurrence and a higher 5-year survival rate, 3.9 years and 89%, respectively, as compared to 1.7 years and 48% of progressed HCC [5, 19, 41].

Morphologically, early HCC is recognized by its well-differentiated, vaguely nodular appearance, whereas progressed HCC is moderately differentiated and has distinct nodular pattern often with evidence of microvascular invasion [5, 19, 42].

11.3.4 Early HCC

Also called small well-differentiated HCC of vaguely nodular type or HCC with indistinct margins

The international consensus in 2009 defines early HCC as a vaguely nodular, well-differentiated lesion with a combination of the following histological features: increased cellularity of greater than two times the surrounding tissue, increased nuclear to cytoplasmic ratio, irregular trabecular pattern, varying number of portal tracts within the nodule, pseudoglandular pattern, diffuse and frequent steatosis (seen in approximately 40% of the cases), and variable number of unpaired arteries [1, 19]. The tumor cells in early HCC grow by replacing the non-neoplastic hepatic cords without forming a tumor capsule; thus, the margins of early HCC is usually indistinct [5, 19].

Early HCC neither have the ability to invade the vessels nor metastasize in contrast to classical HCC. Therefore it may represent an entity between in situ carcinoma and invasive carcinoma similar to microinvasion in other organs [1]. Early HCC, similar to DNs, usually appears to be isovascular or hypovascular compared to classical HCC, which is often hypervascular in the arterial phase of contrast-enhanced imaging [19]. This can be explained by more developed unpaired arteries and arterial neovascularization in classical HCC in contrast to early HCC and DNs [1, 21].

The reticulin framework may be reduced compared to adjacent normal parenchyma but is not completely lost as one can appreciate in progressed HCC [1, 5].

It has been shown that early HCC is a precursor lesion for progressed HCC and interestingly at the periphery of some cases of progressed HCC; a focus of well-differentiated HCC has been identified, suggesting a multistep sequence of events in hepatocellular carcinoma pathogenesis [1].

The morphologic features of early HCC can be diffuse or may be limited to a subnodule (nodule in nodule). It is very important to note that all the features of early HCC can be found in H-DNs. However, stromal invasion into portal tracts or fibrous septa is considered to be the most valuable diagnostic feature in distinguishing early HCC from H-DNs [19, 43, 44]. As discussed earlier, immunohistochemical staining for CK7/19 can be useful to identify areas of ductular reaction which is present around dysplastic nodules and absent in areas of stromal invasion in HCC [32].

11.3.5 Progressed HCC

Also called progressed HCC or HCC of distinctly nodular type or HCC with distinct margin:

Progressed HCC may arise from dysplastic foci, nodules, or an early HCC. The subset that arises within a DN or early HCC often forms the so-called nodule in nodule appearance [5, 42]. Progressed HCCs are often moderately differentiated and rimmed by a condensed fibrotic capsule [5]. Portal tracts are not present within the nodule [45]. They are rarely steatotic which can be explained by more advanced neoarterialization. Almost a third of cases show portal vein invasion, and 10% show intrahepatic metastases [1]. Unpaired arteries are more developed than DNs and early HCC, and as a result, they appear hypervascular in the arterial phase of enhanced hepatic imaging [19].

11.4   The Use of Immunohistochemistry in Hepatic Nodules

The utility of immunohistochemical stains is limited in regard to diagnosing dysplasia. There is some utility in the use of IHC when differentiating dysplasia from well-differentiated HCC as discussed below.

11.4.1 Stains of Moderate Utility

Cytokeratins 7 and 19
Stromal invasion, defined as the presence of tumor cells in the portal tract or fibrous septa, is the most useful feature in distinguishing H-DNs from early well-differentiated HCC [19]. Immunostaining for cytokeratin 7 and/or cytokeratin 19 can identify areas of ductular reaction around regenerating, nonmalignant nodules (pseudoinvasion), while this pattern of staining is absent in areas of true stromal invasion [1, 5, 32].

Glypican 3
Glypican 3 (GPC3), a cell surface heparin sulfate proteoglycan, is a serum and tissue marker for HCC with sensitivity and specificity of 77% and 96%, respectively [19, 21, 46–48]. Staining can be cytoplasmic, membranous, or canalicular [1]. In a study by Di Tommaso et al., GPC3 immunoreactivity was reported in 81% of

moderate to poorly differentiated HCCs, in 69% of well-differentiated HCCs and in 9% of H-DNs. None of the L-DNs showed immunoreactivity. Of note, GPC3 staining has been identified in regenerative hepatocytes of chronic hepatitis [3, 49].

Heat Shock Protein 70

Heat shock protein 70 (HSP70) is a stress protein involved in regulation of cell cycle progression and apoptosis [50, 51]. Chuma et al., in their study of 12,600 genes, reported HSP70 as the most abundantly upregulated gene in early HCC [52]. Significant overexpression of HSP70 was also reported in progressed HCC in comparison to early HCC and in early HCC in comparison to precancerous lesions [3, 49]. HSP70 immunohistochemistry shows nuclear and cytoplasmic staining [1]. The stain is considered positive when more than 10% of the cells show immunoreactivity. HSP70 immunoreactivity has been reported in a higher percentage of well-differentiated HCCs, 78%, when compared to 67% of moderately and poorly differentiated HCCs. Only 5% of H-DNs are positive for HSP70, and L-DNs are reported to be negative [3, 49]. Normal hepatocytes do not react with HSP70. The biliary epithelial cells of ductular reaction are immunoreactive for HSP70 and can serve as an internal positive control [1].

Glutamine Synthetase

Glutamine synthetase (GS) is the β-catenin target gene [19]. Overexpression of beta catenin is associated with a mutation of β-catenin or activation of this pathway. Upregulation of GS has been reported in HCC with a progressive increase in GS immunoreactivity from precancerous lesions to early HCC to progressed HCC [53, 54]. In addition, GS is the catalyzing enzyme in the synthesis of glutamine from glutamate and ammonia in the liver, mainly in pericentral/periseptal hepatocytes. Glutamine is the major source of energy for tumor cells [3, 49, 55]. As normal liver surrounding the terminal hepatic venules also stains for GS, the pattern of immunostaining should be strong and diffuse in malignant hepatocytes in order to increase its specificity [1]. This pattern has been shown in about 60% of well-differentiated HCCs and approximately 90% of moderately to poorly differentiated HCCs in resected specimens. Fourteen percent (14%) of H-DNs were also reported to show moderate and focal staining [3, 49].

β-catenin-activated hepatocellular adenoma (B-HCAs) and β-catenin-activated HCCs have been also reported to show diffuse GS immunoreactivity [56, 57].

The Combination of GPC3, HSP70, and GS

The use of single marker for detection of well-differentiated and early HCC lacks both sensitivity and specificity [1]. Using a combination of markers has shown an increase in the overall accuracy in both biopsies and resected specimens. The positivity of any two immunomarkers out of these three (GPC3, HSP70, and GS) has a reported specificity of 100% and a sensitivity of 72% for detection of well-differentiated HCC. The sensitivity was reported to be lower in biopsies (57%); however it can still be useful in difficult cases when stromal invasion is not apparent [3, 49].

11.4.2 Less Useful Markers

CD34 and Ki-67

CD34 can detect unpaired arteries and capillarized sinusoids which are the features showing a gradual increase from L-DNs, H-DNs, early HCCs to progressed HCCs [1, 31].

Similarly, proliferative activity and Ki67 show a gradual increase from L-DNs, H-DNs, early HCCs to progressed HCCs [1]. Given the absence of any definite cutoff values for each of these lesions, these two stains are not very helpful in differentiating H-DNs from well-differentiated HCC [1].

Alpha-Fetoprotein

Serum alpha-fetoprotein, the most widely used serum marker for detection of HCC, is rarely elevated in early HCC and is not detected in DNs [1, 58]. Because of its low sensitivity (about 30%), alpha-fetoprotein is not a useful tissue marker even in less differentiated HCCs [19].

P53

Mutation of p53 occurs later in the process of hepatocarcinogenesis. Progressed and less differentiated HCC show nuclear staining with p53 immunohistochemistry [1].

11.4.3 Molecular Analysis

Although many DNA structural abnormalities have been identified in precancerous lesions and HCCs, as discussed above, their use for diagnostic purposes is not yet established [21].

Some studies have shown that some chromosomal gains, such as 1q and 8q, can be detected by fluorescent in situ hybridization and can be of use in distinguishing well-differentiated HCC from hepatocellular adenoma [21, 59, 60].

11.5   Liver Biopsy Role and Interpretation in Regard to Dysplasia

The American Association for the Study of Liver Diseases recommends that biopsy should only be performed for the lesions that are less than 2.0 cm and do not have typical radiologic finding of HCC. Biopsy is not necessary in lesions with characteristic radiologic finding [19, 34].

Biopsy diagnosis of moderately to poorly differentiated carcinomas is usually easily made. The challenge remains for the distinction between DNs and well-differentiated HCCs [1, 19]. The detection of stromal invasion, unpaired arteries, mitoses, and immunohistochemical markers is difficult in minute biopsies due to sampling errors [19].

Stromal invasion, the most useful histologic marker for diagnosis of HCC, can be very difficult to assess in small biopsies as the biopsy may not include the intratumoral portal tracts. Likewise, the detection of unpaired arteries, mitoses, and also interpretation of immunohistochemical markers are difficult in small biopsies due to sampling errors. To avoid some of the sampling errors, sampling of both intralesional and extralesional tissues is recommended. This sampling provides the possibility of comparing these two regions [1].

The use of combination of GPC3, HSP70, and GS, as discussed above, has been shown to be useful in diagnosing well-differentiated HCCs in liver biopsies with sensitivity and specificity of 60 and 100% [3, 49]. Because the gross morphology is not available and only a small portion of the lesion is available when the liver biopsies are being interpreted, correlation with clinical and radiological finding is recommended [1].

11.6 Summary

To summarize, there is evidence to support a progression from dysplasia to malignancy in the development of HCC. Dysplasia can be diagnosed as a dysplastic focus, characterized by small cell or large cell change, or as a dysplastic nodule of either low or high grade. The ability to detect a liver lesion in its premalignant (dysplastic) state can have a significant clinical impact. Caution should be taken not to falsely believe that every nodule in cirrhosis is malignant. Correlation of clinical, radiological, and pathological finding in individual basis is valuable to identify patients who require treatment with local ablation, surgical resection, or liver transplant (H-DNs, small HCCs, both early and progressed.) and to decrease the possibility of premature transplantation of patients who do not have HCC [5, 19].

References

1. Park YN. Update on precursor and early lesions of hepatocellular carcinomas. Arch Pathol Lab Med. 2011;135(6):704–15.
2. Jemal A, Bray F, Center MM, Ferlay J, Ward E, Forman D. Global cancer statistics. CA Cancer J Clin. 2011;61(2):69–90.
3. Koo JS, Kim H, Park BK, et al. Predictive value of liver cell dysplasia for development of hepatocellular carcinoma in patients with chronic hepatitis B. J ClinGastroenterol. 2008;42(6):738–43.
4. Marquardt JU, Andersen JB, Thorgeirsson SS. Functional and genetic deconstruction of the cellular origin in liver cancer. Nat Rev Cancer. 2015;15(11):653–67.
5. Roncalli M, Terracciano L, Di Tommaso L, et al. Liver precancerous lesions and hepatocellular carcinoma: the histology report. Dig Liver Dis. 2011;43(Suppl 4):S361–72.
6. Sherman M. Hepatocellular carcinoma: epidemiology, surveillance, and diagnosis. Semin Liver Dis. 2010;30(1):3–16.
7. Borzio M, Bruno S, Roncalli M, et al. Liver cell dysplasia is a major risk factor for hepatocellular carcinoma in cirrhosis: a prospective study. Gastroenterology. 1995;108(3):812–7.

8. Röcken C, Carl-McGrath S. Pathology and pathogenesis of hepatocellular carcinoma. Dig Dis. 2001;19(4):269–78.
9. Schulze K, Imbeaud S, Letouzé E, et al. Exome sequencing of hepatocellular carcinomas identifies new mutational signatures and potential therapeutic targets. Nat Genet. 2015;47(5):505–11.
10. Nault JC, Calderaro J, Di Tommaso L, et al. Telomerase reverse transcriptase promoter mutation is an early somatic genetic alteration in the transformation of premalignant nodules in hepatocellular carcinoma on cirrhosis. Hepatology. 2014;60(6):1983–92.
11. Nault JC. Pathogenesis of hepatocellular carcinoma according to aetiology. Best Pract Res Clin Gastroenterol. 2014;28(5):937–47.
12. Sung WK, Zheng H, Li S, et al. Genome-wide survey of recurrent HBV integration in hepatocellular carcinoma. Nat Genet. 2012;44(7):765–9.
13. Levrero M, Zucman-Rossi J. Mechanisms of HBV-induced hepatocellular carcinoma. J Hepatol. 2016;64(1):S84–S101.
14. Bressac B, Kew M, Wands J, Ozturk M. Selective G to T mutations of p53 gene in hepatocellular carcinoma from southern Africa. Nature. 1991;350(6317):429–31.
15. Anthony PP, Vogel CL, Barker LF. Liver cell dysplasia: a premalignant condition. J Clin Pathol. 1973;26(3):217–23.
16. Watanabe S, Okita K, Harada T, et al. Morphologic studies of the liver cell dysplasia. Cancer. 1983;51(12):2197–205.
17. Adachi E, Hashimoto H, Tsuneyoshi M. Proliferating cell nuclear antigen in hepatocellular carcinoma and small cell liver dysplasia. Cancer. 1993;72(10):2902–9.
18. International Working Party. Terminology of nodular hepatocellular lesions. Hepatology. 1995;22(3):983–93.
19. Neoplasia ICGfH. Pathologic diagnosis of early hepatocellular carcinoma: a report of the international consensus group for hepatocellular neoplasia. Hepatology. 2009;49(2):658–64.
20. Hytiroglou P, Park YN, Krinsky G, Theise ND. Hepatic precancerous lesions and small hepatocellular carcinoma. Gastroenterol Clin North Am. 2007;36(4):867–87, vii.
21. Robert D, Odze JRG. Surgical pathology of the GI tract, liver, biliary tract and pancreas, vol 44. 3rd ed. New York: Elsevier; 2014. p. 1192–6.
22. Marchio A, Terris B, Meddeb M, et al. Chromosomal abnormalities in liver cell dysplasia detected by comparative genomic hybridisation. Mol Pathol. 2001;54(4):270–4.
23. Zondervan PE, Wink J, Alers JC, et al. Molecular cytogenetic evaluation of virus-associated and non-viral hepatocellular carcinoma: analysis of 26 carcinomas and 12 concurrent dysplasias. J Pathol. 2000;192(2):207–15.
24. Terris B, Ingster O, Rubbia L, et al. Interphase cytogenetic analysis reveals numerical chromosome aberrations in large liver cell dysplasia. J Hepatol. 1997;27(2):313–9.
25. Roncalli M, Borzio M, Brando B, Colloredo G, Servida E. Abnormal DNA content in liver-cell dysplasia: a flow cytometric study. Int J Cancer. 1989;44(2):204–7.
26. Park YN, Roncalli M. Large liver cell dysplasia: a controversial entity. J Hepatol. 2006;45(5):734–43.
27. Ganne-Carrié N, Chastang C, Chapel F, et al. Predictive score for the development of hepatocellular carcinoma and additional value of liver large cell dysplasia in Western patients with cirrhosis. Hepatology. 1996;23(5):1112–8.
28. Plentz RR, Park YN, Lechel A, et al. Telomere shortening and inactivation of cell cycle checkpoints characterize human hepatocarcinogenesis. Hepatology. 2007;45(4):968–76.
29. Kim H, BK O, Roncalli M, et al. Large liver cell change in hepatitis B virus-related liver cirrhosis. Hepatology. 2009;50(3):752–62.
30. Deugnier YM, Charalambous P, Le Quilleuc D, et al. Preneoplastic significance of hepatic iron-free foci in genetic hemochromatosis: a study of 185 patients. Hepatology. 1993;18(6):1363–9.
31. Park YN, Yang CP, Fernandez GJ, Cubukcu O, Thung SN, Theise ND. Neoangiogenesis and sinusoidal "capillarization" in dysplastic nodules of the liver. Am J Surg Pathol. 1998;22(6):656–62.

32. Park YN, Kojiro M, Di Tommaso L, et al. Ductular reaction is helpful in defining early stromal invasion, small hepatocellular carcinomas, and dysplastic nodules. Cancer. 2007;109(5):915–23.
33. Forner A, Vilana R, Ayuso C, et al. Diagnosis of hepatic nodules 20 mm or smaller in cirrhosis: prospective validation of the noninvasive diagnostic criteria for hepatocellular carcinoma. Hepatology. 2008;47(1):97–104.
34. Bruix J, Sherman M, Practice Guidelines Committee AeAftSoLD. Management of hepatocellular carcinoma. Hepatology. 2005;42(5):1208–36.
35. Theise ND, Park YN, Kojiro M. Dysplastic nodules and hepatocarcinogenesis. Clin Liver Dis. 2002;6(2):497–512.
36. Nam SW, Park JY, Ramasamy A, et al. Molecular changes from dysplastic nodule to hepatocellular carcinoma through gene expression profiling. Hepatology. 2005;42(4):809–18.
37. Tornillo L, Carafa V, Sauter G, et al. Chromosomal alterations in hepatocellular nodules by comparative genomic hybridization: high-grade dysplastic nodules represent early stages of hepatocellular carcinoma. Lab Investig. 2002;82(5):547–54.
38. Sun M, Eshleman JR, Ferrell LD, et al. An early lesion in hepatic carcinogenesis: loss of heterozygosity in human cirrhotic livers and dysplastic nodules at the 1p36-p34 region. Hepatology. 2001;33(6):1415–24.
39. BK O, Jo Chae K, Park C, et al. Telomere shortening and telomerase reactivation in dysplastic nodules of human hepatocarcinogenesis. J Hepatol. 2003;39(5):786–92.
40. Lee YH, BK O, Yoo JE, et al. Chromosomal instability, telomere shortening, and inactivation of p21(WAF1/CIP1) in dysplastic nodules of hepatitis B virus-associated multistep hepatocarcinogenesis. Mod Pathol. 2009;22(8):1121–31.
41. Takayama T, Makuuchi M, Hirohashi S, et al. Early hepatocellular carcinoma as an entity with a high rate of surgical cure. Hepatology. 1998;28(5):1241–6.
42. Kojiro M, Nakashima O. Histopathologic evaluation of hepatocellular carcinoma with special reference to small early stage tumors. Semin Liver Dis. 1999;19(3):287–96.
43. Kondo F, Kondo Y, Nagato Y, Tomizawa M, Wada K. Interstitial tumour cell invasion in small hepatocellular carcinoma. Evaluation in microscopic and low magnification views. J Gastroenterol Hepatol. 1994;9(6):604–12.
44. Nakano M, Saito A, Yamamoto M, Doi M, Takasaki K. Stromal and blood vessel wall invasion in well-differentiated hepatocellular carcinoma. Liver. 1997;17(1):41–6.
45. Nakashima Y, Nakashima O, Hsia CC, Kojiro M, Tabor E. Vascularization of small hepatocellular carcinomas: correlation with differentiation. Liver. 1999;19(1):12–8.
46. Capurro M, Wanless IR, Sherman M, et al. Glypican-3: a novel serum and histochemical marker for hepatocellular carcinoma. Gastroenterology. 2003;125(1):89–97.
47. Libbrecht L, Severi T, Cassiman D, et al. Glypican-3 expression distinguishes small hepatocellular carcinomas from cirrhosis, dysplastic nodules, and focal nodular hyperplasia-like nodules. Am J SurgPathol. 2006;30(11):1405–11.
48. Wang XY, Degos F, Dubois S, et al. Glypican-3 expression in hepatocellular tumors: diagnostic value for preneoplastic lesions and hepatocellular carcinomas. Hum Pathol. 2006;37(11):1435–41.
49. Di Tommaso L, Franchi G, Park YN, et al. Diagnostic value of HSP70, glypican 3, and glutamine synthetase in hepatocellular nodules in cirrhosis. Hepatology. 2007;45(3):725–34.
50. Garrido C, Gurbuxani S, Ravagnan L, Kroemer G. Heat shock proteins: endogenous modulators of apoptotic cell death. Biochem Biophys Res Commun. 2001;286(3):433–42.
51. Jolly C, Morimoto RI. Role of the heat shock response and molecular chaperones in oncogenesis and cell death. J Natl Cancer Inst. 2000;92(19):1564–72.
52. Chuma M, Sakamoto M, Yamazaki K, et al. Expression profiling in multistage hepatocarcinogenesis: identification of HSP70 as a molecular marker of early hepatocellular carcinoma. Hepatology. 2003;37(1):198–207.
53. Christa L, Simon MT, Flinois JP, Gebhardt R, Brechot C, Lasserre C. Overexpression of glutamine synthetase in human primary liver cancer. Gastroenterology. 1994;106(5):1312–20.

54. Osada T, Sakamoto M, Nagawa H, et al. Acquisition of glutamine synthetase expression in human hepatocarcinogenesis: relation to disease recurrence and possible regulation by ubiquitin-dependent proteolysis. Cancer. 1999;85(4):819–31.
55. Reitzer LJ, Wice BM, Kennell D. Evidence that glutamine, not sugar, is the major energy source for cultured HeLa cells. J Biol Chem. 1979;254(8):2669–76.
56. Bioulac-Sage P, Rebouissou S, Thomas C, et al. Hepatocellular adenoma subtype classification using molecular markers and immunohistochemistry. Hepatology. 2007;46(3):740–8.
57. Lee JM, Yang J, Newell P, et al. β-Catenin signaling in hepatocellular cancer: implications in inflammation, fibrosis, and proliferation. Cancer Lett. 2014;343(1):90–7.
58. Zhao YJ, Ju Q, Li GC. Tumor markers for hepatocellular carcinoma. Mol Clin Oncol. 2013;1(4):593–8.
59. Wilkens L, Bredt M, Flemming P, et al. Diagnostic impact of fluorescence in situ hybridization in the differentiation of hepatocellular adenoma and well-differentiated hepatocellular carcinoma. J Mol Diagn. 2001;3(2):68–73.
60. Kakar S, Chen X, Ho C, et al. Chromosomal abnormalities determined by comparative genomic hybridization are helpful in the diagnosis of atypical hepatocellular neoplasms. Histopathology. 2009;55(2):197–205.

Locoregional Therapies for Hepatocellular Carcinoma

12

Beau Toskich

12.1 Introduction

Despite the widespread implementation of surveillance programs for populations with chronic liver disease, more than half of patients with hepatocellular carcinoma (HCC) are diagnosed outside of criteria for curative treatment [1]. Many who receive therapy are subject to new or recurrent disease as a result of an underlying malignant hepatic parenchymal field defect [2]. Management of liver cancer is further complicated by variable hepatic substrate function which, in advanced disease, may pose greater threat to life than HCC [3]. Unlike traditional TNM staging systems, HCC treatment algorithms must factor physiologic reserve, patient performance, and expected disease control rates after transplantation. The Barcelona Clinic Liver Cancer (BCLC) classification is generally adopted in Western nations as the standard protocol to manage patients with HCC as endorsed by the European Association for the Study of the Liver (EASL) and the American Association for the Study of Liver Diseases (AASLD) [3, 4].

Given the complexities involved in managing cancer within a diseased organ, most regimens require multidisciplinary input which typically involves a hepatologist, a transplant surgeon, an interventional radiologist with experience in interventional oncology, and a patient care coordinator who will ascertain and manage the patient's nonmedical support structure. Institutional protocols help guide decisions based on established societal guidelines and local standards of practice. Considerations will include the benefits and disadvantages of surgical resection, liver transplantation with or without bridging or downstaging interventions, locoregional therapy, systemic therapy, clinical trials, and best supportive care.

Locoregional therapy (LRT) is a broad term that encompasses the fundamental principle of in situ tumor destruction while preserving adjacent hepatic tissue and

B. Toskich, M.D.
Department of Radiology, University of Florida College of Medicine,
Gainesville, FL, USA
e-mail: toskib@radiology.ufl.edu

© Springer International Publishing AG 2018
C. Liu (ed.), *Precision Molecular Pathology of Liver Cancer*,
Molecular Pathology Library, https://doi.org/10.1007/978-3-319-68082-8_12

viscera. Tumor cells, once destroyed, remain within the patient and ultimately undergo necrosis and immune-mediated fibrosis. While most surgical resection is based on excision of hepatic segments based on vascular supply, LRT is performed almost entirely by targeting indirect evidence of tumors via imaging modalities. Successful locoregional therapy requires evaluation of the patient's ability to tolerate treatment, ascertaining disease stage, obtaining an adequate margin, mitigating physiologic or technical deficiencies that diminish treatment effect, and minimizing collateral damage to uninvolved tissue.

12.2 Diagnosis

Most cases of symptomatic HCC are advanced at presentation with the majority of curable tumors detected either incidentally or via screening programs [1]. Serum tumor markers which can indicate the presence of HCC such as alpha-fetoprotein (AFP), prothrombin induced by vitamin K absence (PIVKA) 2, and carcinoembryonic antigen (CEA) are unreliable screening instruments due to both false-negative and false-positive rates in nonsecreting lesions and hepatic inflammatory states, respectively. While many reports suggest that AFP elevations greater than 400 ng/dL are specific to the presence of HCC, the most practical use for tumor marker surveillance lies in monitoring treatment response [5].

The AASLD recommends a screening hepatic ultrasound (US) every 6 months for at-risk populations. The sensitivity and specificity of US is 60% and 85%, respectively, due to variabilities in operator skill and the sonographic quality of the patient's abdomen [6]. Routine screening of patients with multiphase contrast-enhanced computed tomography (CT) or magnetic resonance imaging (MRI) is currently impractical from both an economic standpoint and a large volume of anticipated false-positive results [5]. CT is the most commonly utilized modality to further evaluate sonographic abnormalities given a favorable cost profile and readily reproducible image quality. MRI provides the most sensitive (81%) data for the diagnosis of HCC and has become standard of care for many experienced institutions. The benefits of MRI include superior contrast resolution, ability to discern regenerating nodules from dysplasia and carcinoma, identify malignant vascular invasion, distinguish intact hepatocellular function using hepatospecific paramagnetic gadolinium-based contrast agents, and quantify liver fibrosis using elastography to aid in risk stratification based on predicted liver reserve [7, 8]. Ultimately, a tumor's size, location, demarcation, vascular or adjacent structural invasion, and presence of satellite lesions must all be examined prior to engaging in LRT to determine the best approach.

12.3 Local Ablative Therapies

12.3.1 Percutaneous Ethanol Injection

The destruction of liver cancer via transabdominal instrumentation was first well established with percutaneous ethanol injection (PEI). Prior to PEI, nonsurgical candidates with HCC had limited systemic therapy options and were often offered supportive care only. Ethanol is a highly caustic agent that results in local tissue dehydration, protein denaturation, and vascular thrombosis that is inexpensive and well tolerated in patients with cirrhosis. The technique of PEI involves direct visualization of the HCC lesion with US and the insertion of low-profile needles directly into the tumor. An estimated volume of 100% dehydrated ethanol is then infused throughout the tumor using $V = (4/3)\pi(r + 0.5)^3$ as a general dose guideline where V = volume of ethanol and r = the tumor radius. Multiple sessions are typically required for each lesion. PEI efficacy is variable based on operator experience and tumor tissue composition limiting uniform ethanol distribution [9]. PEI has shown inferior performance compared to RFA and has largely been replaced by thermal ablation based on RCT data [10]. While thermal ablation has become standard of practice for nonresectable disease at most institutions [11], current EASL recommendations for PEI include treatment of small HCCs in anatomic territory where RFA would result in substantial collateral damage, such as the hepatic hilum [12]. Given the minimal required instrumentation, PEI provides options to patients with major comorbidities precluding general anesthesia or conscious sedation.

12.3.2 Radiofrequency Ablation

Radiofrequency ablation (RFA) represents the benchmark ablation technology for the treatment of HCC as it possesses the most data and widespread usage. RFA generates thermal damage via the placement of an electrode producing medium frequency alternating current (350–500 kHz) within target tissue completing an ionic circuit through the body toward remotely placed grounding pads or a second electrode. This current generates resistive heating as a function of tissue impedance, typically less than 100 °C, which propagates into adjacent tissues resulting in tumor cell death at temperatures greater than 60 °C [13]. Advantages to RFA include a fairly predictable and reproducible ablation zone as well as a short learning curve. Disadvantages center on several points of failure: as ablated tissue desiccates and carbonizes, it decreases ionic conductivity and stagnates growth of the ablation zone. Monopolar electrode designs do not allow for multiple probe placements which can limit effectiveness in challenging anatomy and lesions that lack spherical morphology. Several RFA probe designs utilize multiple tines to enlarge the ablation zone which may damage adjacent structures such as the lung or bowel. Finally, RFA is susceptible to intrinsic vascular-mediated cooling of tissues known as "heat sink," and incomplete ablations surrounding blood vessels greater than 3 mm in diameter are not uncommon [13].

Given the well-investigated experience with RFA, it is recommended by both EASL and AASLD guidelines for early-stage HCC in patients who are not eligible for surgery or who are anticipated to await more than 6 months for liver transplantation [3, 12]. A Cochrane Database review suggested that RFA was inferior to hepatic resection of HCC when considering recurrence-free and overall survival but superior to resection with regard to procedure-related complications and quality of life [14]. While two randomized control trials comparing RFA to hepatic resection for healthy patients with limited tumor generated conflicting evidence regarding overall survival and disease-free survival rates, a definitive conclusion would require a massive sample size to demonstrate a minor added survival benefit for either treatment [15].

While RFA has been shown to not complicate subsequent transplant surgery [16], there is concern for inadvertent tumor upstaging via withdrawal of malignant cells through the hepatic capsule into the peritoneal cavity or body wall. This process, referred to as "seeding," occurs in approximately 1% of cases [17] and may preclude future liver transplantation. While subscapular tumor location, directed tumor puncture without intervening parenchyma, and rapid tissue heating have been implicated as causes for seeding [18], aggressive tumor biology is most likely responsible and may occur regardless of changes in ablation technique [3].

12.3.3 Microwave Ablation

Initially introduced in the early 2000s, microwave is currently the most rapidly developing ablation technology as it accrues more comparative data to RFA and increased adoption by both surgeons and interventional radiologists. Microwave generates tissue destruction by applying an alternating electromagnetic field, typically 915 MHz or 2.45 GHz, to imperfectly dielectric tissue forcing water molecules to oscillate out of phase and generate local temperatures that can surpass 130 °C (Fig. 12.1). The higher the water content and effective conductivity of the target tissue, the more heat generation and transfer is achieved.

While MWA shares the basics of thermal-based tumor destruction with RFA, several advantages are emerging. MWA is not limited to the insulating effects of charring and appears to resist heat sink given its higher temperature profile [19], both of which are limitations to RFA. All microwave ablation systems allow placement of multiple probes with differing ablation fields, powering each individual probe with separate wattage, to best match the lesion morphology and neighboring anatomy. Most MWA sessions are performed concomitantly in all probe stations within 10 min or less which is considerably shorter than RFA.

EASL-EORTC and AASLD guidelines have not yet sanctioned the use of MWA for HCC given the lack of large-scale randomized trials comparing its efficacy to RFA and PEI. Multi-institutional analyses demonstrate comparable results for MWA and RFA with regard to overall survival, local progression, and the degree of local tumor ablation for HCC < 3 cm [20]. A recent study demonstrated complete tumor ablation rates of approximately 94% as assessed by histology after resection with a reported median recurrence-free survival of 25 months and a complication rate of approximately 11% [21].

12.3.4 Cryotherapy

Cryotherapy of malignant tissue was first reported in 1819 with the successful use of crushed ice and sodium chloride for reduction of pain and hemorrhage associated with tumors [22]. The basic principle of cryotherapy relies on the volumetric

Fig. 12.1 (**a**) Contrast-enhanced abdominal CT demonstrating a 4 cm biopsy-proven HCC in hepatic segment 4A of the liver in a patient with portal hypertension who was denied resection. (**b**) Intraprocedural noncontrast CT showing placement of a microwave probe along the base of the tumor and vaporized water within the entirety of the lesion as a result of internal temperatures reaching over 130 °C. (**c**) A 3-month follow-up contrast-enhanced abdominal CT showing no residual tumor

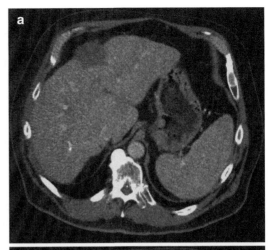

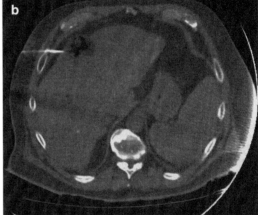

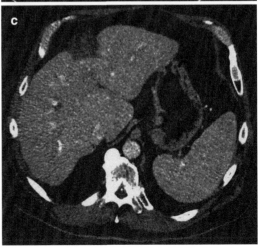

expansion of water as it transitions from liquid to solid within tumor cells disrupting cell membranes, denaturing proteins, and causing microvascular thrombosis. Low water content and acellular tissues, such as the collagenous network of the extracellular matrix and connective tissue, sustain less damage reducing regional soft tissue complications [23]. Temperatures within the ablation field are referred to as isotherms which are lethal at −20 to −40 °C, frequently administered in two or three freeze and thaw cycles per session.

Current cryoprobes rely on the Joule-Thomson effect of expanding gases, usually argon, transitioning from a constrained to an expanded chamber to generate probe temperatures that can reach −160 °C transferring heat from adjacent tissues via passive thermal diffusion. The reduction in water density as it crystalizes at the zero degree isotherm is visible under CT guidance allowing for accurate real-time intraprocedural observation of the ablation zone. Disadvantages to cryoablation include smaller ablation fields which typically require several probes as well as the highest susceptibility to heat sink of all thermal technologies.

Early experience with hepatic cryoablation observed incidences of post ablation hemodynamic compromise subsequently referred to as cryoshock in approximately 1% of cases. This was felt to be a function of large volume interleukin-6 and tumor necrosis factor-α exposure during the thaw cycle of treatment that was eliminated by reducing treatment volumes [24]. Cryotherapy may also result in increased post-procedural hemorrhage rates given the intrinsic preservation of larger blood vessels within the tumor which is addressed with preoperative embolization or utilizing hybrid probes that convert to low-energy RFA and coagulate the tract during probe removal [25].

The only Cochrane Database review for cryoablation in the treatment of HCC concludes there is insufficient evidence for recommendation [26]. Single center experiences report promising local tumor control rates, low complication rates, and a 10-year survival of 9% in patients with cirrhosis [27].

12.3.5 Irreversible Electroporation

Reversible electroporation has been utilized since the mid-1970s as means of inducing a temporary collapse of the cell wall barrier as a means of infusing high-dose regional chemotherapy. The cell wall if perforated by producing electrical impulses across the lipid bilayer produces innumerable nanscopic microchannels resulting in dysautoregulation of homeostasis [28]. When greater voltage and pulse frequency are applied, the nanochannels remain patent after current cessation and irreversible electroporation (IRE) ensues. Tissue temperatures average less than 60 °C, and cell death is brought upon predominantly by apoptosis [29].

IRE is impervious to heat sink and provides theoretical safety in areas of critical anatomy such as the portal triad, pancreas, bowel, or urinary collecting system. Interestingly, IRE of peripheral nerves has demonstrated preservation of the neuronal scaffold allowing axonal regeneration and functional recovery in animal models [30]. Disadvantages to IRE include a higher technical demand for near exact parallel placement of probes in monopolar systems, variability of ablation zones, the necessity for neuromuscular paralysis during ablation, and a potential risk for cardiac arrhythmias [31].

IRE has seen significant development since its FDA approval in 2007 as an adjuvant or to pancreatic resection for primary adenocarcinoma [32], but its utility for the treatment of HCC remains to be determined. A multi-institutional prospective registry of patients undergoing IRE for HCC in proximity to vital structures demonstrated a 100% initial complete response rate with a local recurrence-free survival at 12 months of 59%, predominantly on lesions larger than 4 cm [33]. A prospective phase II multicenter clinical trial showed complete response rates of 77% with a low incidence of major complications suggesting that IRE is a valuable option for unresectable HCC, particularly in anatomy that precludes thermal ablation [34].

12.3.6 Laser-Induced Thermotherapy

Laser is a well-established tool in multiple medical specialties given its ability to generate precise tissue charring with an immediate hemostatic effect and minimal penetration. These attributes are usually avoided when designing a visceral ablation device as charring limits the size of the ablation zone and the lack of penetration increases the number of probes that are required for treatment. The benefit of laser-induced thermotherapy (LITT) is the ability to perform MRI-guided procedure ablation for tumors that are inconspicuous on US or CT due to the nonferromagnetic probe. A single retrospective report on LITT of 113 patients with HCC has described favorable response in lesions less than 2 cm [35]. Prospective and randomized data is currently unavailable.

12.3.7 Transarterial Chemoembolization

First introduced by Yamada in the 1980s, transarterial chemoembolization (TACE) represents the landmark catheter-based therapy for unresectable HCC. Unlike standard liver perfusion which receives 70–80% of its perfusion from the portal vein, tumors ranging from 3 to 10 mm will develop preferential vascular supply from the hepatic artery [36]. Translational studies in hepatic neoplasms have also demonstrated increased chemotherapeutic uptake in hypoxic tissues compared to normal oxygen tension [37]. As such, iatrogenically induced arterial ischemia will preferentially damage tumor in patients without advanced portal hypertension. TACE capitalizes on this relationship by combining both high-dose intra-arterial chemoinfusion and embolization. Conventional TACE involves the transarterial delivery of local high-dose chemotherapy, such as doxorubicin, cisplatin, or mitomycin-C, with micellized iodinated poppy seed oil. Subsequent tumor arterial inflow reduction is achieved with embolization using occlusive agents such as gelatin slurry. This incites an intense local ischemic inflammatory response described as post-embolization syndrome in up to 50% within 24 h manifested by fever, abdominal pain, nausea, and rigors which is usually self-limited [38].

Despite multiple reports of complete tumor response [39], TACE is considered a palliative procedure due to its inability to overcome fundamental tumor reparative biology. HCC cell colonies have both a great metabolic demand for blood supply and ensuing capability to enact local vascular recruitment via hypoxic ischemic factor (HIF) and vascular endothelial growth factor (VEGF) neoangiogenic pathways [40]. When HCC sustains an infarct, an avascular core of completed ischemia and a peripheral zone of marginal perfusion develop; the characteristics of which may be highly variable based on collateral blood supply, watershed anatomy, and tumor biology. While adjunctive regional high-dose chemotherapy serves to damage the surviving at-risk tissue, a lethal chemotoxic margin is difficult to achieve [41]. Challenges to TACE also include a risk for liver infarction in patients with main branch portal invasion and tumor vascular conduit reduction with multiple embolizations limiting additional therapy [42].

Level 1A evidence supports the use of TACE for unresectable, intermediate stage HCC, in patients with preserved liver function with two prospective randomized trials showing superior overall survival when compared to large particle bland embolization and supportive care. A landmark prospective study by Llovet et al. demonstrated TACE benefit versus bland arterial embolization alone with nearly a 25% and 36% increase in survival probability at 1 and 2 years, respectively [43]. Lo et al. showed a 25% and 20% increase in survival as compared to supportive care at 1 and 2 years, respectively [44]. TACE has become a well-tolerated treatment for patients with moderate liver disease either as a bridge to transplantation or palliative cytoreduction allowing overall prognosis to be determined by hepatic substrate as opposed to progressive tumor burden.

12.3.8 Drug-Eluting Bead Chemoembolization

Conventional TACE (cTACE) technique was modified with the development of drug-eluting bead TACE (DEB-TACE) in which millions of hydrogel microspheres, specifically designed to adsorb chemotherapeutic agents, provide increased local drug delivery and peripheral occlusion of tumor blood supply (Fig. 12.2) [45]. Randomized studies of DEB-TACE vs. cTACE have shown decreased treatment-related toxicity, improved safety, higher disease control (63% vs. 52%), and slightly higher complete response (27% vs. 22%) rates favoring DEB-TACE [46]. Although survival benefits remain under investigation, DEB-TACE has become well adopted in the clinical setting due to its safety profile. Patients with low-volume disease and marginal liver function may benefit from super selective administrations of DEB-TACE within fourth-order or smaller vessels that would have otherwise sustained early central occlusion with higher-volume cTACE infusions.

12.3.9 Bland Embolization

Bland embolization encompasses a wide range of substances used to occlude vascular supply to the liver or hepatic tumors, including gelatin, polyvinyl alcohol, microspheres, and n-butyl cyanoacrylate. Reduction of blood supply induces ischemic

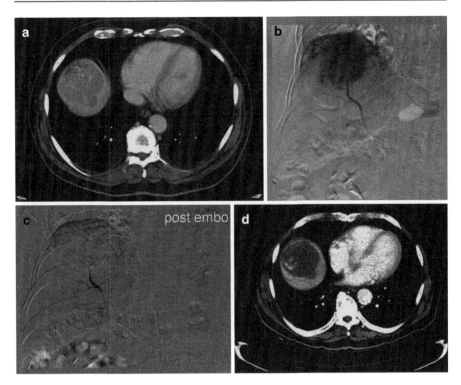

Fig. 12.2 (**a**) Abdominal CT scan demonstrating a 6 cm right hepatic dome hepatocellular carcinoma with a well-delineated pseudocapsule. (**b**) Selective hepatic angiography showing avid tumor neovascular arterial enhancement. (**c**) Post epirubicin DEB-TACE angiogram demonstrating no residual arterial supply to the lesion. (**d**) Post-embolization abdominal CT scan obtained at 1 month showing a necrotic tumor with retained contrast and foci of gas secondary to tumor infarction. Despite the excellent imaging response, there was a faint rim of viable tumor present at explanation due to sublethal ischemic penumbra

tissue loss in the tumor; the more peripheral an occlusion occurs, the more ischemic the resulting vascular deficit becomes. The majority of available data for TAE in HCC has been generated by phase II studies and cannot compete with TACE or DEB-TACE. As such, most societal practice guidelines do not recommend bland transarterial embolization (TAE) of HCC over transarterial chemoembolization. A prospective randomized comparison of DEB-TACE and TAE demonstrated complete response 26.8% vs. 14% in favor of the DEB-TACE arm with higher 12-month recurrences in the bland arm. A more recent retrospective case control study of liver explants in matched patients treated with TAE and TACE demonstrated no significant difference in complete response, 3-year recurrence-free survival, and overall survival rates. Ultimately, the literature has remained somewhat conflicted regarding the role of TAE due to lack of technique uniformity, mainly as a result of variable operator experience and preference.

Bland portal vein embolization (PVE) has been used as an adjunct to transarterial embolization [47] but predominantly provides benefit as a neoadjuvant to surgical resection in patients with anticipated inadequate future liver remnant (FLR). In patients with normal liver function, PVE is indicated when the FLR is <20% and up to 40% in cirrhotics. Preoperative occlusion of the portal supply to the lobe undergoing resection approximately 1 month prior to surgery stimulates circulation of trophic factors due to gradual parenchymal atrophy. Within 2 weeks, PVE will induce hyperplasia of the contralateral liver in patients with normal liver function at a rate of 12–21 cm^3/day, compared to 9 cm^3/day in cirrhotic patients [48]. While results are evident in as early as 6 days to 1 month, the trophic factors may inadvertently stimulate growth of the primary tumor and potentially compromise its respectability leading to a race between adequate post resection liver reserve and disease progression [49]. More specific application of PVE will be discussed in detail within the hepatic surgery section of this book.

12.3.10 Radioembolization

Hepatic transarterial brachytherapy, also known as radioembolization (RE), was first introduced in the 1960s but remained generally underexplored until the FDA granted a humanitarian device exemption for the treatment of unresectable HCC in 1999. HCC radiotherapy has been historically limited by the poor tolerance of the liver to traditional external beam radiation; whole-liver intensity-modulated radiotherapy doses are limited to 30 Gy while minimal tumoricidal doses exceed 50 Gy [50]. The rate of tumor response in relation to the normal tissue complication probability, also referred to as the therapeutic ratio, continues to limit even current technology such as stereotactic and proton-based external beam therapies when whole-liver treatment is required. In contrast, RE safely delivers tumor doses ranging from 120 to more than 1500 Gy [51] by exploiting local redistribution of radioactive elements via upregulated neovascular arterial conduit relative to the background hepatic parenchyma. Millions of radioactive glass or resin microspheres delivered via the hepatic artery irradiate the tumor bed over approximately 2 weeks with negligible effect on the liver substrate [52]. The most commonly used isotope, yttrium-90 (y90), emits a constant stream of β particles that penetrate liver tissue at a range of 2–11 mm providing an added treatment margin, irrespective of blood supply, which cannot be achieved with embolic therapies.

Perhaps the more intriguing advancement brought by RE is the flexibility of both treatment volume and administered radiation dose to best suit the distribution of disease and treatment intent. Administrations can be lobar, sublobar, segmental, or even subsegmental based on the liver tissue supplied by the selected blood vessel. These vascular territories, or angiosomes, can be accurately determined with the utilization of angiographic suite fluoroscopic CT acquisition, or cone beam CT, while injecting contrast via selective catheterization of the suspected arterial supply (Fig. 12.3). Dosimetry is then calculated using either the Body Surface Area (BSA) method, which relies on an assumed volume of liver based on the patient's ideal body weight in relation to the volume of tumor, partition model, or the Medical Internal Radiation Dose (MIRD) method which relegates a given activity to the

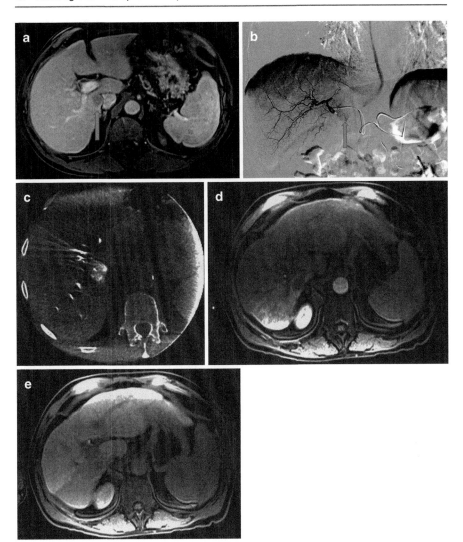

Fig. 12.3 (**a**) Inconspicuous HCC adjacent to the caudate that was best visualized on the delayed venous phase of MRI (blue arrow). (**b**) Lesion is faintly identified during selective angiography (blue arrow). (**c**) Cone beam CT scan performed while injecting contrast through the suspected angiosome of the lesion shows complete supply arising from the hepatic segment 7 artery. (**d**) Arterial phase MRI 3 months after radiation segmentectomy showing enhancement within the treated angiosome but not contrast uptake within the lesion. (**e**) Twenty-minute hepatobiliary contrast agent shows retraction and nonviability of the angiosome as well as the tumor and no hepatic decompensation

measured involved volume of the liver. The operator may choose to administer either a hepatocyte sparing dose which will maintain liver function or escalate to an ablative dose which will abolish both tumor and normal liver within the angiosome. When ablative doses are utilized, the treated liver will slowly decrease in volume over 3–6 months, become nearly completely fibrotic, and demonstrate absent hepatocyte function that approaches surgical resection.

The principal limitations to RE are mainly inadequate and inhomogeneous intralesional blood supply which create regions of subtherapeutic radiation exposure referred to as radiation watershed. Both BSA and MIRD dosimetry assume uniform distribution of spheres within a lesion and are unable to account for the limitations of radiation watershed. Conceptually, the y90 β particle emission radii (up to 11 mm) are directly proportional to particle's energy level (up to 2.3 MeV) and follow a distribution curve with approximately 66% of particles in the 2 mm range. More emissions within a treatment bed will equal a greater probability of high-energy 11 mm particles present within the angiosome both simultaneously contributing to a wider lethal margin and mitigating radiation watershed. This flexibility in dosimetry allows for RE to mimic the results of TACE for non-ablative lobar applications and approach surgical resection when ablative doses are administered to a tumor encompassing angiosome [54]. The later has been referred to as a radiation segmentectomy and is currently under investigation with early promising results for early HCC showing complete response rates or 95% per EASL criteria [53] and explant pathology revealing 100% and 50–99% necrosis in 52% and 48% of treated patients, respectively [54].

A common contraindication to surgery has been the presence of vascular invasion due to the probability of contemporaneous metastases [55]. Unfortunately, the inability to adequately stage these patients with either tumor markers or imaging has allowed their pretest probability for extrahepatic disease to dictate treatment rather than tumor biology. This is illustrated in the BCLC staging system where patients with portal invasion are anticipated to live approximately 11 months and only offered systemic chemotherapy or palliation. However, HCC that invades the portal or hepatic vein derives the majority of its blood supply from the artery, despite its location, and remains equally vulnerable to transarterial RE with early studies showing a 16.6-month (51% increase) improved survival rate with branch invasion based on BCLC stage, 20% conversion to surgery, and 4% conversion to transplantation [56, 57]. In patients with vascular invasive HCC that would otherwise be candidates for resection, ablative dose RE may permit an extended surveillance period to more accurately stage metastatic burden and allow conversion of consolidated disease to resection or ablation.

Ablative lobar doses, referred to as radiation lobectomies, have also shown promising early results in generating neoadjuvant of the anticipated FLR in an effort to diminish the probability of postoperative liver failure (Fig. 12.4). The degree of hypertrophy is greater than traditional portal vein embolization but requires approximately 3–9 months [58, 59]. Vouche et al. demonstrated that 85% of patients who underwent radiation lobectomy were ultimately understaged in the FLR at the time of presentation which may have deterred surgery altogether [59]. In distinction to PVE, radiation lobectomies provide control of the primary tumor site during FLR growth and theoretically preserve hepatic pedicles during resection by sterilizing tumor margins within the angiosome. Furthermore, radiation lobectomies are not contraindicated in the setting of central portal venous invasion.

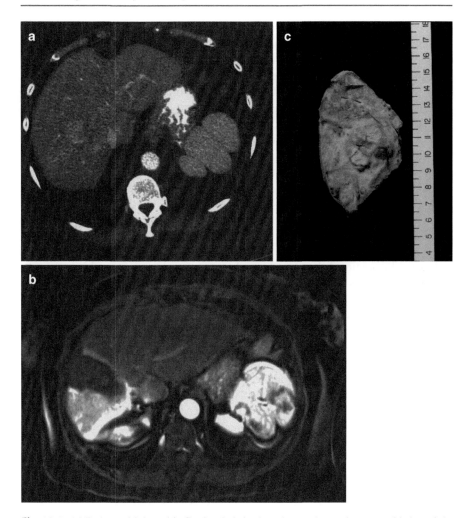

Fig. 12.4 (**a**) Patient with hepatitis C-related cirrhosis and a previous microwave ablation of the left hepatic lobe presents with a new 4 cm lesion in the right hepatic lobe. Patient was interested in surgery, but there was insufficient future liver remnant to safely offer resection. (**b**) A hybrid dose radiation lobectomy was performed with a supratherapeutic ablative dose within the angiosome encompassing the tumor (non-enhancing right liver tissue) and a reduced ablative dose within the remaining right hepatic lobe resulting in a radiation lobectomy. The patient's left hepatic lobe was monitored and allowed to hypertrophy for 6 months sowing no evident field progression. Patient successfully underwent right hepatic lobe escharectomy without change in liver function despite her cirrhosis. (**c**) Pathology revealed a T0 result with no viable disease

The high degree of fibrotic contraction observed in treated livers suggests an immense immune response that currently has an indeterminate effect on tumor volume but warrants analysis. Although further investigation is warranted, ablative lobar radioembolization provides an encouraging alternative to the established shortcomings of PVE.

The clinical role for RE is rapidly accelerating as collective understating continues to grow and with current level 2A evidence to support its use in HCC [60], particularly in patients with vascular invasion [57, 61]. Although large retrospective studies have shown at least similar efficacy between TACE and RE—with RE outperforming TACE in downstaging HCC from UNOS T3 to T2 [62], reduced systemic toxicity [63], and on quality of life scores [64]—a randomized controlled trial is in place to more accurately equate the two modalities [65]. RE provides a broad spectrum of valuable treatment options ranging from palliative whole-liver cytoreduction in advanced disease to potentially surgical grade catheter-based hepatectomy for both operative neoadjuvant and locoregional curative intent.

12.3.11 Hybrid Therapy

Individual locoregional therapies have shown synergism when used in combination [66]. The most commonly utilized technique, other than TACE which combines intra-arterial chemotherapy with an embolic agent, is neoadjuvant bland embolization or TACE prior to thermal ablation (Fig. 12.5). This effect may be a function of occluded vasculature preventing interstitial heat sink and weakening of cells which otherwise would have achieved sublethal temperatures. Meta-analyses have shown improved 1- and 3-year survival when compared with the RFA alone [67], lower complication rates, and comparable overall and disease-free survival to hepatic resection in tumors <2 cm [68]. Malluccio et al. demonstrated no survival difference in those treated with RFA plus TAE versus HR in HCC less than 7 [69]. Patients with advanced HCC treated with TACE and concurrent sorafenib in a phase II multicenter prospective trial demonstrated a median time to progression of 16.4 months and overall survival of 20.1 months which was of uncertain benefit [70]. Synergistic properties of chemoradiation are well established, and a phase I trial of radiosensitizing capecitabine dose escalations with concurrent RE for hepatic metastases and cholangiocarcinoma has shown an acceptable safety profile [71], but similar studies are currently lacking for HCC. Prospective trials of radioembolization with and without sorafenib have shown no significant clinical benefit and increased biliary complication rate in one study [72, 73]. Ablative dosing radioembolization may conceptually benefit from hyperbaric oxygenation although, currently, there is no available data.

12.4 Treatment Evaluation

Traditional methods of evaluating treatment response via tumor size are usually inapplicable to LRT due to coinciding necrosis, hemorrhage, and fibrosis. The modified response evaluation criteria in solid tumors (mRECIST) [74] and EASL [75] criteria were created as a means to specifically gauge tumor viability when treated with LRT. Residual HCC is defined by its arterial enhancement using bidimensional

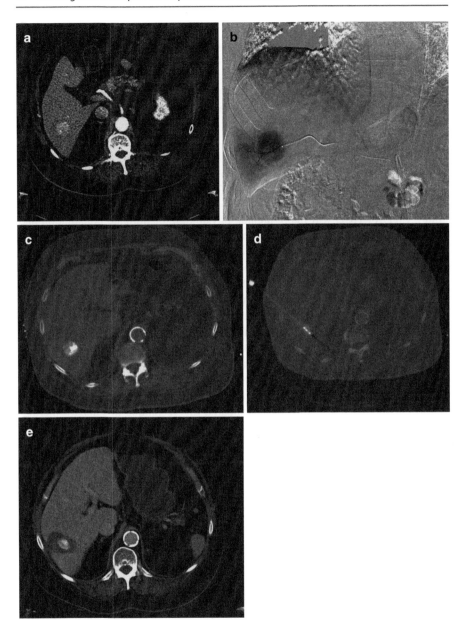

Fig. 12.5 (**a**) Arterial CT of the abdomen demonstrates a well-circumscribed arterially enhancing lesion in hepatic segment 6 in a patient with chronic hepatitis C infection most consistent with early e = hepatocellular carcinoma. (**b**) Selective hepatic segment 6 angiography demonstrating the vascular angiosome supplying the tumor prior to bland embolization. (**c**) Noncontrast liver CT prior to ablation showing uptake of the transarterial ethiodized oil within the no conspicuous tumor. (**d**) Microwave probe within the center of tumor mass and visible low-density gas margin. (**e**) Twelve-month portovenous phase CT scan demonstrating the retained ethiodized oil within the fibrotic ablation zone and no viable tumor

or longest diameter measurements in the EASL and mRECIST criteria, respectively. These do not apply to the liver in its entirety and synchronous disease must be ascertained separately. Benign changes that retain tissue enhancement, such as granulation tissue seen in the periphery of lesions treated with RE, may be falsely characterized as having an incomplete response, and a more accurate means of evaluating ablative RE will be required. Despite their limitations, both mRECIST and EASL provide benefit over WHO, and criteria have become incorporated in the vernacular of most interdisciplinary teams.

12.5 Developing Locoregional Therapies

Future LRT for HCC will likely include physiologic or immune potentiation and will avoid mechanical instrumentation or ionizing radiation. While stereotactic body radiotherapy has shown early benefit in the treatment of HCC while avoiding classical radiation-induced liver disease [76], it remains constrained by many of the anatomic limitations that limit thermal ablation. There are randomized phase III studies in place to determine whether treatment with vaccinia virus-based immunotherapy followed by sorafenib increases survival compared to treatment with sorafenib in patients with advanced hepatocellular carcinoma who have not received prior systemic therapy (NCT02562755). High-intensity focused ultrasound (HIFU) is a developing modality that uses compression waves to liquefy tumor. Lack of availability and long procedure times are the current major limitations to HIFU, but reported experiences have demonstrated promising safety and efficacy for unresectable HCC, though few studies have compared this technique to standard thermal ablation [77]. Light-activated drug therapy, which uses light-emitting diodes to initiate intravenously infused talaporfin within HCC, is currently being evaluated with a phase III study (NCT00355355).

Conclusion

Interventional oncology has established itself as the fourth pillar of cancer therapy and has progressed to the forefront in the management of hepatocellular carcinoma. Locoregional therapy provides well-tolerated curative and palliative solutions for patients with HCC who are surgically inoperable and may augment surgical outcomes as a neoadjuvant. Innovation is expected to accelerate as the American Board of Medical Specialties has recently recognized interventional radiology as an independent medical specialty. As more interventionalists expand on the data foundation which is currently under construction—likely with the formation of large registries, interventional oncology fellowships, advances in imaging, and molecular level instruments—treatments will undoubtedly approach first-line applications. Patients may no longer be required to choose between best overall survival and the quality of life provided by minimally invasive therapies.

References

1. Kim WR, Gores GJ, Benson JT, Therneau TM, Melton LJ. Mortality and hospital utilization for hepatocellular carcinoma in the United States. Gastroenterology. 2005;129(2):486–93.
2. Cucchetti A, Piscaglia F, Caturelli E, Benvegnù L, Vivarelli M, Ercolani G, et al. Comparison of recurrence of hepatocellular carcinoma after resection in patients with cirrhosis to its occurrence in a surveilled cirrhotic population. Ann Surg Oncol. 2009;16(2):413–22. Available from: http://www.ncbi.nlm.nih.gov/pubmed/19034578
3. Bruix J, Sherman M. AASLD PRACTICE GUIDELINE Management of hepatocellular carcinoma : an update. Hepatology. 2010;42:1–35. Available from: http://www.ncbi.nlm.nih.gov/pubmed/21374666
4. Bruix J, Sherman M, Llovet JM, Beaugrand M, Lencioni R, Burroughs AK, et al. Clinical management of hepatocellular carcinoma. Conclusions of the barcelona-2000 EASL conference. European Association for the Study of the Liver. J Hepatol. 2001;35(3):421–30.
5. Bialecki ES, Di Bisceglie AM. Diagnosis of hepatocellular carcinoma. HPB (Oxford). 2005;7(1):26–34.
6. Singal A, Volk ML, Waljee A, Salgia R, Higgins P, Rogers MA, Marrero JA, et al. Meta-analysis: surveillance with ultrasound for early-stage hepatocellular carcinoma in patients with cirrhosis. Aliment Pharmacol Ther. 2009;30(1):37–47.
7. McEvoy SH, McCarthy CJ, Lavelle LP, Moran DE, Cantwell CP, Skehan SJ, et al. Hepatocellular carcinoma: illustrated guide to systematic radiologic diagnosis and staging according to guidelines of the American Association for the Study of Liver Diseases. Radiographics. 2013;33(6):1653–68. Available from: http://www.ncbi.nlm.nih.gov/pubmed/24108556/nhttp://radiographics.rsna.org/content/33/6/1653.short
8. Erhardt A, Lörke J, Vogt C, Poremba C, Willers R, Sagir A, et al. [Transient elastography for diagnosing liver cirrhosis]. Dtsch Med Wochenschr. 2006;131(49):2765–9. Available from: http://www.ncbi.nlm.nih.gov/pubmed/17136655
9. Shiina S, Tateishi R, Imamura M, Teratani T, Koike Y, Sato S, et al. Percutaneous ethanol injection for hepatocellular carcinoma: 20-year outcome and prognostic factors. Liver Int. 2012;32(9):1434–42. Available from: http://www.pubmedcentral.nih.gov/articlerender.fcgi?artid=3466412&tool=pmcentrez&rendertype=abstract
10. Bouza C, López-Cuadrado T, Alcázar R, Saz-Parkinson Z, Amate J. Meta-analysis of percutaneous radiofrequency ablation versus ethanol injection in hepatocellular carcinoma. BMC Gastroenterol. 2009;9(1):31. Available from: http://www.pubmedcentral.nih.gov/articlerender.fcgi?artid=3224700&tool=pmcentrez&rendertype=abstract
11. Gervais DA, Goldberg SN, Brown DB, Soulen MC, Millward SF, Rajan DK. Society of Interventional Radiology position statement on percutaneous radiofrequency ablation for the treatment of liver tumors. J Vasc Interv Radiol. 2009;20(7):S342–7. https://doi.org/10.1016/j.jvir.2009.04.029
12. Dufour JF, Greten TF, Raymond E, Roskams T, De T, Ducreux M, et al. Clinical Practice Guidelines EASL – EORTC Clinical Practice Guidelines: management of hepatocellular carcinoma European Organisation for Research and Treatment of Cancer. J Hepatol. 2012;56(4):908–43. Available from: http://www.ncbi.nlm.nih.gov/pubmed/22424438
13. Brace CL. Radiofrequency and microwave ablation of the liver, lung, kidney, and bone: what are the differences? Curr Probl Diagn Radiol. 2009;38(3):135–43. https://doi.org/10.1067/j.cpradiol.2007.10.001
14. Weis S, Franke A, Mössner J, Jakobsen JC, Schoppmeyer K. Radiofrequency (thermal) ablation versus no intervention or other interventions for hepatocellular carcinoma. Cochrane database Syst Rev. 2013;12:CD003046. Available from: http://www.ncbi.nlm.nih.gov/pubmed/24357457.
15. Lencioni R, Crocetti L. Local-regional treatment of hepatocellular carcinoma. Radiology. 2012;262(1):43–58. Available from: http://www.ncbi.nlm.nih.gov/pubmed/22190656

16. Feng K, Ma K-S. Value of radiofrequency ablation in the treatment of hepatocellular carcinoma. World J Gastroenterol. 2014;20(20):5987–98. Available from: http://www.pubmedcentral.nih.gov/articlerender.fcgi?artid=4033438&tool=pmcentrez&rendertype=abstract

17. Stigliano R, Marelli L, Yu D, Davies N, Patch D, Burroughs AK. Seeding following percutaneous diagnostic and therapeutic approaches for hepatocellular carcinoma. What is the risk and the outcome? Seeding risk for percutaneous approach of HCC. Cancer Treat Rev. 2007;33(5):437–47. Available from: http://www.ncbi.nlm.nih.gov/pubmed/17512669

18. Kumar N, Gaba RC, Knuttinen MG, Omene BO, Martinez BK, Owens CA, et al. Tract seeding following radiofrequency ablation for hepatocellular carcinoma: prevention, detection, and management. Semin Intervent Radiol. 2011;28:187–92.

19. Brace CL. Microwave tissue ablation: biophysics, technology, and applications. Crit Rev Biomed Eng. 2010;38(1):65–78. Available from: http://www.pubmedcentral.nih.gov/articlerender.fcgi?artid=3058696&tool=pmcentrez&rendertype=abstract

20. Zhang L, Wang N, Shen Q, Cheng W, Qian GJ. Therapeutic efficacy of percutaneous radiofrequency ablation versus microwave ablation for hepatocellular carcinoma. PLoS One. 2013;8(10):1–8.

21. Groeschl RT, Pilgrim CHC, Hanna EM, Simo KA, Swan RZ, Sindram D, et al. Microwave ablation for hepatic malignancies: a multiinstitutional analysis. Ann Surg. 2014;259(6):1195–200. Available from: http://www.ncbi.nlm.nih.gov/pubmed/24096760

22. Gage AA. History of cryosurgery. Semin Surg Oncol. 1998;14(2):99–109. Available from: http://www.ncbi.nlm.nih.gov/pubmed/10940055

23. Yiu WK, Basco MT, Aruny JE, Cheng SWK, Sumpio BE. Cryosurgery: a review. Int J Angiol. 2007;16(1):1–6.

24. Seifert JK, Stewart GJ, Hewitt PM, Bolton EJ, Junginger T, Morris DL. Interleukin-6 and tumor necrosis factor-alpha levels following hepatic cryotherapy: association with volume and duration of freezing. World J Surg. 1999;23(10):1019–26. Available from: http://www.ncbi.nlm.nih.gov/pubmed/10512941

25. Kariappa SM, Morris DL. Cryotherapy—a mature ablation technique. HPB (Oxford). 2006;8(3):179–81. Available from: http://www.pubmedcentral.nih.gov/articlerender.fcgi?artid=2131681&tool=pmcentrez&rendertype=abstract

26. Awad T, Thorlund K, Gluud C. Cryotherapy for hepatocellular carcinoma. Cochrane Database Syst Rev. 2009;7(4):CD007611.

27. Rong G, Bai W, Wang C. Cryotherapy for cirrhosis-based hepatocellular carcinoma: a single center experience from 1595 treated cases. Front Med. 2015;9(1):63–71.

28. Granot Y, Rubinsky B. Mass transfer model for drug delivery in tissue cells with reversible electroporation. Int J Heat Mass Transf. 2008;51(23–24):5610–6. https://doi.org/10.1016/j.ijheatmasstransfer.2008.04.041

29. Faroja M, Ahmed M, Appelbaum L, Ben-David E, Moussa M, Sosna J, et al. Irreversible electroporation ablation: is all the damage nonthermal? Radiology. 2013;266(2):462–70.

30. Onik G, Mikus P, Rubinsky B. Irreversible electroporation: implications for prostate ablation. Technol Cancer Res Treat. 2007;6:295–300.

31. Scheffer HJ, Nielsen K, De Jong MC, Van Tilborg AA, Vieveen JM, Bouwman A, et al. Irreversible electroporation for nonthermal tumor ablation in the clinical setting: a systematic review of safety and efficacy. J Vasc Interv Radiol. 2014;25(7):997–1011. https://doi.org/10.1016/j.jvir.2014.01.028

32. Martin RCG. Irreversible electroporation of locally advanced pancreatic head adenocarcinoma. J Gastrointest Surg. 2013;17(10):1850–6.

33. Cannon R, Ellis S, Hayes D, Narayanan G, Martin RCG. Safety and early efficacy of irreversible electroporation for hepatic tumors in proximity to vital structures. J Surg Oncol. 2013;107(5):544–9.

34. Lencioni R, Izzo F, Vilgrain V, Crocetti L, Ricke J, Bruix J. Irreversible electroporation for the treatment of early-stage hepatocellular carcinoma: a prospective multicenter phase II clinical trial. J Vasc Interv Radiol. 2012;23 (6):853.e3. Available from: http://ovidsp.ovid.com/ovidweb.cgi?T=JS&CSC=Y&NEWS=N&PAGE=fulltext&D=emed10&AN=70810653\nhttp://sfx.ucl.ac.uk/

sfx_local?sid=OVID:embase&id=pmid:&id=doi:10.1016/j.jvir.2012.04.029&issn=1051-0443&isbn=&volume=23&issue=6&spage=853&pages=853.e3&date=2012&ti

35. Eichler K, Zangos S, Gruber-Rouh T, Vogl TJ, Mack MG. Magnetic resonance-guided laser-induced thermotherapy in patients with oligonodular hepatocellular carcinoma: long-term results over a 15-year period. J Clin Gastroenterol. 2012;46(9):796–801. Available from: http://www.ncbi.nlm.nih.gov/pubmed/22955262

36. Kennedy A, Nag S, Salem R, Murthy R, McEwan AJ, Nutting C, et al. Recommendations for radioembolization of hepatic malignancies using yttrium-90 microsphere brachytherapy: a consensus panel report from the radioembolization brachytherapy oncology consortium. Int J Radiat Oncol Biol Phys. 2007;68(1):13–23. Available from: http://www.ncbi.nlm.nih.gov/pubmed/17448867

37. Kruskal JB, Hlatky L, Hahnfeldt P, Teramoto K, Stokes KR, Clouse ME. In vivo and in vitro analysis of the effectiveness of doxorubicin combined with temporary arterial occlusion in liver tumors. J Vasc Interv Radiol. 1993;4(6):741–7. Available from: http://www.ncbi.nlm.nih.gov/pubmed/8280994

38. Lewandowski RJ, Mulcahy MF, Kulik LM, Riaz A, Ryu RK, Baker TB, et al. Chemoembolization for hepatocellular carcinoma: comprehensive imaging and survival analysis in a 172-patient cohort. Radiology. 2010;255(3):955–65. Available from: http://www.pubmedcentral.nih.gov/articlerender.fcgi?artid=2948657&tool=pmcentrez&rendertype=abstract

39. Nicolini A, Martinetti L, Crespi S, Maggioni M, Sangiovanni A. Transarterial chemoembolization with Epirubicin-eluting beads versus transarterial embolization before liver transplantation for hepatocellular carcinoma. J Vasc Interv Radiol. 2010;21(3):327–32. https://doi.org/10.1016/j.jvir.2009.10.038

40. Luo D, Wang Z, Wu J, Jiang C, Wu J. The role of hypoxia inducible factor-1 in hepatocellular carcinoma. Biomed Res Int. 2014;2014:409272. Available from: http://www.pubmedcentral.nih.gov/articlerender.fcgi?artid=4101982&tool=pmcentrez&rendertype=abstract

41. Gurney H. How to calculate the dose of chemotherapy. Br J Cancer. 2002;86:1297–302.

42. Quirk M, Yun K, Saab S. Management of hepatocellular carcinoma with portal vein thrombosis. World J Gatroenterol. 2015;21(12):3462–71.

43. Llovet JM, Real MI, Montaña X, Planas R, Coll S, Aponte J, et al. Arterial embolisation or chemoembolisation versus symptomatic treatment in patients with unresectable hepatocellular carcinoma: a randomised controlled trial. Lancet (London, England). 2002;359(9319):1734–9. Available from: http://www.ncbi.nlm.nih.gov/pubmed/12049862

44. Lo C-M, Ngan H, Tso W-K, Liu C-L, Lam C-M, Poon RT-P, et al. Randomized controlled trial of transarterial lipiodol chemoembolization for unresectable hepatocellular carcinoma. Hepatology. 2002;35(5):1164–71. Available from: http://www.ncbi.nlm.nih.gov/pubmed/11981766

45. Varela M, Real MI, Burrel M, Forner A, Sala M, Brunet M, et al. Chemoembolization of hepatocellular carcinoma with drug eluting beads: efficacy and doxorubicin pharmacokinetics. J Hepatol. 2007;46(3):474–81. Available from: http://www.sciencedirect.com/science/article/pii/S0168827806006295

46. Lammer J, Malagari K, Vogl T, Pilleul F, Denys A, Watkinson A, et al. Prospective randomized study of doxorubicin-eluting-bead embolization in the treatment of hepatocellular carcinoma: results of the PRECISION v study. Cardiovasc Intervent Radiol. 2010;33(1):41–52.

47. Aoki T, Imamura H, Hasegawa K, Matsukura A, Sano K, Sugawara Y, et al. Sequential preoperative arterial and portal venous embolizations in patients with hepatocellular carcinoma. Arch Surg. 2004;139(7):766–74.

48. May BJ, Madoff DC. Portal vein embolization: rationale, technique, and current application. Semin Intervent Radiol. 2012;29(212):81–9.

49. Ribero D, Abdalla E. Tumor progression after preoperative portal vein embolization. Br J Surg. 2007;256(5):812–7; discussion 817–8. Available from: http://onlinelibrary.wiley.com/doi/10.1002/bjs.5836/full

50. Kataria T, Rawat S, Sinha SN, Negi PS, Garg C, Bhalla NK, et al. Intensity modulated radiotherapy in abdominal malignancies: our experience in reducing the dose to normal structures

as compared to the gross tumor. J Cancer Res Ther. 2006;2(4):161–5. Available from: http://www.ncbi.nlm.nih.gov/pubmed/17998698

51. Cremonesi M, Chiesa C, Strigari L, Ferrari M, Botta F, Guerriero F, et al. Radioembolization of hepatic lesions from a radiobiology and dosimetric perspective. Front Oncol. 2014;4:210. Available from: http://www.pubmedcentral.nih.gov/articlerender.fcgi?artid=4137387&tool=pmcentrez&rendertype=abstract

52. Lewandowski RJ, Salem R. Yttrium-90 radioembolization of hepatocellular carcinoma and metastatic disease to the liver. Semin Intervent Radiol. 2006;23(1):64–72.

53. Padia SA, Kwan SW, Roudsari B, Monsky WL, Coveler A, Harris WP. Superselective yttrium-90 radioembolization for hepatocellular carcinoma yields high response rates with minimal toxicity. J Vasc Interv Radiol. 2014;25(7):1067–73. Available from: https://doi.org/10.1016/j.jvir.2014.03.030\nhttp://www.ncbi.nlm.nih.gov/pubmed/24837982\nhttp://www.sciencedirect.com/science/article/pii/S105104431400400X

54. Vouche M, Habib A, Ward TJ, Kim E, Kulik L, Ganger D, et al. Unresectable solitary hepatocellular carcinoma not amenable to radiofrequency ablation: multicenter radiology-pathology correlation and survival of radiation segmentectomy. Hepatology. 2014;60(1):192–201.

55. Thuluvath P. Vascular invasion is the most important predictor of survival in HCC, but how do we find it? J Clin Gastroenterol. 2009;2(43):101–2.

56. Pracht M, Edeline J, Lenoir L, Latournerie M, Mesbah H, Audrain O, et al. Lobar hepatocellular carcinoma with ipsilateral portal vein tumor thrombosis treated with yttrium-90 glass microsphere radioembolization: preliminary results. Int J Hepatol. 2013;2013:827649. Available from: http://www.pubmedcentral.nih.gov/articlerender.fcgi?artid=3586521&tool=pmcentrez&rendertype=abstract

57. Lau W-Y, Sangro B, Chen P-J, Cheng S-Q, Chow P, Lee R-C, et al. Treatment for hepatocellular carcinoma with portal vein tumor thrombosis: the emerging role for radioembolization using yttrium-90. Oncology. 2013;84(5):311–8. Available from: http://www.ncbi.nlm.nih.gov/pubmed/23615394

58. Siddiqi NH, Devlin PM. Radiation lobectomy-a minimally invasive treatment model for liver cancer: case report. J Vasc Interv Radiol. 2009;20(5):664–9. https://doi.org/10.1016/j.jvir.2009.01.023

59. Vouche M, Lewandowski RJ, Atassi R, Memon K, Gates VL, Ryu RK, et al. Radiation lobectomy: time-dependent analysis of future liver remnant volume in unresectable liver cancer as a bridge to resection. J Hepatol. 2013;59(5):1029–36. https://doi.org/10.1016/j.jhep.2013.06.015

60. Hilgard P, Hamami M, Fouly AE, Scherag A, Müller S, Ertle J, et al. Radioembolization with yttrium-90 glass microspheres in hepatocellular carcinoma: European experience on safety and long-term survival. Hepatology. 2010;52(5):1741–9. Available from: http://www.ncbi.nlm.nih.gov/pubmed/21038413

61. Kulik LM, Carr BI, Mulcahy MF, Lewandowski RJ, Atassi B, Ryu RK, et al. Safety and efficacy of 90Y radiotherapy for hepatocellular carcinoma with and without portal vein thrombosis. Hepatology. 2008;47(1):71–81.

62. Lewandowski RJ, Kulik LM, Riaz A, Senthilnathan S, Mulcahy MF, Ryu RK, et al. A comparative analysis of transarterial downstaging for hepatocellular carcinoma: chemoembolization versus radioembolization. Am J Transplant. 2009;9:1920–8.

63. Salem R, Lewandowski RJ, Kulik L, Wang E, Riaz A, Ryu RK, et al. Radioembolization results in longer time-to-progression and reduced toxicity compared with chemoembolization in patients with hepatocellular carcinoma. Gastroenterology. 2011;140(2):497–507.e2. https://doi.org/10.1053/j.gastro.2010.10.049

64. Salem R, Gilbertsen M, Butt Z, Memon K, Vouche M, Hickey R, et al. Increased quality of life among hepatocellular carcinoma patients treated with radioembolization, compared with chemoembolization. Clin Gastroenterol Hepatol. 2013;11(10):1358–65.e1. Available from: http://www.ncbi.nlm.nih.gov/pubmed/23644386

65. Seinstra BA, Defreyne L, Lambert B, Lam MGEH, Verkooijen HM, van Erpecum KJ, et al. Transarterial radioembolization versus chemoembolization for the treatment of hepatocellular carcinoma (TRACE): study protocol for a randomized controlled trial. Trials. 2012;13:144. Available from: /pmc/articles/PMC3493260/?report=abstract

66. Yan S, Xu D, Sun B. Combination of radiofrequency ablation with transarterial chemoembolization for hepatocellular carcinoma: a meta-analysis. Dig Dis Sci. 2013;58(7):2107–13. Available from: http://www.ncbi.nlm.nih.gov/pubmed/23361576

67. Jiang G, Xiaojun X, Sontgao R. Combining transarterial chemoembolization with radiofrequency ablation for hepatocellular carcinoma. Tumor Biol. 2014;35(4):3405–8.

68. Lu Z, Wen F, Guo Q, Liang H, Mao X, Sun H. Radiofrequency ablation plus chemoembolization versus radiofrequency ablation alone for hepatocellular carcinoma: a meta-analysis of randomized-controlled trials. Eur J Gastroenterol Hepatol. 2012;25(2):187–94. Available from: http://www.ncbi.nlm.nih.gov/pubmed/23134976

69. Maluccio M, Covey AM, Gandhi R, Gonen M, Getrajdman GI, Brody LA, et al. Comparison of survival rates after bland arterial embolization and ablation versus surgical resection for treating solitary hepatocellular carcinoma up to 7 cm. J Vasc Interv Radiol. 2005;16(7):955–61. Available from: http://www.ncbi.nlm.nih.gov/pubmed/16002503

70. Erhardt A, Kolligs F, Dollinger M, Schott E, Wege H, Bitzer M, et al. TACE plus sorafenib for the treatment of hepatocellular carcinoma: results of the multicenter, phase II SOCRATES trial. Cancer Chemother Pharmacol. 2014;74(5):947–54. Available from: http://ovidsp.ovid.com/ovidweb.cgi?T=JS&PAGE=reference&D=medl&NEWS=N&AN=25173458

71. Hickey R, Mulcahy MF, Lewandowski RJ, Gates VL, Vouche M, Habib A, et al. Chemoradiation of hepatic malignancies: prospective, phase 1 study of full-dose capecitabine with escalating doses of yttrium-90 radioembolization. Int J Radiat Oncol Biol Phys. 2014;88(5):1025–31. Available from: http://www.ncbi.nlm.nih.gov/pubmed/24661655

72. Ricke J, Bulla K, Kolligs F, Peck-Radosavljevic M, Reimer P, Sangro B, et al. Safety and toxicity of radioembolization plus Sorafenib in advanced hepatocellular carcinoma: analysis of the European multicentre trial SORAMIC. Liver Int. 2014;35:620–6.

73. Kulik L, Vouche M, Koppe S, Lewandowski RJ, Mulcahy MF, Ganger D, et al. Prospective randomized pilot study of Y90+/−sorafenib as bridge to transplantation in hepatocellular carcinoma. J Hepatol. 2014;61(2):309–17. Available from: http://www.ncbi.nlm.nih.gov/pubmed/24681342

74. Lencioni R, Llovet JM. Modified RECIST (mRECIST) assessment for hepatocellular carcinoma. Semin Liver Dis. 2010;30(1):52–60. Available from: http://www.ncbi.nlm.nih.gov/pubmed/20175033

75. Riaz A, Memon K, Miller FH, Nikolaidis P, Kulik LM, Lewandowski RJ, et al. Role of the EASL, RECIST, and WHO response guidelines alone or in combination for hepatocellular carcinoma: radiologic-pathologic correlation. J Hepatol. 2011;54(4):695–704. Available from: http://www.sciencedirect.com/science/article/pii/S0168827810009104

76. Bibault J-E, Dewas S, Vautravers-Dewas C, Hollebecque A, Jarraya H, Lacornerie T, et al. Stereotactic body radiation therapy for hepatocellular carcinoma: prognostic factors of local control, overall survival, and toxicity. PLoS One. 2013;8(10):e77472. Available from: http://www.pubmedcentral.nih.gov/articlerender.fcgi?artid=3795696&tool=pmcentrez&rendertype=abstract

77. Chan ACY, Cheung TT, Fan ST, Chok KSH, Chan SC, Poon RTP, et al. Survival analysis of high-intensity focused ultrasound therapy versus radiofrequency ablation in the treatment of recurrent hepatocellular carcinoma. Ann Surg. 2013;257(4):686–92. Available from: http://www.ncbi.nlm.nih.gov/pubmed/23426335

The Future Prospect of Targeted Therapy in Hepatocellular Carcinoma

13

Stephanie H. Greco, Kristen Spencer, and Darren R. Carpizo

13.1 Introduction

Liver cancer is the sixth most common cancer and the second leading cause of cancer death worldwide, accounting for 6% of all diagnosed cancers and approximately 745,000 deaths [1]. Hepatocellular carcinoma (HCC) accounts for up to 90% of all liver cancer cases [1]. More striking, however, is that the incidence has risen over the past several decades in numerous countries, including the United States [2, 3]. Only 30–40% of patients have early HCC at the time of diagnosis and are eligible for potentially curative therapies such as surgical resection, liver transplantation, radiofrequency ablation (RFA), or transarterial chemoembolization (TACE). Furthermore, recurrence remains the leading cause of death after curative resection, occurring in greater than 50% of patients [4]. Cytotoxic chemotherapy has had only modest benefit in advanced disease, and effectiveness is frequently limited by underlying hepatic dysfunction.

To date, sorafenib, a multiple kinase inhibitor is the only therapy to have shown an overall survival benefit in advanced disease, with an improvement from 7.9 to 10.7 months with a favorable toxicity profile. This finding has established sorafenib as the standard of care in this setting [5]. With only a modest benefit offered by sorafenib, there is a pressing need to develop additional therapies to improve outcomes in this disease.

In recent years, HCC has been shown to have a diverse array of phenotypic and genetic alterations, although a few common molecular alterations have been identified that provide an opportunity to develop targeted therapies. These targets include receptors for vascular endothelial growth factor (VEGF), epidermal growth factor

S.H. Greco, M.D. • K. Spencer, M.D. • D.R. Carpizo, M.D. (✉)
Rutgers Cancer Institute of New Jersey, New Brunswick, NJ, USA
e-mail: carpizdr@cinj.rutgers.edu

© Springer International Publishing AG 2018
C. Liu (ed.), *Precision Molecular Pathology of Liver Cancer*,
Molecular Pathology Library, https://doi.org/10.1007/978-3-319-68082-8_13

(EGF), fibroblast growth factor (FGF), and platelet-derived growth factor (PDGF), as well as mammalian target of rapamycin (mTOR) and histone deacetylases (HDACs). Several phase III studies of therapies targeted toward these alterations have followed; however, none has shown a significant survival benefit. This chapter will review our current understanding of the molecular targeted pathways at play in HCC, as well as ongoing clinical trials of targeted agents, and the future direction for therapy in the treatment of HCC.

13.2   Systemic Chemotherapy for the Treatment of HCC

Despite many effective cytotoxic chemotherapy regimens in other tumor types, there remains no effective chemotherapeutic strategy for the treatment of HCC. HCC has long been considered a chemotherapy-refractory tumor through multiple mechanisms: enhanced cellular efflux mechanisms associated with an increase in drug transporter proteins such as MDR1 and P-gp [6], increased expression of TP53 mutations [7] and heat shock proteins (HSPs) [8], DNA damage repair, epithelial-mesenchymal transition (EMT), hypoxia-inducible factor 1 alpha (HIF-1α), and others [9]. Historically, response rates for any chemotherapeutic agent have been low, ranging from approximately 10 to 20% [10]. Because the majority of HCC occurs in the setting of cirrhosis, it is often difficult to determine the survival benefit of these therapies because the ability of patients to tolerate these treatments is often limited by hepatic dysfunction. Several studies have shown that systemic chemotherapy has low efficacy in patients with significant cirrhosis, particularly in those with a bilirubin >2, poor performance status, ascites, or portal vein thrombus [11]. Nonetheless, a large number of studies have been performed using both single agents and combination regimens, resulting in a wide range of responses. Additionally, many of these studies were performed in distinct patient populations (Asian, European), which likely results in important differences between study populations such as hepatitis B or C etiology, or age, thereby making the results less applicable to a more uniform population.

13.2.1 Monotherapy

The most studied single agent has been the anthracycline doxorubicin. The earliest phase II trial was done in 1975 and showed an objective response rate of 79% [12]. However, subsequent studies using the same dose of 75 mg/m^2 failed to corroborate these results and suggested that the true response rate is actually 20% or less [13–17]. Despite this discrepancy, one study has demonstrated a survival benefit with doxorubicin as compared to the best supportive care alone [18]. Lower doses have even lower reported response rates [19, 20].

Many other agents have been evaluated as monotherapies in phase III trials including mitoxantrone, epirubicin, pegylated liposomal doxorubicin, gemcitabine, irinotecan, and thalidomide, all of which have similar or even lower response rates as compared to doxorubicin [21–26]. 5-FU and its oral equivalent, capecitabine, have low toxicity and can be administered more easily in the setting of hepatic dysfunction. Studies evaluating the efficacy of 5-FU monotherapy, with or without leucovorin, show response rates no higher than 28% [27, 28]. Capecitabine has been evaluated in very small trials with mixed populations of both previously treated and untreated patients, with median overall survival rates of about 10 months [29, 30]. Most patients had stable disease with a low number of partial or complete responses. However, a recent phase II trial showed superior median overall survival and progression-free survival in patients treated with sorafenib versus capecitabine, thereby making the role of capecitabine in the treatment of HCC unclear [31].

13.2.2 Combination Chemotherapy

Several different combination chemotherapy regimens using cisplatin or gemcitabine backbones have been tested in patients with advanced HCC. Gemcitabine has been used in combination with several different agents including cisplatin, pegylated liposomal doxorubicin, and oxaliplatin (GEMOX). In phase II trials, the reported overall responses rates were 20% [32], 24% [33], and 18% [34], respectively. However, median overall survival remained dismal, anywhere from 11.5 to 22.5 months, with the addition of significant toxicities including thrombocytopenia, anemia, neutropenia, and neuropathy. Additionally, numerous cisplatin, oxaliplatin, and irinotecan-based regimens have been studied, including XELOX, FOLFOX (infusional fluorouracil, leucovorin, and oxaliplatin), and FOLFOX4, all of which have not had promising results [35, 36]. The PIAF regimen (cisplatin, interferon, doxorubicin, and 5-FU) initially appeared to have some efficacy in patients with unresectable HCC after a phase II trial found a median overall survival of 8.9 months [37]. However, in a randomized phase III trial comparing PIAF to doxorubicin monotherapy, no significant survival benefit was found [17].

Overall, an abundance of cytotoxic chemotherapy regimens have been tested without convincing evidence of a survival benefit. The evaluation of these regimens has been limited by the use of small, single-arm trials with heterogenous patient populations, lack of appropriate controls, and lack of patient risk stratification. As such, there is insufficient data for the routine use of any chemotherapy regimen in HCC. Subsequently, the emergence of targeted agents such as sorafenib has since become the focus of treatment for patients with advanced HCC.

13.3   Molecular Pathogenesis of HCC

In order to develop effective targeted molecular agents, it is critical to understand the molecular pathogenesis of HCC. The most common etiologies of HCC include hepatitis B (HBV), hepatitis C (HCV), chronic alcohol consumption, and aflatoxin toxicity. Nonalcoholic fatty liver disorders (NALFD) have also been shown to contribute to the development of HCC [38]. Importantly, the underlying disease process

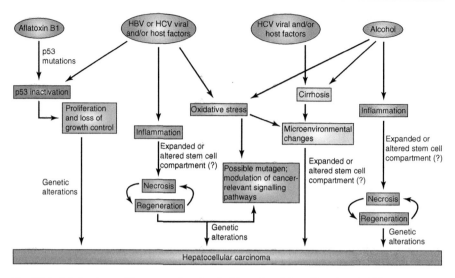

Fig. 13.1 Mechanisms of hepatocarcinogenesis (Reproduced from Farazi et al. 2006)

dictates the specific molecular changes that promote carcinogenesis in HCC and is responsible for the great genomic heterogeneity associated with HCC tumors. For example, alcohol induces significant inflammation with cycles of necrosis and proliferation, whereas aflatoxin contributes to hepatocarcinogenesis specifically via p53 mutations (Fig. 13.1) [39].

However, in general, hepatocarcinogenesis is a multistep process which evolves in the setting of chronic liver disease. It often develops over a prolonged time period of up to 30 years, preceded by the chronic inflammation and pre-dysplastic processes resulting from cirrhosis and chronic hepatitis. Injury induced by these processes leads to a continuous cycle of hepatocyte necrosis and regeneration, which involves proliferation of the stem cell compartment of the liver leading to DNA mutations and genomic instability [39]. In the setting of liver damage, hepatic mesenchymal cells called stellate cells are activated and participate in extracellular matrix production and chemotaxis. Chronic liver damage leads to recurrent activation of stellate cells, resulting in alteration of the extracellular matrix and fibrosis [40]. Additionally, throughout these processes, various growth factors are secreted, which can each contribute to oncogenesis on their own through processes such as angiogenesis.

Overall, the molecular pathogenesis and specific genomic alterations that lead to the development of HCC are extremely complex and are not fully understood. However, the key mechanism appears to be formation of genomic instability in the setting cirrhosis. Specifically, telomere shortening and telomerase reactivation are key features of hepatocarcinogenesis along with loss or mutation of the p53 tumor suppressor gene [39]. Several studies have shown that there is a broad mutational profile in HCC, with approximately 30–40 mutations per tumor, among which 5–8 function as driver mutations while the rest are passenger mutations that do not contribute significantly to tumorigenesis [41–45]. Nonetheless, despite the vast heterogeneity of HCC tumors, there are several common molecular themes and pathways which are known to play prominent roles in the pathogenesis of HCC.

13.3.1 Genetic Mutations and Drivers

Comprehensive genomic analyses are essential to identify mutational signatures in heterogeneous HCC tumors which can help associate them with specific risk factors and improve personalized treatment with molecular targeted agents. Several studies have helped elucidate the most common genetic profiles and driver genes of HCC through exome sequencing analyses. Schulze et al. analyzed whole coding sequences of 243 liver tumors in three European countries [46]. Approximately, 41% were associated with alcohol, 26% with HCV, 18% with nonalcoholic steatohepatitis (NASH), and 14% with HBV. Approximately 49% of tumors were from cirrhotic livers. The authors found a median of 21 silent and 64 non-silent mutations per tumor with 8 signature patterns and 161 driver genes (Fig. 13.2). The most common gene alterations were *TERT* (60%), *CTNNB1* (37%), *TP53* (24%), and *ARID1A* (13%). They performed copy number analysis and were able to correlate focal copy number alterations (CNAs) and mutations to identify the 11 most commonly associated molecular pathways affecting: telomerase expression (60%), cellular inflammation and proliferation via WNT-β-catenin (54%), and PI3-AKT-mTOR (51%). The three most common clusters of alterations centered on *CTNNB1*, *AXIN1*, and *TP53*. Finally, the authors were able to correlate genetic profiles with specific risk factors.

For example, alcohol-related HCCs were enriched in *CTNNB1* and *TERT* alterations, whereas HCV infection was associated with more TP53 mutations. Overall 28% of patients harbored at least one molecular alteration that is targetable by an FDA-approved drug.

Other studies have reported similar findings. Gouichard et al. performed copy number analysis on 125 HCC tumors with whole exome sequencing on 24 tumors primarily associated with alcohol intake [42]. They found that the most common alterations were related to β-catenin (*CTNNB1* (32.8%), *AXIN1* (15.2%), *APC* (1.6%)), cell cycle control (*TP53* (20.8%), *CDKN2A* (7.2%), *IRF2* (4.8%)), chromatin remodeling (*ARID1A* (16.8%), *ARID2* (5.6%)), P13K/Ras signaling (*RPS6KA3* (9.6%)), and oxidative stress (*NFE2L2* (6.4%)). Inactivation of the tumor suppressor IRF2 was exclusively found in HBV-related tumors and led to impaired TP53 function. Mutations in chromatin-remodeling genes were more frequently associated with alcohol-related tumors.

Overall, the most common oncogene amplifications include *TERT*, *CCNB1*, *MET*, *MYC*, *FGF19*, and *VEGFA*, whereas the most frequent homozygous deletions are *CDKN2A*, *TP53*, *Rb1*, and *AXIN1* [5, 41, 45–49]. Additionally, *HDAC2*, a histone deacetylase (HDAC) enzyme that participates in chromatin remodeling, has been found to be upregulated in patients with HCC and is associated with poor survival [50, 51]. The functional classification of these genes has led to the

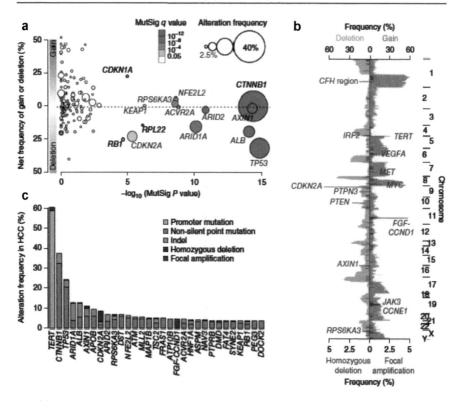

Fig. 13.2 Driver genes, copy number alterations, and most frequent gene alterations in HCC (reproduced from Schulze et al. [46] with the following caption). (**a**) The 161 putative driver genes identified by integrating mutations and focal CNAs are presented, with log-transformed mutation significance on the x axis and the net frequency of gains and deletions on the y axis. The size and color of each circle represent the alteration frequency and MutSig q value, respectively. Significantly mutated genes ($q < 0.05$) are labeled. (**b**) Frequency of CNAs along the genome. The top axis indicates the frequency of low-amplitude changes (gains and losses); the bottom axis indicates the frequency of high-amplitude changes (focal amplifications and homozygous deletions). Genes targeted by recurrent amplifications and homozygous deletions are labeled. (**c**) Bar plot indicating the number and type of events for the most frequently altered genes (≥4% of samples)

identification of several key signaling pathways involved in the pathogenesis of HCC and serve as potential therapeutic targets. A selection of these will be discussed below.

13.3.2 Signaling Pathways

p53

The p53 tumor suppressor is an important driver in HCC, with a mutation rate of 18–50%, depending on the underlying etiology [52]. For example, aflatoxin B1-associated HCC is more common in Southeast Asia and Sub-Saharan Africa and causes a missense mutation at codon 249 (R249S) on exon 7 in 90% of cases [53, 54]. The mutated protein promotes hepatocarcinogenesis through inhibition of apoptosis and cellular proliferation. Mutations at codon 249 are suggested by some to be driver mutations, since they are also found in normal liver tissue after aflatoxin exposure [55]. However, at the same time, other studies have some that these mutations were related to tumor stage and may therefore reflect late molecular changes [56]. TP53 mutations are also prevalent in HBV and HCV HCC and may serve as a biomarker for HCC as well as chemoresistance [7, 56, 57]. A recent meta-analysis has shown that HCC patients with upregulated mutant p53 expression have a shorter overall survival than those with wild type p53 [58]. Other mutations that commonly alter p53 function include G:C to T:A transversions at codon 249 and C:G to A:T and C:G to T:A transversions at codon 250 [59].

WNT/β-Catenin

Dysregulation of the Wnt/β-catenin pathway is known to be crucial in hepatocarcinogenesis [60]. About 50% of patients with HCC have activation of this pathway through either mutations of *CTNNB1*, inactivation of cadherin-1, or overexpression of frizzled receptors [61]. Mutations in *AXIN1*, a negative regulator of Wnt/β--catenin, are also common. These mutations affect many cellular processes including homeostasis, mobility, angiogenesis, proliferation, and apoptosis. In addition, disruption of the adenomatous polyposis coli (APC) gene leads to activation of this pathway and promotes inflammation and early oncogenesis. This pathway is significantly involved in alcoholic and HBV- and HCV-related HCC [59]. Specifically, activation of this pathway leads to transcription of a variety of genes including cyclin D1, COX2, matrix metalloproteinase 7 (MMP7), COX2, and MYC, all of which are pro-tumorigenic. β-catenin signaling leads to activation of NF-κβ which also promotes inflammation and cell death [62, 63].

PI3K/AKT/mTOR

The phosphatidylinositol 3-kinase (PI3K/AKT/mTOR) pathway affects cellular processes such as cell proliferation and survival and is upregulated in 40–50% of HCC [64]. mTOR (mammalian target of rapamycin) is targeted by rapamycin (sirolimus), which was first discovered as an important immunosuppressant after kidney transplant. Important tyrosine kinase receptors such as vascular endothelial growth factor receptor (VEGFR), platelet-derived growth factor receptor (PDGFR), epidermal growth factor receptor (EGFR), and insulin-like growth factor receptor (IGFR) activate this pathway, while phosphatase and tensin homologue (PTEN) inhibits it. There are now numerous PI3K inhibitors in clinical trials [65]. Upregulation of PI3K/AKT/mTOR is associated with decreased overall survival, aggressive tumor behavior, and early recurrence [66–68].

RAS/MAPK

Over 50% of patients with early-stage HCC and nearly 100% of patients with advanced HCC have activation of the RAS/MAPK pathway, which is stimulated by several receptors including EGFR, fibroblast growth factor receptor (FGFR), and c-mesenchymal-epithelial transition factor-1 (c-MET) [69, 70]. The Ras protein belongs to a family of GTPases, which once activated, recruit Raf-1 kinase, which in turn phosphorylates MEK1 and MEK2 and ultimately ERK 1 and ERK2 [71]. It is known that both the Hbx and HCV core proteins can activate this pathway, which plays an important role in cellular proliferation and survival [72, 73]. Several studies have demonstrated increased expression of MEK and ERK proteins in both animal and human liver cancer [71]. Additionally, increased expression of Raf is associated with poor prognosis and is an independent marker of tumor recurrence in human HCC [74]. Although mutations in Raf and Ras proteins are highly prevalent in cancers such as pancreatic cancer, these genes are rarely mutated in human HCC [69]. Alternatively, downregulation of inhibitors of this pathway, such as DUSP1, RKIP, Spred, and Sprouty proteins, appears to play a prominent role in hepatocarcinogenesis [71].

JAK/STAT

The JAK/STAT pathway consists of a cell surface receptor, a Janus kinase (JAK), and a signal transducer and activator of transcription (STAT) protein. The pathway is activated by a variety of growth factors, hormones, and cytokines. Ligand binding activates JAK, ultimately resulting in phosphorylation of STAT, which then translocates to the cell nucleus and induces transcription of target genes. JAK/STAT signaling promotes cell proliferation, migration, and differentiation. Dysregulation of STAT is associated with HCC, and alterations in JAK/STAT signaling occur with a prevalence of 1.5% based on deep-sequencing analyses [44, 69]. Further, the suppressors of cytokine signaling proteins (SOCS) are negative regulators of this pathway and when altered lead to over-activation of the pathway and oncogenesis. Inactivation of SOCS-1 has also been demonstrated in HCC [52, 69].

Notch

Notch signaling via its ligands Jagged (Jag-1, Jag-2) and Delta-like (Dl-1, Dl-3, and Dl-4) is important in cell fate and differentiation. Studies have shown that Notch is involved in hepatocarcinogenesis through activation of Sox9- and K19-positive liver progenitor cells [75]. Genomic studies have shown activation of Notch in about 30% of human HCC, thereby implicating this pathway as a potential therapeutic target [76].

HDACs

Histone deacetylases are critical regulators of gene expression. Numerous studies have demonstrated aberrant expression of HDACs in human cancers, and they have been associated with an either better or worse prognosis, depending on the type of cancer [77]. HDAC inhibitors (HDACis) cause acetylation of histone and non-histone proteins leading to destabilization of various proteins and suppression of transcriptional activity [78]. They are potent inducers of apoptosis, autophagy, cell cycle arrest, and inhibition of tumor angiogenesis [79]. They have become a prominent part of cancer therapy. Upregulation of HDAC 1, 3, 4, 5, and 10 has been found in HCC tumors, although the prognosis of these markers in HCC is unclear [78, 80]. One study found that HDAC 3 was a useful biomarker for HBV-HCC recurrence after liver transplantation [81].

Other

There are multiple other molecular pathways and mechanisms known to play a strong role in HCC. These include the tumor suppressor retinoblastoma (Rb) pathway which is activated by cyclin-dependent kinases (CDKs) and induces G1/S cell cycle transition [82]. Alteration in expression or inactivation of various CDK inhibitors such as p16INK4A, p21(WAF1/CIP1), and p27Kip1 is associated with early hepatocarcinogenesis [59]. Additionally, the transforming growth factor beta (TGF-β) pathway is known to play a role in inflammation and fibrosis leading to the development of HCC. Studies have correlated late rather than early molecular alterations in TGF-β signature with poor prognosis and tumor recurrence which is likely due to TGF-β stimulation of epithelial-mesenchymal transition, which is essential for metastasis [83]. Finally, the hepatocyte growth factor (HGF)/c-mesenchymal-epithelial transition factor-1 (c-MET) pathway is associated with angiogenesis, invasion, and tumor growth. Increased expression of MET gene signature is associated with poor prognosis [84, 85]. Multiple other receptor tyrosine kinase receptors which activate the RAS/MAPK and PI3/AKT/mTOR pathways are very important in the pathogenesis of HCC as well and include the receptors for insulin-like growth factor (IGF), epidermal growth factor (EGF), platelet-derived growth factor (PDGF), vascular endothelial growth factor (VEGF), and fibroblast growth factor (FGF). The latter two growth factors play a significant role in angiogenesis as discussed below. Finally, other mediators of the cellular stress response including heat shock proteins and genes involved in oxidative stress that contribute to cellular mutations and damage in HCC are also potential targets for therapeutic intervention.

13.4 Molecular Targeted Therapies for the Treatment of HCC

Hepatocellular carcinoma is a hypervascular tumor, which frequently invades local vasculature. As a result, angiogenesis is thought to play a key role in the progression of HCC. This process is mediated by a variety of growth factors which activate many of the aforementioned molecular pathways, including VEGF. Higher circulating levels of VEGF are associated with a poor prognosis and decreased overall survival in patients with HCC and correlate with worse outcomes including tumor recurrence after surgery or local ablative procedures [86, 87]. Therefore, this receptor was one of the first targets of molecular therapy. In addition, PDGFR and FGFR are additional targets of angiogenesis which are currently being explored.

13.4.1 Anti-VEGF Agents

Sorafenib

Sorafenib is an oral multiple tyrosine kinase inhibitor that targets the Raf kinases, including VEGF receptors 1–3 and PDGF receptor (PDGFR) via the Raf-MEK-ERK pathway. In 2008, sorafenib became the first approved molecular targeted agent for the treatment of patients with advanced HCC based on positive data from the SHARP trial, a multicenter European phase III trial of sorafenib in 602 patients with advanced (unresectable) HCC and Child-Pugh Class A cirrhosis. Patients were randomly assigned to receive either sorafenib 400 mg twice daily or placebo, with the primary endpoints of overall survival and time to symptomatic progression, as measured by a 4-point decrease in the FACT hepatobiliary symptom index questionnaire. Secondary endpoints included time to radiographic progression based on the Response Evaluation Criteria in Solid Tumors (RECIST), disease control rate, and safety. Sorafenib resulted in a significant overall survival benefit (10.7 vs. 7.9 months) and an improvement in time to radiologic progression (5.5 vs. 2.8 months). However, objective response rates according to the RECIST criteria were low [5]. Seventy-one percent of patients had a partial response, with no complete responses. The survival benefit is likely due to delayed disease progression. Overall there was a low toxicity profile with primarily grade 1 and grade 2 adverse events. Grade 3 events included diarrhea, hand-foot reaction, hypertension, and abdominal pain [5].

Cheng et al. conducted a second phase II trial in the Asian-Pacific population using the same dose of sorafenib in patients with primarily HBV-related HCC and Child-Pugh Class A cirrhosis. They also found improved overall survival in the sorafenib group (6.5 vs. 4.2 months) as well as improved time to tumor progression (2.8 vs. 1.4 months) [88]. Again, sorafenib was well tolerated with similar grade 3 and 4 toxicities as in the SHARP trial. The difference in the survival benefit between the SHARP and Cheng studies may be due to the difference in the etiology of HCC, as the SHARP trial included patients with a more uniform distribution of HBV-, HCV-, and alcohol-related cirrhosis. In fact, a subgroup analysis in the SHARP trial showed that the median overall benefit was greatest in patients with hepatitis C-related cirrhosis [89]. The results of both of these studies were extremely significant and exciting at the time, as there had been no consistent survival benefits of any anti-HCC drugs in the previous decades. Therefore, sorafenib became the standard of care and benchmark to demonstrate superior or non-inferiority in future trials of molecular targeted agents for HCC.

Sorafenib has also been tested in combination with transarterial chemoembolization (TACE), as well as in combination with chemotherapy. TACE is the only transarterial treatment that has been shown to have a survival benefit as compared to placebo in randomized studies [90, 91]. Llovet et al. showed an increased overall survival of 63% vs. 27% at 2 years in patients with HCC and Child-Pugh Class A or B treated with repeated chemoembolization as compared to controls [90]. Several studies, including phase III trials, have evaluated the efficacy of sorafenib in combination with TACE. An initial phase III showed no difference in overall survival in 458 patients with unresectable HCC assigned to placebo or sorafenib (400 mg twice daily) after TACE [92]. However, the median study dose of sorafenib was only 386 mg daily due to dose reductions, much lower than the current standard of 400 mg twice daily. A subsequent phase II trial (SPACE) randomly assigned 307 to sorafenib or placebo with repeated doses of TACE with doxorubicin-eluting beads [93]. It found better trends toward TTP in the sorafenib group but no statistical differences in TTP or overall survival. Finally, there is no known benefit of using sorafenib in combination with systemic chemotherapeutic agents such as doxorubicin [94].

Currently, sorafenib remains first-line therapy for patients with unresectable HCC. However, further studies are needed to further characterize predictive biomarkers of response to sorafenib. The SHARP trial has served as a template for the design of trials investigating other targeted therapies, and several important design features have been replicated in subsequent studies. First, the majority of patients being enrolled have Child-Pugh Class A cirrhosis, thereby eliminating the risk of patients dying as a result of liver decompensation. Also, patients with advanced HCC who do not qualify for curative therapies such as resection or transplant, or those who progress after conventional therapies such as TACE, are good candidates for clinical trials. Lastly, overall survival and time to progression are more frequently serving as primary endpoints, as progression-free survival may be confounded by outcomes related to the severity of liver dysfunction.

Sunitinib

Sunitinib is another oral tyrosine kinase inhibitor that targets VEGFR as well as PDGFR, c-Kit, rearranged during transfection (RET), and fms-like tyrosine receptor kinases (FLT3). In several phase II trials, sunitinib resulted in high levels of grade 3 and 4 toxicities, such as thrombocytopenia, neutropenia, and hand-foot skin reaction. More importantly, sunitinib has repeatedly resulted in minimal objective responses [95, 96]. A phase III trial of over 1000 patients with previously untreated advanced HCC comparing sunitinib to sorafenib was closed prematurely due to the inferiority of sunitinib. At the time of trial cessation, the median survival of patients was 7.9 months in the sunitinib group versus 10.2 months in the sorafenib group. Treatment-related deaths accounted for 3.3% of patients versus 0.3% of patients, respectively. Additionally, the median OS was shorter in HCV-infected patients [97].

Regorafenib

Similar to sorafenib, regorafenib also targets VEGF receptors 1 and 3, in addition to other kinases that promote tumor growth and angiogenesis. The recent RESORCE trial has preliminarily suggested a benefit with regorafenib as compared to placebo in 573 patients with Child-Pugh Class A cirrhosis who had radiologic progression on sorafenib. Regorafenib was associated with improved median overall survival (10.6 versus 7.8 months) and objective response rate (11% vs. 4%) [98]. This study is still ongoing. This has suggested that regorafenib may be a reasonable second-line therapy in patients who progress on or are intolerant of sorafenib.

Bevacizumab

Bevacizumab (Avastin) is an anti-VEGF monoclonal antibody which was first approved in 2004 for the treatment of metastatic colon cancer in combination with chemotherapy. Several phase I/II trials have shown that it is safe and potentially effective against HCC at doses of 5–10 mg/kg in several trials [99, 100]. However, these trials had small sample sizes of only 30–45 patients. Therefore, the efficacy of bevacizumab either alone or in combination needs to be further evaluated in phase III randomized trials. Additionally, studies have shown this agent to have a moderate effect on objective response rate, progression-free survival, and median overall survival when combined with gemcitabine and oxaliplatin (GEMOX) [101] or in combination with capecitabine with or without oxaliplatin [102, 103]. Outcomes of bevacizumab when combined with erlotinib, which targets EGFR, are discussed below. Lastly, bevacizumab may diminish neo-vessel formation after TACE due to its anti-angiogenesis effects [104].

Brivanib

Brivanib is an oral inhibitor of both VEGF and FGF signaling pathways, which was first tested as a second-line agent in patients who progressed or were intolerant of sorafenib. However, results of a phase III randomized trial did not show that brivanib improved overall survival [105]. Subsequently, the BRISK-FL phase III trial randomized 1150 patients with advanced HCC and no prior systemic treatment to receive either sorafenib 400 mg twice daily or brivanib 800 mg daily. The primary endpoint was median overall survival which was 9.9 months in the sorafenib group and 9.5 months in the brivanib group. However, although the study did not meet its primary endpoint of non-inferiority, the objective response rates and TTP were similar. Patients on brivanib had a higher rate of discontinuation due to adverse events (43 vs. 33%) [106]. Despite the trend toward increased OS in the brivanib, the drug could not meet approval for first-line therapy, owing to the strict requirements of non-inferiority trials, which required a hazard ratio for survival with 95% confidence interval between 1 and 1.08.

Others

Several other anti-VEGF agents have been evaluated in both phase II and phase III trials, some of which are still ongoing (Tables 13.1 and 13.2). These include axitinib, ramucirumab, and lenvatinib. Overall, despite the promise of some of these agents such as brivanib, none has shown a clinically significant improvement in overall survival as compared to either placebo or sorafenib.

13.4.2 Anti-PDGF Agents

Linifanib

Linifanib is a more potent targeted inhibitor of both VEGFR and PDGFR than sorafenib. In a phase II trial of 44 patients with advanced or metastatic HCC, treatment with linifanib yielded a median overall survival of 9.7 months, suggesting possible clinical efficacy. Patients were primarily Asian (89%), Child-Pugh Class A (86%), and HBV infected (61%) [107]. However, the phase III head-to-head trial of linifanib versus sorafenib in over 1000 patients failed to meet non-inferiority boundaries, and the overall survival rates were 9.1 versus 9.8 months, respectively. Linifanib also appeared to be more toxic with adverse events in 54% of patients versus 38% with sorafenib [108].

Table 13.1 Molecular targeted agents for HCC in early-phase clinical trials

Drug	Trial phase(s)	Targets	Trials (*n*)	Biomarker	Primary outcome(s)
Anti-angiogenesis					
AMG 386	II	Angiopoietin-1/2	1	No	PFS
Anlotinib	II	VEGFR, PDGFR, FGFR, c-Kit, RET	1	No	PFS
Axitinib	II	VEGFR/c-Kit/PDGFR	3	No	DCR
Bevacizumab	II	VEGF	3	No	DCR
Cediranib	II	VEGFR	1	No	OS at 6 months
Foretinib	I	VEGF2, MET	1	No	MTD
Nintedanib	I, II	VEGFR, PDGFR, FGFR	3	No	MTD, TTP
Orantinib (TSU-68)	I, II	VEGFR2, PDFR, FGFR	1	No	DLT, ORR
Pazopanib	II	VEGFR, PDGFR, FGFR, c-Kit	1	No	MTD
Tivozanib	I, II	VEGFR	1	No	PFS
TRC 105	I, II	Endoglin	1	No	MTD, TTP
Vandetanib	II	VEGFR, EGFR, RET	1	No	ORR
Inhibitors of cell cycle/proliferation					
ABC294640	II	Sphingosine kinase-2	1	No	ORR
AZD8055	I	mTOR	1	No	DLT
Bavituximab	I, II	Phosphatidylserine	1	No	TTP
BGJ398	II	FGFR1–4	1	*FGFR mutation*	ORR
BIIB022	I	IGF-1R	1	No	DLT
CC-122	I	Pleiotropy	2	No	DLT, ORR
CC-223	I, II	mTOR	1	No	DLT
Cixutumumab	II	IGF-1R	3	No	PFS
DCR-MYC	I, II	MYC	1	No	MTD
DENSPM	I	Polyamines	1	No	MTD
Dovitinib	II	FGFR3	1	No	OS
ENMD-2076	II	Aurora kinases	1	No	PFS
Enzalutamide	I, II	Androgen receptor	2	No	PFS, OS
Galunisertib	II	TGFβR1	2	No	TTP
Gefitinib	II	EGFR	2	No	PFS
H3B-6527	I	FGFR4	1	No	DLT
INC280	II	MET	2	*MET mutations*	TTP, ORR
Lapatinib	II	EGFR, Her2/neu	2	No	ORR
LDE225	I	Hedgehog	1	No	DLT
LEE011	II	CDK4/6	1	No	PFS
LY2157299	II	TGF-β	3	No	OS
LY2875358	I, II	MET/VEGFR	1	No	DLT
MEDI-573	I	IGF-1/2	1	No	DLT
MK2206	II	AKT (protein kinase B)	1	No	ORR
MLN0128	I, II	mTOR	1	No	MTD, TTP

(continued)

Table 13.1 (continued)

Drug	Trial phase(s)	Targets	Trials (n)	Biomarker	Primary outcome(s)
MSC2156119J	I, II	MET	2	*MET* mutations	DLT, TTP
Napabucasin (BBI608)	I, II	STAT	2	No	DLT, ORR
OMP-54F28	I	WNT	1	No	DLT, MTD
Onartuzumab	I	MET	1	No	DLT
Pimasertib	I	MEK1/MEK2	1	No	DLT
Refametinib	II	MEK	1	*RAS* mutations	ORR
RO5323441	I	Placenta growth factor	1	No	DLT
Selumetinib (AZD624)	I, II	MEK	2	No	MTD, ORR
Sirolimus	I, II	mTOR	2	No	MTD, RFS
TAC-101	II	Retinoic acid receptor	4	No	OS
Temsirolimus	I, II	mTOR	4	No	TTP
TKM-080301	I, II	PLK1	1	No	MTD
Trametinib	I, II	MEK1/MEK2	2	No	MTD, OS
U3-1784	I	FGFR4	1	No	AE
[Met5]-enkephalin	I	Opioid growth factor	1	No	MTD
Epigenetic modulators					
AEG35156	I, II	XIAP mRNA	1	No	MTD, PFS
Belinostat	I, II	Histone deacetylase	1	No	DLT, ORR
Cinobufacin	II	miR-494	1	No	ORR
CUDC-101	I	Histone deacetylase/ EGFR/HER2	1	No	Safety
MRX34	I	miR-34	1	No	MTD
MTL-CEBPA	I	CEPBA	1	No	DLT
Panobinostat	I	Histone deacetylase	1	No	MTD
Resminostat (4SC-201)	I, II	Histone deacetylase	1	No	DLT, TTP, PFSR
SGI-110	II	DNMT	1	No	DCR
Tefinostat	I, II	Histone deacetylase	1	No	DLT, PFS
Vorinostat	I	Histone deacetylase	1	No	MTD
Immunomodulators					
OPC-18	II	Interferon-α receptor	1	No	ORR
AZD9150	I	STAT3	1	No	MTD
Dalantercept	I, II	TGF-β	1	ALK1, BMP 9/10	DLT, PFS, OS, DCR
GLYCAR T cells	I	T cells	1	No	DLT
Icaritin	II	STAT3	1	No	TTP
Ipilimumab	I, II	CTLA-4	1	No	DLT, ORR
NGR-hTNF	II	TNF-α	1	No	PFS
OPB-31121	I, II	STAT3	1	No	DLT

Table 13.1   (continued)

Drug	Trial phase(s)	Targets	Trials (*n*)	Biomarker	Primary outcome(s)
OPB-111,077	I	STAT3	1	No	MTD
PDR001	I, II	PD-1	1	No	MTD, DLT, ORR
SHR1210	I, II	PD-1	1	No	OS
Tasquinimod	II	Protein S100A9	1	No	PFS
Tremelimumab (CP 675,206)	II	CTLA-4	1	No	ORR
Proapoptotic or DNA-damaging agents					
ABT-888	I, II	PARP	1	No	ORR
Mapatumumab	I, II	TRAIL-R1	2	No	TTP
Navitoclax	I	BCL2, BCLX	1	No	MTD
STA-9090	I	Hsp90	1	No	DLT
Tigatuzumab (CS-1008)	II	TRAIL-R2	1	No	TTP
Veliparib (ABT-888)	II	PARP1/2	1	No	ORR
Miscellaneous					
ABT-751	I	β-tubulin	1	No	MTD
BBI608/BBI503	I, II	Cancer stem cells	1	No	ORR
Bortezomib	II	Proteasome	2	No	ORR
CF102	II	Adenosine receptor	2	No	OS
Darinaparsin	II	Unknown	1	No	ORR
Dasatinib	II	BCR/Abl	2	No	ORR,PFS
GC33	I, II	GPC3	3	No	DLT, PFS
Ispinesib	II	Kinesin spindle protein	1	No	ORR
Lenalidomide	I	Ubiquitin E3 ligase/ proteasome	1	No	PFS
Oprozomib	I, II	Proteasome	1	No	TTP
RO5137382	II	Glypican-3	1	Glypican-3 on IHC	PFS
T900607	II	Microtubule	1	No	ORR
Z-208	I, II	Unknown	1	No	MTD, ORR

Data accessed in October 2016 on clinicaltrials.gov using search criteria "hepatocellular carcinoma" OR "liver cancer" "drug" NOT "procedure" phase 0–2 to identify relevant clinical trials either completed, ongoing, or terminated with results, not withdrawn or terminated due to adverse effects. Table adapted from Table 3 Llovet et al. [65]. *PFS* progression-free survival, *DCR* disease control rate, *OS* overall survival, *MTD* maximum-tolerated dose, *TTP* time to progression, *ORR* objective response rate, *DLT* dose-limiting toxicity, *RFS* relapse-free survival, *AE* adverse events, *PFSR* progression-free survival rate

13.4.3   Anti-FGF Agents

FGFR signaling has a role in both proliferation and angiogenesis which contributes to hepatocarcinogenesis [109]. Studies in pancreatic tumors have suggested that resistance to VEGF-targeted therapy may be mediated by upregulation of FGFR

Table 13.2 Molecular targeted agents for HCC in phase III clinical trials

Trial name or ID#	Agents	Molecular targets	Biomarker enrichment	Primary outcome(s)	N	Median OS	P value	HR
SHARP	Sorafenib	VEGFR, PDGFR, BRAF		OS, TTSP	602	10.7	0.001	0.69
	Placebo					7.9		
Cheng et al. [88]	Sorafenib	VEGFR, PDGFR, BRAF		OS	226	6.5	0.01	0.68
	Placebo					4.2		
STORM	Sorafenib	VEGFR, PDGFR, BRAF		RFS	1114	33.4	0.94	0.26
	Placebo					33.8		
Cheng et al. [97]	Sunitinib	VEGFR, PDGFR, c-Kit		OS	1074	7.9	0.001	1.3
	Sorafenib					10.2		
RESORCE[a]	Regorafenib	VEGFR, PDGFR, FGFR, BRAF, RET		OS	573	10.6	0.001	0.62
	Sorafenib					7.8		
BRISK-FL	Brivanib	VEGFR, FGFR		Non-inferiority, OS	1155	9.5	1.06	0.31
	Sorafenib					9.9		
BRISK-PS	Brivanib	VEGFR, FGFR		OS	395	9.4	0.89	0.33
	Placebo					8.2		
REACH	Ramucirumab	VEGRF2		OS	553	9.2	0.14	0.87
	Placebo					7.6		
REACH-2[a]	Ramucirumab + BSC	VEGRF2	AFP	OS				
	Placebo + BSC							
LIGHT	Linifanib	VEGFR, PDGFR		Non-inferiority, OS	1035	9.1	1.04	0.52[#]
	Sorafenib					9.8		
SEARCH[a]	Erlotinib + Sorafenib	EGFR		OS	720	9.5	0.92	0.4
	Sorafenib					8.5		
CELESTIAL[a]	Cabozantinib	MET, VEGFR2		OS	760[b]			
	Placebo							
JET-HCC[a]	Tivantinib (ARQ197)	MET		PFS				
	Placebo							

Trial	Drug	MET	MET	OS				
METIV-HCC[a]	Tivantinib (ARQ197)	MET		OS				
	Placebo							
EVOLVE-1	Everolimus	mTOR		OS	546	7.6	1.05	0.68
	Placebo					7.3		
NCT02576509[a]	Nivolumab	PD-1		OS, TTP				
	Placebo							
NCT02645981[a]	Donafenib	BRAF		OS				
	Sorafenib							
NCT01761266[a]	Lenvatinib	VEGFR2/3, FGFR, c-Kit, RET		OS				
	Sorafenib							
ADI-PEG 20[a]	Pegylated arginine deiminase	Arginine deiminase		OS				
	Placebo							
BOOST[a]	Sorafenib		Child-Pugh Class B	OS				
	BSC							
ORIENTAL[a]	Orantinib (TSU-568) + TACE	VEGFR2, PDGFR, FGFR, c-Kit		OS				
	Placebo							
KEYNOTE-240[a]	Pembrolizumab	PD-1		OS, PFS				
	BSC							
NCT02329860[a]	Apatinib	VEGFR2		OS				
	Placebo							
NCT01640808[a]	Peretinoin	Retinoic acid receptor	HCV	RFS				

Data accessed in October 2016 on clinicaltrials.gov using search criteria "hepatocellular carcinoma" OR "liver cancer" "drug" NOT "procedure" phase III to identify ongoing relevant clinical trials

[a] Trial ongoing no results available

[b] Trial is designed to enroll 760 patients; HR hazard ratio

[#] calculated by Llovet et al (ref 65) based on HR and CI in the original report (ref 108)

signaling [110]. Thus, it was hypothesized that brivanib, mentioned above, might have increased efficacy in treatment of HCC by targeting both VEGFR and FGFR. Since the phase III non-inferiority trial of sorafenib versus brivanib did not demonstrate a clear clinical effect, there has been focus on the development of more specific FGFR agents and biomarkers which may demonstrate response to treatment. FGF19 is one such potential biomarker, amplified in 5–10% of HCC, which may predict response to targeted FGF therapy [47, 48]. In addition, blocking FGFR4 may help prevent hepatic tumor formation by interfering with the FGR19 signaling axis [111]. As a result, several generations of targeted FGFR agents have been developed and are underway in clinical studies. The first generation of these drugs were either pan-FGFR inhibitors or those with weak activity against FGFR4, including LY-2874455, ponatinib, BGJ398, and AZD4547 [112]. Currently, there are only a few phase I/II studies underway evaluating specific FGFR inhibitors (Table 13.1). Recent development of another selective FGFR4 inhibitor, BLU9931, may have promise as a future therapy for HCC [113].

13.4.4 Anti-EGRF Agents

Erlotinib

Erlotinib inhibits the tyrosine kinase domain of EGFR and has demonstrated antitumor activity and a median overall survival of 11–13 (11–13 months) in phase II clinical trials of patients with unresectable HCC [114, 115]. Expanding upon this earlier study, the phase III SEARCH trial included 720 patients with advanced HCC who were randomized to receive either sorafenib and erlotinib or sorafenib and placebo [116]. The trial did not show a significant benefit of combination therapy with erlotinib and sorafenib as compared to sorafenib alone (OS 9.5 vs. 8.5 months), and the addition of erlotinib resulted in increased toxicity resulting in shorter durations of treatment. Additionally, a phase II trial of erlotinib plus bevacizumab failed to validate the use of this combination strategy [117]. Other phase II trials of erlotinib and bevacizumab are underway.

13.4.5 Newer Drugs Under Development

MET

As previously mentioned, MET is part of the HGF signaling pathway, and expression of MET signature phenotype is correlated with tumor progression and metastasis [84]. Therefore, MET is a target of new drug development for treatment of HCC. Cabozantinib, which inhibits both MET and VEGFR2, has been shown to suppress tumor growth and metastasis both in vitro and in vivo [118]. This same study also showed high levels of activated MET that are associated with poor response to sorafenib, making this an attractive target for intervention. A phase III randomized trial (the CELESTIAL trial) of cabozantinib versus placebo in advanced HCC is still ongoing (Table 13.2). Tivantinib (ARQ197) which selectively targets c-MET may also be a valuable drug for second-line therapy. A randomized phase II trial of tivantinib versus placebo showed that patients with MET-high tumors who received tivantinib had median OS of 7.2 months, compared to 3.8 months for MET-high patients who received the placebo (HR, 0.38) [119]. A Japanese phase III trial (JET-HCC) with this drug is underway (Table 13.2).

TGF-β

TGF-β signaling is associated with cirrhosis, fibrosis, and inflammation as mentioned previously resulting in epithelial-to-mesenchymal transition and hepatocarcinogenesis [120]. Furthermore, late TGF-β signature correlates to tumor invasiveness and recurrence [83]. Therefore, it is hypothesized that inhibition of TGF-β in HCC will block both inflammation related to liver cirrhosis and HCC tumor metastasis. However, in many cancers, TGF-β has been shown to have both tumor suppressor and tumor promotor functions [121], making it difficult to develop novel inhibitors for therapy. LY2157299 (galunisertib) is a TGF-β inhibitor that has been shown to block HCC tumor invasion and angiogenesis in preclinical studies [122]. Preliminary results of a phase II trial demonstrated tolerable toxicity and increased TTP in patients with declines in serum alpha-fetoprotein and TGF-β levels [123]. Phase II clinical trials of galunisertib alone or in combination with sorafenib are ongoing (Table 13.1). Identification of biomarkers which are predictive of response will be useful for development of anti-TGF-β agents.

RAS/MAPK

Selective inhibitors of the RAS/MAPK pathway, which affects cellular proliferation, include those targeting MEK and RAF. A phase II trial of the MEK inhibitor, refametinib (BAY 86-9766), was conducted in 95 Asian, primary HBV-infected patients assigned to receive refametinib 50 mg twice daily and sorafenib 200 mg (morning)/400 mg (evening), with dose escalation to sorafenib 400 mg twice daily if tolerated. Disease control rate was 44.8% with median TTP of 122 days. Interestingly, the best clinical responders had RAS mutations, suggesting efficacy of this treatment in selected RAS-mutated patients. Unfortunately, dose modifications due to adverse events such as diarrhea, nausea, and vomiting occurred in most patients, which may limit the benefit of this therapeutic combination [124]. Additionally, a low proportion of HCC patients are known to have Ras mutation, thus limiting the feasibility of MEK inhibitors. Additionally, BRAF inhibitors, such as dabrafenib, are under early investigation for treatment in HCC. Many of these drugs are already FDA approved for treatment of advanced melanoma, which commonly harbors BRAF mutations (Table 13.1).

Antiproliferative/Cell Cycle

Cyclin-dependent kinases (CDK) are critical regulators of cell cycle control and apoptosis which are known to be deregulated in cancer [125]. CDKS are known to be altered in HCC, through gene deletions such as *CDKN2A*, which control CDK inhibitory proteins such as p16Ink4, p21, p27, and p57 [126]. Thus CDK inhibitors that can halt cell cycle progression are another potential therapeutic intervention in the treatment of HCC. Examples of this are currently in preclinical phases of development and include xylocydine, an inhibitor of CDK 1, 2, 7, and 9 which has shown the ability to suppress growth of HCC xenografts in nude mice [127]. Additionally, CDK4/6 inhibition can block proliferation in hepatoma cell lines [128]. A third study showed that treatment of xenografted HCC with the novel compounds BA-12 and BP-14 that antagonize CDK1/2/5/7 and CDK9 decreased tumor formation. It also diminished diethylnitrosamine (DEN)-induced hepatoma development in mice, suggesting a role for efficacy in the treatment of HCC [129].

PI3K/mTOR Inhibitors

Everolimus is an mTOR inhibitor which has been shown to improve survival and prevent tumor progression in preclinical models [130]. After success of early clinical studies [131], everolimus was tested in a phase III randomized controlled trial (EVOLVE-1) of 546 patients with sorafenib-refractory or intolerant advanced HCC. There was no difference in median OS in patients who received everolimus as compared to placebo (7.6 vs. 7.3 months). Interestingly, patients with HBV infection fared better than those with HCV (HR 0.63 vs. 0.93). Furthermore, the authors show that HBV-infected patients were more likely to have tuberous sclerosis 2 (TSC2)-null phenotype. This is significant since previous studies have shown that this phenotype is a predictive biomarker for response to everolimus [132]. Therefore, further studies are needed to validate the use of mTOR inhibitors in selected HCC patients.

HDACis

Histone deacetylases (HDAC) are important in chromatin remodeling, and epigenetic dysregulation plays a key role in HCC as previously described. HDAC inhibitors have become important in cancer therapy. They mediate cell death through a variety of mechanisms including cell growth arrest, induction of apoptosis, induction of autophagy, and anti-angiogenesis [80]. In an early phase I/II trial, 42 patients with unresectable HCC received intravenous dosing of belinostat, an HDAC inhibitor which is FDA approved for the treatment of peripheral T-cell lymphoma. The study found that belinostat was well tolerated and resulted in disease stabilization. Also, expression of HR23B, which is known to increase sensitivity to HDAC inhibitors [133], was associated with improved disease stabilization [134]. Currently, several phase I and II trials are underway evaluating the use of different HDAC inhibitors alone or in combination with sorafenib (Table 13.1).

Immunomodulators

Immune checkpoint inhibitors have shown tremendous therapeutic activity in the treatment of advanced melanoma [135]. These include antibodies against cytotoxic T-lymphocyte protein (CTLA-4) and programmed cell death protein 1 (PD-1) and its ligand (PD-L1). CTLA-4 is expressed on regulatory T cells (Tregs) and serves as an inhibitory signal to activated T cells. Cancer cells protect themselves against activated T cells in part by expressing PD-L1 which interacts with PD-1 to attenuate T-cell responses. Therefore, inhibition of these immune checkpoints will improve tumor-associated immune responses. Thus far, results in clinical trials are promising. A phase I/II trial of nivolumab (anti-PD-1 antibody) showed that it was safe at doses up to 10 mL/kg. A total of 47 patients with noninfected HBV- and HCV-related HCC were examined, of whom 70% had extrahepatic metastasis. Most patients had failed sorafenib therapy. The overall objective response rate was 19%, with two patients (5%) demonstrating a complete response. Moreover, the dose escalation part of the study assessed the efficacy of nivolumab at doses between 0.1 and 10 mL/kg. Most importantly, patients demonstrated stable or improved response over time without the development of drug resistance [136]. This trial is still ongoing, and results were recently presented at the ASCO meeting in 2016. Currently, a phase III trial of nivolumab in HCC is underway (Table 13.2), as are other phase I and II trials of CTLA-4 and PD-1 antibodies (Table 13.1).

13.5   Future Directions

Overall there have been substantial developments in understanding the molecular pathogenesis of HCC. Unfortunately, this has not yet translated into more robust therapeutic advances other than sorafenib. For patients with HCC not amenable to potentially curative therapies such as resection, transplant, or ablation, there remain limited options. For early-stage patients who are able to undergo potentially curative resection, the majority (70%) recur with no proven adjuvant therapy [137]. Even sorafenib has failed to have success in the adjuvant setting. In the STORM randomized controlled phase III trial, over 1000 patients with early HCC who had a complete radiologic response to surgical resection or local ablation were treated with sorafenib 400 mg twice daily or placebo for up to 4 years. There was no difference in overall median recurrence-free survival between the two groups (33.7 vs. 33.3 months) [138]. These findings suggest that sorafenib may not prevent progression of early undetected tumor clones or de novo hepatocarcinogenesis. This highlights the fact that further research is indicated to better understand the molecular pathways and signatures which are associated with tumor recurrence.

Many promising drugs have failed to meet primary endpoints in phase II or phase III clinical trials based on the failure to show objective response rates based on the RECIST criteria. However, these criteria can be misleading and may underestimate response to immunotherapy or molecular targeted agents. As a result, the modified RECIST criteria have been developed which characterizes active tumor tissue based on arterial phase enhancement on imaging. These new criteria should be applied to future trials and can be enhanced through identification of other markers of tumor activity as opposed to just tumor size.

Other reasons for the lack of success in molecular targeted therapy thus far include the highly heterogeneic nature of HCC which encompasses numerous alterations in genetic pathways and epigenetic changes. Basket trials designed to enroll patients based on a specific molecular alteration in their tumor may be a more promising strategy to evaluate targeted agents in clinical trials such has been done with vemurafenib in V600E BRAF mutant cancers [139].

Further improvements in targeted therapy for HCC will focus on gaining a better understanding of molecular drivers and, most importantly, designing specific therapy for each patient based on molecular classification and/or etiology of his or her individual tumor(s). In addition, identification of biomarkers which will help identify responder from nonresponder to a specific therapy is also critical. Other promising avenues for research in the therapeutics of HCC include epigenetic modifiers and miRNA-based therapies and agents that target HCC tumor-initiating cells (the so-called cancer stem cells). Ultimately, the development of molecular targeted agents for HCC hinges on more effective translational research that will be able to show which agents are effective for which types of HCC.

References

1. Ferlay J, Soerjomataram I, Dikshit R, et al. Cancer incidence and mortality worldwide: sources, methods and major patterns in GLOBOCAN 2012. Int J Cancer. 2015;136:E359–86.
2. Nordenstedt H, White DL, El-Serag HB. The changing pattern of epidemiology in hepatocellular carcinoma. Dig Liver Dis. 2010;42(Suppl 3):S206–14.
3. Torre LA, Bray F, Siegel RL, et al. Global cancer statistics, 2012. CA Cancer J Clin. 2015;65:87–108.
4. Shah SA, Cleary SP, Wei AC, et al. Recurrence after liver resection for hepatocellular carcinoma: risk factors, treatment, and outcomes. Surgery. 2007;141:330–9.
5. Llovet JM, Ricci S, Mazzaferro V, et al. Sorafenib in advanced hepatocellular carcinoma. N Engl J Med. 2008;359:378–90.
6. Huang C, Xu D, Xia Q, et al. Reversal of P-glycoprotein-mediated multidrug resistance of human hepatic cancer cells by Astragaloside II. J Pharm Pharmacol. 2012;64:1741–50.
7. Chan KT, Lung ML. Mutant p53 expression enhances drug resistance in a hepatocellular carcinoma cell line. Cancer Chemother Pharmacol. 2004;53:519–26.
8. Wang C, Zhang Y, Guo K, et al. Heat shock proteins in hepatocellular carcinoma: molecular mechanism and therapeutic potential. Int J Cancer. 2016;138:1824–34.
9. Wen L, Liang C, Chen E, et al. Regulation of multi-drug resistance in hepatocellular carcinoma cells is TRPC6/calcium dependent. Sci Rep. 2016;6:23269.
10. Deng GL, Zeng S, Shen H. Chemotherapy and target therapy for hepatocellular carcinoma: new advances and challenges. World J Hepatol. 2015;7:787–98.
11. Nagahama H, Okada S, Okusaka T, et al. Predictive factors for tumor response to systemic chemotherapy in patients with hepatocellular carcinoma. Jpn J Clin Oncol. 1997;27:321–4.
12. Olweny CL, Toya T, Katongole-Mbidde E, et al. Treatment of hepatocellular carcinoma with adriamycin. Preliminary communication. Cancer. 1975;36:1250–7.
13. Chlebowski RT, Brzechwa-Adjukiewicz A, Cowden A, et al. Doxorubicin (75 mg/m2) for hepatocellular carcinoma: clinical and pharmacokinetic results. Cancer Treat Rep. 1984;68:487–91.
14. Choi TK, Lee NW, Wong J. Chemotherapy for advanced hepatocellular carcinoma. Adriamycin versus quadruple chemotherapy. Cancer. 1984;53:401–5.
15. Ihde DC, Kane RC, Cohen MH, et al. Adriamycin therapy in American patients with hepatocellular carcinoma. Cancer Treat Rep. 1977;61:1385–1.
16. Nerenstone SR, Ihde DC, Friedman MA. Clinical trials in primary hepatocellular carcinoma: current status and future directions. Cancer Treat Rev. 1988;15:1–31.
17. Yeo W, Mok TS, Zee B, et al. A randomized phase III study of doxorubicin versus cisplatin/interferon alpha-2b/doxorubicin/fluorouracil (PIAF) combination chemotherapy for unresectable hepatocellular carcinoma. J Natl Cancer Inst. 2005;97:1532–8.
18. Lai CL, PC W, Chan GC, et al. Doxorubicin versus no antitumor therapy in inoperable hepatocellular carcinoma. A prospective randomized trial. Cancer. 1988;62:479–83.

19. Gish RG, Porta C, Lazar L, et al. Phase III randomized controlled trial comparing the survival of patients with unresectable hepatocellular carcinoma treated with nolatrexed or doxorubicin. J Clin Oncol. 2007;25:3069–75.

20. Sciarrino E, Simonetti RG, Le Moli S, et al. Adriamycin treatment for hepatocellular carcinoma. Experience with 109 patients. Cancer. 1985;56:2751–5.

21. Boige V, Taieb J, Hebbar M, et al. Irinotecan as first-line chemotherapy in patients with advanced hepatocellular carcinoma: a multicenter phase II study with dose adjustment according to baseline serum bilirubin level. Eur J Cancer. 2006;42:456–9.

22. Dunk AA, Scott SC, Johnson PJ, et al. Mitozantrone as single agent therapy in hepatocellular carcinoma. A phase II study. J Hepatol. 1985;1:395–404.

23. Halm U, Etzrodt G, Schiefke I, et al. A phase II study of pegylated liposomal doxorubicin for treatment of advanced hepatocellular carcinoma. Ann Oncol. 2000;11:113–4.

24. Kubicka S, Rudolph KL, Tietze MK, et al. Phase II study of systemic gemcitabine chemotherapy for advanced unresectable hepatobiliary carcinomas. Hepato-Gastroenterology. 2001;48:783–9.

25. Lin AY, Brophy N, Fisher GA, et al. Phase II study of thalidomide in patients with unresectable hepatocellular carcinoma. Cancer. 2005;103:119–25.

26. Pohl J, Zuna I, Stremmel W, et al. Systemic chemotherapy with epirubicin for treatment of advanced or multifocal hepatocellular carcinoma. Chemotherapy. 2001;47:359–65.

27. Porta C, Moroni M, Nastasi G, et al. 5-Fluorouracil and d,l-leucovorin calcium are active to treat unresectable hepatocellular carcinoma patients: preliminary results of a phase II study. Oncology. 1995;52:487–91.

28. Tetef M, Doroshow J, Akman S, et al. 5-fluorouracil and high-dose calcium leucovorin for hepatocellular carcinoma: a phase II trial. Cancer Investig. 1995;13:460–3.

29. Brandi G, De Rosa F, Agostini V, et al. Metronomic capecitabine in advanced hepatocellular carcinoma patients: a phase II study. Oncologist. 2013;18:1256–7.

30. Patt YZ, Hassan MM, Aguayo A, et al. Oral capecitabine for the treatment of hepatocellular carcinoma, cholangiocarcinoma, and gallbladder carcinoma. Cancer. 2004;101:578–86.

31. Abdel-Rahman O, Abdel-Wahab M, Shaker M, et al. Sorafenib versus capecitabine in the management of advanced hepatocellular carcinoma. Med Oncol. 2013;30:655.

32. Parikh PM, Fuloria J, Babu G, et al. A phase II study of gemcitabine and cisplatin in patients with advanced hepatocellular carcinoma. Trop Gastroenterol. 2005;26:115–8.

33. Lombardi G, Zustovich F, Farinati F, et al. Pegylated liposomal doxorubicin and gemcitabine in patients with advanced hepatocellular carcinoma: results of a phase 2 study. Cancer. 2011;117:125–33.

34. Louafi S, Boige V, Ducreux M, et al. Gemcitabine plus oxaliplatin (GEMOX) in patients with advanced hepatocellular carcinoma (HCC): results of a phase II study. Cancer. 2007;109:1384–90.

35. Boige V, Raoul JL, Pignon JP, et al. Multicentre phase II trial of capecitabine plus oxaliplatin (XELOX) in patients with advanced hepatocellular carcinoma: FFCD 03-03 trial. Br J Cancer. 2007;97:862–7.

36. Qin S, Bai Y, Lim HY, et al. Randomized, multicenter, open-label study of oxaliplatin plus fluorouracil/leucovorin versus doxorubicin as palliative chemotherapy in patients with advanced hepatocellular carcinoma from Asia. J Clin Oncol. 2013;31:3501–8.

37. Leung TW, Patt YZ, Lau WY, et al. Complete pathological remission is possible with systemic combination chemotherapy for inoperable hepatocellular carcinoma. Clin Cancer Res. 1999;5:1676–81.

38. Farrell GC, Larter CZ. Nonalcoholic fatty liver disease: from steatosis to cirrhosis. Hepatology. 2006;43:S99–S112.

39. Farazi PA, Depinho RA. Hepatocellular carcinoma pathogenesis: from genes to environment. Nat Rev Cancer. 2006;6:674–87.

40. Yin C, Evason KJ, Asahina K, et al. Hepatic stellate cells in liver development, regeneration, and cancer. J Clin Invest. 2013;123:1902–10.

41. Ahn SM, Jang SJ, Shim JH, et al. Genomic portrait of resectable hepatocellular carcinomas: implications of RB1 and FGF19 aberrations for patient stratification. Hepatology. 2014;60:1972–82.

42. Guichard C, Amaddeo G, Imbeaud S, et al. Integrated analysis of somatic mutations and focal copy-number changes identifies key genes and pathways in hepatocellular carcinoma. Nat Genet. 2012;44:694–8.
43. Kan Z, Zheng H, Liu X, et al. Whole-genome sequencing identifies recurrent mutations in hepatocellular carcinoma. Genome Res. 2013;23:1422–33.
44. Llovet JM, Villanueva A, Lachenmayer A, et al. Advances in targeted therapies for hepatocellular carcinoma in the genomic era. Nat Rev Clin Oncol. 2015;12:436.
45. Villanueva A, Llovet JM. Liver cancer in 2013: mutational landscape of HCC—the end of the beginning. Nat Rev Clin Oncol. 2014;11:73–4.
46. Schulze K, Imbeaud S, Letouze E, et al. Exome sequencing of hepatocellular carcinomas identifies new mutational signatures and potential therapeutic targets. Nat Genet. 2015;47:505–11.
47. Chiang DY, Villanueva A, Hoshida Y, et al. Focal gains of VEGFA and molecular classification of hepatocellular carcinoma. Cancer Res. 2008;68:6779–88.
48. Sawey ET, Chanrion M, Cai C, et al. Identification of a therapeutic strategy targeting amplified FGF19 in liver cancer by oncogenomic screening. Cancer Cell. 2011;19:347–58.
49. Totoki Y, Tatsuno K, Covington KR, et al. Trans-ancestry mutational landscape of hepatocellular carcinoma genomes. Nat Genet. 2014;46:1267–73.
50. Kramer OH. HDAC2: a critical factor in health and disease. Trends Pharmacol Sci. 2009;30:647–55.
51. Lee JS, Chu IS, Heo J, et al. Classification and prediction of survival in hepatocellular carcinoma by gene expression profiling. Hepatology. 2004;40:667–76.
52. Dhanasekaran R, Bandoh S, Roberts LR. Molecular pathogenesis of hepatocellular carcinoma and impact of therapeutic advances. F1000Res. 2016;5:879.
53. Gouas DA, Shi H, Hautefeuille AH, et al. Effects of the TP53 p.R249S mutant on proliferation and clonogenic properties in human hepatocellular carcinoma cell lines: interaction with hepatitis B virus X protein. Carcinogenesis. 2010;31:1475–82.
54. Hamid AS, Tesfamariam IG, Zhang Y, et al. Aflatoxin B1-induced hepatocellular carcinoma in developing countries: geographical distribution, mechanism of action and prevention. Oncol Lett. 2013;5:1087–92.
55. Ozturk M. p53 mutation in hepatocellular carcinoma after aflatoxin exposure. Lancet. 1991;338:1356–9.
56. Lunn RM, Zhang YJ, Wang LY, et al. p53 mutations, chronic hepatitis B virus infection, and aflatoxin exposure in hepatocellular carcinoma in Taiwan. Cancer Res. 1997;57:3471–7.
57. Kasprzak A, Adamek A, Przybyszewska W, et al. p53 immunocytochemistry and TP53 gene mutations in patients with chronic hepatitis C virus (HCV) infection. Folia Histochem Cytobiol. 2009;47:35–42.
58. Liu J, Ma Q, Zhang M, et al. Alterations of TP53 are associated with a poor outcome for patients with hepatocellular carcinoma: evidence from a systematic review and meta-analysis. Eur J Cancer. 2012;48:2328–38.
59. Aravalli RN, Steer CJ, Cressman EN. Molecular mechanisms of hepatocellular carcinoma. Hepatology. 2008;48:2047–63.
60. Lachenmayer A, Alsinet C, Savic R, et al. Wnt-pathway activation in two molecular classes of hepatocellular carcinoma and experimental modulation by sorafenib. Clin Cancer Res. 2012;18:4997–5007.
61. Llovet JM, Chen Y, Wurmbach E, et al. A molecular signature to discriminate dysplastic nodules from early hepatocellular carcinoma in HCV cirrhosis. Gastroenterology. 2006;131:1758–67.
62. Elsharkawy AM, Mann DA. Nuclear factor-kappaB and the hepatic inflammation-fibrosis-cancer axis. Hepatology. 2007;46:590–7.
63. Luedde T, Schwabe RF. NF-kappaB in the liver—linking injury, fibrosis and hepatocellular carcinoma. Nat Rev Gastroenterol Hepatol. 2011;8:108–18.
64. Matter MS, Decaens T, Andersen JB, et al. Targeting the mTOR pathway in hepatocellular carcinoma: current state and future trends. J Hepatol. 2014;60:855–65.
65. Llovet JM, Villanueva A, Lachenmayer A, et al. Advances in targeted therapies for hepatocellular carcinoma in the genomic era. Nat Rev Clin Oncol. 2015;12:408–24.

66. Baba HA, Wohlschlaeger J, Cicinnati VR, et al. Phosphorylation of p70S6 kinase predicts overall survival in patients with clear margin-resected hepatocellular carcinoma. Liver Int. 2009;29:399–405.
67. Villanueva A, Chiang DY, Newell P, et al. Pivotal role of mTOR signaling in hepatocellular carcinoma. Gastroenterology. 2008;135:1972–1983, 1983 e1–11.
68. Zhou L, Huang Y, Li J, et al. The mTOR pathway is associated with the poor prognosis of human hepatocellular carcinoma. Med Oncol. 2010;27:255–61.
69. Calvisi DF, Ladu S, Gorden A, et al. Ubiquitous activation of Ras and Jak/Stat pathways in human HCC. Gastroenterology. 2006;130:1117–28.
70. Newell P, Toffanin S, Villanueva A, et al. Ras pathway activation in hepatocellular carcinoma and anti-tumoral effect of combined sorafenib and rapamycin in vivo. J Hepatol. 2009;51:725–33.
71. Delire B, Starkel P. The Ras/MAPK pathway and hepatocarcinoma: pathogenesis and therapeutic implications. Eur J Clin Investig. 2015;45:609–23.
72. Nakamura H, Aoki H, Hino O, et al. HCV core protein promotes heparin binding EGF-like growth factor expression and activates Akt. Hepatol Res. 2011;41:455–62.
73. Zhang X, Zhang H, Ye L. Effects of hepatitis B virus X protein on the development of liver cancer. J Lab Clin Med. 2006;147:58–66.
74. Chen L, Shi Y, Jiang CY, et al. Expression and prognostic role of pan-Ras, Raf-1, pMEK1 and pERK1/2 in patients with hepatocellular carcinoma. Eur J Surg Oncol. 2011;37:513–20.
75. Morell CM, Strazzabosco M. Notch signaling and new therapeutic options in liver disease. J Hepatol. 2014;60:885–90.
76. Villanueva A, Alsinet C, Yanger K, et al. Notch signaling is activated in human hepatocellular carcinoma and induces tumor formation in mice. Gastroenterology. 2012;143:1660.
77. West AC, Johnstone RW. New and emerging HDAC inhibitors for cancer treatment. J Clin Invest. 2014;124:30–9.
78. Lachenmayer A, Toffanin S, Cabellos L, et al. Combination therapy for hepatocellular carcinoma: additive preclinical efficacy of the HDAC inhibitor panobinostat with sorafenib. J Hepatol. 2012;56:1343–50.
79. Witt O, Lindemann R. HDAC inhibitors: magic bullets, dirty drugs or just another targeted therapy. Cancer Lett. 2009;280:123–4.
80. Khan O, La Thangue NB. HDAC inhibitors in cancer biology: emerging mechanisms and clinical applications. Immunol Cell Biol. 2012;90:85–94.
81. LM W, Yang Z, Zhou L, et al. Identification of histone deacetylase 3 as a biomarker for tumor recurrence following liver transplantation in HBV-associated hepatocellular carcinoma. PLoS One. 2010;5:e14460.
82. Harbour JW, Dean DC. The Rb/E2F pathway: expanding roles and emerging paradigms. Genes Dev. 2000;14:2393–409.
83. Coulouarn C, Factor VM, Thorgeirsson SS. Transforming growth factor-beta gene expression signature in mouse hepatocytes predicts clinical outcome in human cancer. Hepatology. 2008;47:2059–67.
84. Kaposi-Novak P, Lee JS, Gomez-Quiroz L, et al. Met-regulated expression signature defines a subset of human hepatocellular carcinomas with poor prognosis and aggressive phenotype. J Clin Invest. 2006;116:1582–95.
85. Llovet JM, Pena CE, Lathia CD, et al. Plasma biomarkers as predictors of outcome in patients with advanced hepatocellular carcinoma. Clin Cancer Res. 2012;18:2290–300.
86. Schoenleber SJ, Kurtz DM, Talwalkar JA, et al. Prognostic role of vascular endothelial growth factor in hepatocellular carcinoma: systematic review and meta-analysis. Br J Cancer. 2009;100:1385–92.
87. Zhang W, Kim R, Quintini C, et al. Prognostic role of plasma vascular endothelial growth factor in patients with hepatocellular carcinoma undergoing liver transplantation. Liver Transplant. 2015;21:101–11.
88. Cheng AL, Kang YK, Chen Z, et al. Efficacy and safety of sorafenib in patients in the Asia-Pacific region with advanced hepatocellular carcinoma: a phase III randomised, double-blind, placebo-controlled trial. Lancet Oncol. 2009;10:25–34.

89. Bruix J, Raoul JL, Sherman M, et al. Efficacy and safety of sorafenib in patients with advanced hepatocellular carcinoma: subanalyses of a phase III trial. J Hepatol. 2012;57:821–9.
90. Llovet JM, Real MI, Montana X, et al. Arterial embolisation or chemoembolisation versus symptomatic treatment in patients with unresectable hepatocellular carcinoma: a randomised controlled trial. Lancet. 2002;359:1734–9.
91. Lo CM, Ngan H, Tso WK, et al. Randomized controlled trial of transarterial lipiodol chemoembolization for unresectable hepatocellular carcinoma. Hepatology. 2002;35:1164–71.
92. Kudo M, Imanaka K, Chida N, et al. Phase III study of sorafenib after transarterial chemoembolisation in Japanese and Korean patients with unresectable hepatocellular carcinoma. Eur J Cancer. 2011;47:2117–27.
93. Lencioni R, Llovet JM, Han G, et al. Sorafenib or placebo plus TACE with doxorubicin-eluting beads for intermediate stage HCC: the SPACE trial. J Hepatol. 2016;64:1090–8.
94. Abou-Alfa GK, Johnson P, Knox JJ, et al. Doxorubicin plus sorafenib vs doxorubicin alone in patients with advanced hepatocellular carcinoma: a randomized trial. JAMA. 2010;304:2154–60.
95. Barone C, Basso M, Biolato M, et al. A phase II study of sunitinib in advanced hepatocellular carcinoma. Dig Liver dis. 2013;45:692–8.
96. Faivre S, Raymond E, Boucher E, et al. Safety and efficacy of sunitinib in patients with advanced hepatocellular carcinoma: an open-label, multicentre, phase II study. Lancet Oncol. 2009;10:794–800.
97. Cheng AL, Kang YK, Lin DY, et al. Sunitinib versus sorafenib in advanced hepatocellular cancer: results of a randomized phase III trial. J Clin Oncol. 2013;31:4067–75.
98. Bruix J, Merle P, Granito A, et al. Efficacy and safety of regorafenib versus placebo in patients with hepatocellular carcinoma progressing on sorafenib: results of the international, randomized phase 3 Resorce trial. Esmo World Congress on Gastrointestinal Cancer. Abstract Lba-03. Presented June 30, 2016.
99. Boige V, Malka D, Bourredjem A, et al. Efficacy, safety, and biomarkers of single-agent bevacizumab therapy in patients with advanced hepatocellular carcinoma. Oncologist. 2012;17:1063–72.
100. Siegel AB, Cohen EI, Ocean A, et al. Phase II trial evaluating the clinical and biologic effects of bevacizumab in unresectable hepatocellular carcinoma. J Clin Oncol. 2008;26:2992–8.
101. Zhu AX, Blaszkowsky LS, Ryan DP, et al. Phase II study of gemcitabine and oxaliplatin in combination with bevacizumab in patients with advanced hepatocellular carcinoma. J Clin Oncol. 2006;24:1898–903.
102. Hsu CH, Yang TS, Hsu C, et al. Efficacy and tolerability of bevacizumab plus capecitabine as first-line therapy in patients with advanced hepatocellular carcinoma. Br J Cancer. 2010;102:981–6.
103. Sun W, Sohal D, Haller DG, et al. Phase 2 trial of bevacizumab, capecitabine, and oxaliplatin in treatment of advanced hepatocellular carcinoma. Cancer. 2011;117:3187–92.
104. Britten CD, Gomes AS, Wainberg ZA, et al. Transarterial chemoembolization plus or minus intravenous bevacizumab in the treatment of hepatocellular cancer: a pilot study. BMC Cancer. 2012;12:16.
105. Llovet JM, Decaens T, Raoul JL, et al. Brivanib in patients with advanced hepatocellular carcinoma who were intolerant to sorafenib or for whom sorafenib failed: results from the randomized phase III BRISK-PS study. J Clin Oncol. 2013;31:3509–16.
106. Johnson PJ, Qin S, Park JW, et al. Brivanib versus sorafenib as first-line therapy in patients with unresectable, advanced hepatocellular carcinoma: results from the randomized phase III BRISK-FL study. J Clin Oncol. 2013;31:3517–24.
107. Toh HC, Chen PJ, Carr BI, et al. Phase 2 trial of linifanib (ABT-869) in patients with unresectable or metastatic hepatocellular carcinoma. Cancer. 2013;119:380–7.
108. Cainap C, Qin S, Huang WT, et al. Linifanib versus Sorafenib in patients with advanced hepatocellular carcinoma: results of a randomized phase III trial. J Clin Oncol. 2015;33:172–9.
109. Sandhu DS, Baichoo E, Roberts LR. Fibroblast growth factor signaling in liver carcinogenesis. Hepatology. 2014;59:1166–73.

110. Casanovas O, Hicklin DJ, Bergers G, et al. Drug resistance by evasion of antiangiogenic targeting of VEGF signaling in late-stage pancreatic islet tumors. Cancer Cell. 2005;8:299–309.
111. French DM, Lin BC, Wang M, et al. Targeting FGFR4 inhibits hepatocellular carcinoma in preclinical mouse models. PLoS One. 2012;7:e36713.
112. Hagel M, Miduturu C, Sheets M, et al. First selective small molecule inhibitor of FGFR4 for the treatment of hepatocellular carcinomas with an activated FGFR4 signaling pathway. Cancer Discov. 2015;5:424–37.
113. Schmidt B, Wei L, Deperalta DK, et al. Molecular subclasses of hepatocellular carcinoma predict sensitivity to fibroblast growth factor receptor inhibition. Int J Cancer. 2016;138:1494–505.
114. Philip PA, Mahoney MR, Allmer C, et al. Phase II study of Erlotinib (OSI-774) in patients with advanced hepatocellular cancer. J Clin Oncol. 2005;23:6657–63.
115. Thomas MB, Chadha R, Glover K, et al. Phase 2 study of erlotinib in patients with unresectable hepatocellular carcinoma. Cancer. 2007;110:1059–67.
116. Zhu AX, Rosmorduc O, Evans TR, et al. SEARCH: a phase III, randomized, double-blind, placebo-controlled trial of sorafenib plus erlotinib in patients with advanced hepatocellular carcinoma. J Clin Oncol. 2015;33:559–66.
117. Philip PA, Mahoney MR, Holen KD, et al. Phase 2 study of bevacizumab plus erlotinib in patients with advanced hepatocellular cancer. Cancer. 2012;118:2424–30.
118. Xiang Q, Chen W, Ren M, et al. Cabozantinib suppresses tumor growth and metastasis in hepatocellular carcinoma by a dual blockade of VEGFR2 and MET. Clin Cancer Res. 2014;20:2959–70.
119. Santoro A, Rimassa L, Borbath I, et al. Tivantinib for second-line treatment of advanced hepatocellular carcinoma: a randomised, placebo-controlled phase 2 study. Lancet Oncol. 2013;14:55–63.
120. Giannelli G, Villa E, Lahn M. Transforming growth factor-beta as a therapeutic target in hepatocellular carcinoma. Cancer Res. 2014;74:1890–4.
121. Neuzillet C, Tijeras-Raballand A, Cohen R, et al. Targeting the TGFbeta pathway for cancer therapy. Pharmacol Ther. 2015;147:22–31.
122. Dituri F, Mazzocca A, Fernando J, et al. Differential inhibition of the TGF-beta signaling pathway in HCC cells using the small molecule inhibitor LY2157299 and the D10 monoclonal antibody against TGF-beta receptor type II. PLoS One. 2013;8:e67109.
123. Faivre SJ, Santoro A, Kelley RK, Merle P, Gane E, Douillard J-Y, Waldschmidt D, Mulcahy MF, Costentin C, Minguez B, Papappicco P, Gueorguieva I, Cleverly A, Desaiah D, Lahn MMF, Murray N, Benhadji KA, Raymond E, Giannelli G. Randomized dose comparison phase II study of the oral transforming growth factor-Beta (Tgf-S) receptor I kinase inhibitor Ly2157299 monohydrate (Ly) in patients with advanced hepatocellular carcinoma (Hcc). Asco gastrointestinal cancers symposium; 2014.
124. Lim HY, Heo J, Choi HJ, et al. A phase II study of the efficacy and safety of the combination therapy of the MEK inhibitor refametinib (BAY 86-9766) plus sorafenib for Asian patients with unresectable hepatocellular carcinoma. Clin Cancer Res. 2014;20:5976–85.
125. Rossi AG, Sawatzky DA, Walker A, et al. Cyclin-dependent kinase inhibitors enhance the resolution of inflammation by promoting inflammatory cell apoptosis. Nat Med. 2006;12:1056–64.
126. Fornari F, Gramantieri L, Ferracin M, et al. MiR-221 controls CDKN1C/p57 and CDKN1B/p27 expression in human hepatocellular carcinoma. Oncogene. 2008;27:5651–61.
127. Cho SJ, Lee SS, Kim YJ, et al. Xylocydine, a novel Cdk inhibitor, is an effective inducer of apoptosis in hepatocellular carcinoma cells in vitro and in vivo. Cancer Lett. 2010;287:196–206.
128. Rivadeneira DB, Mayhew CN, Thangavel C, et al. Proliferative suppression by CDK4/6 inhibition: complex function of the retinoblastoma pathway in liver tissue and hepatoma cells. Gastroenterology. 2010;138:1920–30.
129. Haider C, Grubinger M, Reznickova E, et al. Novel inhibitors of cyclin-dependent kinases combat hepatocellular carcinoma without inducing chemoresistance. Mol Cancer Ther. 2013;12:1947–57.

130. Semela D, Piguet AC, Kolev M, et al. Vascular remodeling and antitumoral effects of mTOR inhibition in a rat model of hepatocellular carcinoma. J Hepatol. 2007;46:840–8.
131. Zhu AX, Abrams TA, Miksad R, et al. Phase 1/2 study of everolimus in advanced hepatocellular carcinoma. Cancer. 2011;117:5094–102.
132. Huynh H, Hao HX, Chan SL, et al. Loss of tuberous sclerosis complex 2 (TSC2) is frequent in hepatocellular carcinoma and predicts response to mTORC1 inhibitor Everolimus. Mol Cancer Ther. 2015;14:1224–35.
133. Khan O, Fotheringham S, Wood V, et al. HR23B is a biomarker for tumor sensitivity to HDAC inhibitor-based therapy. Proc Natl Acad Sci U S A. 2010;107:6532–7.
134. Yeo W, Chung HC, Chan SL, et al. Epigenetic therapy using belinostat for patients with unresectable hepatocellular carcinoma: a multicenter phase I/II study with biomarker and pharmacokinetic analysis of tumors from patients in the Mayo phase II consortium and the cancer therapeutics research group. J Clin Oncol. 2012;30:3361–7.
135. Marquez-Rodas I, Cerezuela P, Soria A, et al. Immune checkpoint inhibitors: therapeutic advances in melanoma. Ann Transl Med. 2015;3:267.
136. El-Khoueiry AB, Ignacio M, Crocenzi TS, et al. Phase I/II safety and antitumor activity of nivolumab in patients with advanced hepatocellular carcinoma (Hcc): CA209-040. J Clin Oncol. 2015;33(Suppl; Abstr Lba101).
137. Llovet JM, Schwartz M, Mazzaferro V. Resection and liver transplantation for hepatocellular carcinoma. Semin Liver Dis. 2005;25:181–200.
138. Bruix J, Takayama T, Mazzaferro V, et al. Adjuvant sorafenib for hepatocellular carcinoma after resection or ablation (STORM): a phase 3, randomised, double-blind, placebo-controlled trial. Lancet Oncol. 2015;16:1344–54.
139. Hyman DM, Puzanov I, Subbiah V, et al. Vemurafenib in multiple nonmelanoma cancers with BRAF V600 mutations. N Engl J Med. 2015;373:726–36.

Index

© Springer International Publishing AG 2018   263
C. Liu (ed.), *Precision Molecular Pathology of Liver Cancer*,
Molecular Pathology Library, https://doi.org/10.1007/978-3-319-68082-8